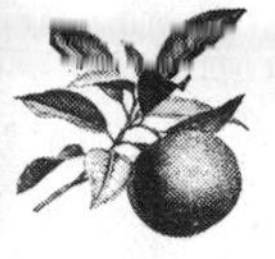

Dr. Jean Mayer's Diet and Nutrition Guide

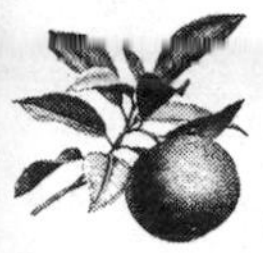

Dr. Jean Mayer's Diet and Nutrition Guide

Jean Mayer, Ph.D., Sc.D.
and
Jeanne P. Goldberg, Ph.D., R.D.

Pharos Books
A Scripps Howard Company
New York

DEDICATION

To Don, Lauren, and Hope who have endured the practice of nutrition with patience and humor. JPG

ACKNOWLEDGMENTS

We would like to thank the many people whose help and insight have contributed to sustaining our syndicated newspaper column over nearly two decades, among them Sara Ash, Dorothy Campbell, Madeline Dalton, Johanna Dwyer, Stanley Gershoff, Elizabeth Lenart, Laura Maloney, Viola Roth, Lynne Vincent Hewes, and our late editor and good friend, William H. White. We would also like to thank William B. Dickinson, Jr. and the staff at the Washington Post Writers' Group for their weekly efforts that keep the column going. Finally, we thank our readers whose questions have kept us attuned to what people really want to know.

First published in 1990.

Library of Congress Cataloging-in-Publication Data

Mayer, Jean, 1920-
[Diet and nutrition guide]
Dr. Jean Mayer's diet and nutrition guide / Jean Mayer and Jeanne P. Goldberg.
p. cm.
ISBN 0-88687-568-4 : $19.95
1. Diet therapy. 2. Nutrition. 3. Food—Composition—Tables.
I. Goldberg, Jeanne P. II. Title
RM216.M445 1990
613.2—dc20 89-27195
CIP

Printed in the United States

Pharos Books
A Scripps Howard Company
200 Park Avenue
New York, NY 10166

Interior design: Bea Jackson
Jacket design: Antler & Baldwin, Inc.

10 9 8 7 6 5 4 3 2 1

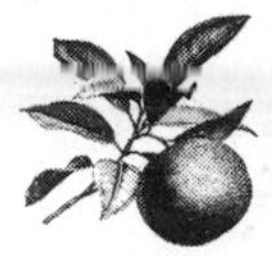

Contents

1 OUR CHANGING DIET

Standing in a modern supermarket with its towering rows of well-stocked shelves, refrigerated cases, and bulging freezers, with foods culled from all over the world, it may surprise you to learn that many Americans—maybe even you—may not be eating as well as people following centuries-old traditional diets quite unlike your own. You would probably think it outrageous if we suggested that our paleolithic ancestors crouching in their caves may have been routinely eating a better diet than do many Americans today.

While we are not recommending a return to the life of the hunter-gatherer, we do believe that those of our early ancestors who lived in temperate climates ate a diet that serves as a model for contemporary healthy living: one that is low in fat, salt, and sugar, with generous amounts of fiber-rich fruits and vegetables and whole grains.

Over the centuries the human diet has been shaped and reshaped by such forces as the domestication of animals, the development of agriculture, and the invention of fishing gear. Consider the fact that while there was some honey in their eras, Jesus, Julius Caesar, and Socrates never tasted sugar, which today supplies as many as 20% of the calories in some American diets. Closer to our own times, in the mid-nineteenth century, refrigeration and the development of transcontinental shipping ushered in an epoch marked by variety and change. Technological innovations over the past century have only accelerated the pace.

Our food supply is constantly changing and is likely to continue to do so. Even in the past 20 years the supermarket has altered dramatically. Along with the flood of new products has come a surge of nutrition-related information—on food labels, and in scientific reports, media stories, and advertising—through which we must sort to make our food choices. Interpreting the relevant terms can be almost as challenging as learning a new language.

Today, people are eating a greater percentage of their meals away from home. They rely on restaurants and take-out shops to prepare their food. Questions have arisen about how this trend affects nutritional intake. Issues have surfaced involving food safety, both of our food supply as a whole and on an individual basis, within our private kitchens, where following safety guidelines can shield our families' health as we prepare food.

In this modern world, the task of feeding ourselves wisely and well sometimes seems to have grown more difficult rather than easier. Yet despite the abundance and complexity of our food supply, by keeping a few selected principles in mind, we can find the age-old pathway to nutritional excellence.

HUNTING AND GATHERING IN THE 20TH CENTURY

Hunting and gathering in the supermarket is as American as apple pie—fresh or frozen. It was here in the United States in the early 1930's that the world's first supermarket, King Kullen, was opened in Jamaica, New York. That was in the early years of the Great Depression. Housewives welcomed the chance to buy foods more cheaply, and they enjoyed the new method of choosing groceries from the shelves, piling them into carts, and wheeling through the checkout. Because shoppers sold themselves more products than clerks in old-fashioned stores ever could, supermarkets were good for business.

Today's spacious, ever-changing emporia, studded with innumerable products, differ greatly from the modest markets of yesteryear. Most Americans now do the bulk of their food shopping in supermarkets, also buying an increasing number of nonfood items there. For consumers who hunt and gather wisely, these large stores can provide both good-tasting food and first-rate nutrition.

When you visit the store, however, you need to turn on your good-sense radar. Supermarkets are laid out in a plan scientifically designed to encourage maximum purchases, gently luring you toward products not always in your best nutritional interest. Lulling muzak and the piped-in aroma of baking bread help create a relaxing atmosphere to encourage you to buy more than you need. Just remember this: the surest course to a healthful diet is through reliance on fresh and lightly processed foods. That awareness, coupled with an effort to limit salt, fat, and sugar, will allow you to get the most nutrition for your dollars.

In most supermarkets, the produce section is located at one end of the store or the other, and you can't go wrong nutritionally by starting out there. In season, locally grown fresh fruits and vegetables are cheaper, better-tasting, and provide more nutrients than canned produce. Make it a point to buy fresh produce in season—especially fruits and vegetables rich in vitamin C and yellow and green vegetables, good sources of vitamin A. But if fresh local fruits and vegetables are not available or are too expensive, don't pass up canned and frozen produce as inferior. Fruits and vegetables, if picked ripe and canned or frozen by modern methods, are frequently higher in nutrients than produce that's been plucked unripe and artificially "improved" while being transported thousands of miles. When buying canned fruit, choose those packed in light syrup, or better yet, "water-packed." With frozen vegetables, mixtures of different kinds are fine if you want the convenience and can pay the premium, but avoid those in prepared sauces: they're often high in fat and calories, and sometimes salt.

Next stop: the meat section. Because the names of cuts vary by region, our advice is to let your eyes guide you. Buy cuts with little visible fat marbling the muscle and only a thin trimming of fat. Use more chicken and less cured meat, especially sausage types which are high in both salt and fat. And save some of the week's purchases for the fish department.

Here are two important tips for the cereal aisle. First, select products made completely or mostly from whole grains, such as whole wheat, all-bran, or rolled oats, for example, or where the second ingredient is either bran or a whole grain. Second, check the ingredients list or nutrition label to make sure the cereal isn't loaded with sugar and saturated fat in the form of palm or coconut oil or hydrogenated shortening. Don't be enticed by a label that promises heavy fortification with a smorgasbord of vitamins and minerals.

In the cracker and cookie aisle, labeling information remains scarce. Among crackers, your best bets include melba rounds, matzos, and flatbreads. Cookies contain considerable sugar, but to satisfy an occasional sweet tooth without extra fat, choose sugar wafers, animal crackers, fig newtons, raisin biscuits, graham crackers, or meringues. Our choices for snack food include unsalted pretzels and plain popcorn—or popcorn kernels that can be popped at home. Unsalted homemade popcorn is cheaper and fresher and will fill your house with a delightful aroma.

Among prepared soups, salt is the issue. Where available, consult nutrition labeling. Otherwise, you'll have to use trial and error, avoiding a second purchase of those soups which taste too salty. Skim off fat floating on any canned soup before you pour it into a pot.

On to frozen foods, where the casefuls of new products may seem overwhelming. Scrutinize nutrition labels; if necessary, use a pocket calculator. Look for entrees where no more than 30% of the calories come from fat and sodium doesn't exceed 1,000 milligrams per serving. Or, check the ingredients list to see if fat is at or near the top. Some prepared foods, like veal parmigiana or fried chicken, are obviously not sound, everyday choices. As for frozen desserts, fruit ices are the wisest choice.

When you come to the bread (or bakery) aisle, remember that a dark bread with a healthy-sounding name is often white bread in disguise. If you're looking for whole grains you must read the ingredients list. Look for the same grains you search for when buying cereals, or for unbolted cornmeal, high on the ingredients list. When "wheat flour" is listed as the first ingredient, you merely have a variation on white bread.

Dairy products are vital to your family's calcium supply. Many, including milk, also contain plenty of protein and high levels of riboflavin. Vitamin D-fortified milk is especially important for small children and pregnant and nursing women. Saturated fat is an issue, however. Skim milk is best, but if you find it too watery, choose one of the low-fat options, the lower in fat the better. Ditto with cottage cheese and yogurt. When it comes to yogurt, choose the plain, low-fat variety and add the fruit or vegetables yourself. Hard cheeses, high in fat, are fine for kids, but adults should only use them sparingly. And, of course, cream, both sweet and sour, is best left for special occasions.

Although today's supermarket is bigger and better lit than old-time stores, the elements of a healthy diet remain the same. Good-tasting, nutritional food is still in style, and most of the basic foods we're recommending were on the shelves of the original King Kullen over 50 years ago.

Questions and Answers

Q. Why are so many produce items coated with a waxy film?
A. There are a couple of reasons. One is cosmetic. Food growers and processors believe that shiny fruits and vegetables have more appeal, a point with which many of today's consumers would take issue.

Waxing is also one way to slow deterioration and retard spoilage. Deterioration proceeds more rapidly once produce has been harvested. First, the rate of respiration, or the intake of oxygen and release of carbon dioxide and moisture through the pores, increases. This can result in a drop in sugar content and a loss of ascorbic acid. Second, washing can increase the loss of water through evaporation. Finally, when commercially raised produce is cleaned with solvent detergents to remove dirt and residues from chemical sprays, the protective wax coating which occurs naturally on many fruits and vegetables may be removed.

Highly sophisticated cold storage techniques and, in some cases, waxing, can retard the aging process and extend storage life. The waxes are applied in a variety of ways: by brushing, fogging, or foaming. Produce may also be passed through a tank of wax emulsion as it travels over a conveyor belt.

Waxes and the components of wax coatings are subject to FDA regulation and must be approved for safety. The FDA sets limits for amounts that can be used. In some cases, regulations detail the specific fruits and vegetables on which a particular wax may be used. These regulations may depend not only on the type of wax but also on whether the waxed skin or shell would normally be eaten.

Incidentally, there is nothing new about using waxes on food. As early as the twelfth or thirteenth century, the Chinese coated oranges and lemons in molten wax to make the fruit ferment.

Q. As a measure of economy, we buy bread and produce on the reduced shelf. I am concerned that these foods are nutritionally inferior and wonder whether we might be better off economizing elsewhere if possible?

A. The vitamin most vulnerable to destruction in overripe fruits and vegetables is vitamin C. There may also be some loss of other vitamins. But, if you eat a varied diet, you should still be getting adequate supplies of essential vitamins.

We would, however, advise particular caution in avoiding foods which show signs of mold. Molds can be perfectly harmless, or, like the mold that provides penicillin, invaluable. But some molds can be potentially harmful. Moreover, trimming away visible mold does not get rid of it. What you see, the "bloom," is only part of the mold. Because roots may be spread throughout a food which only appears moldy on the surface, trimming does not adequately get rid of it. Mold won't make you sick every time you inadvertently happen to consume a bit of it, but it's not a good idea to take chances.

Q. Is it true that homogenized milk contains xanthine oxidase, an enzyme linked to hardening of the arteries, and that goat's milk, which contains less of the enzyme, is a better choice?

A. No. No relationship between xanthine oxidase and heart disease has ever been demonstrated. The xanthine oxidase-heart disease link was proposed more than 15 years ago by Dr. Kurt Oster, who claimed that homogenization was "a procedure which foists unnaturally small particles on the digestive tract." Oster claimed that xanthine oxidase, absorbed from tiny fat droplets in milk, caused tissue damage and set in motion the atherosclerotic process that led to heart disease. Xanthine oxidase supposedly destroyed plasmalogen, a phospholipid found in heart cells.

A review of the evidence gathered for more than a decade after the theory was first put forth found insufficient evidence to support the idea that plasmalogen depletion is a cause of heart disease. Available studies failed to demonstrate that xanthine oxidase is even absorbed from the intestine or that there is a link between consumption of dairy products containing homogenized fat and blood levels of xanthine oxidase. The fact that prolonged intravenous feeding of cow's milk xanthine oxidase to laboratory animals did not destroy arterial or coronary tissue plasmalogens and did not induce plaque formation indicates that even if minute amounts were absorbed, they would have no effect.

These and still other pieces of evidence suggest that the time to bury the xanthine oxidase-heart disease connection is long overdue.

Q. I have often noticed, especially on some of the imported cheeses, a label statement about the minimum fat content, and I am not sure I understand it. What does it mean, for example, when the label says that it contains not less than 45% fat? Is there any way to figure out the actual amount of fat per ounce using this information?

A. The figure for percent fat in a particular cheese refers to the amount of fat in the cheese solids after the moisture has been removed. So, to figure out how much fat a serving of cheese contains, it is necessary to know both the percent of fat in the solids and the usual moisture content of the cheese. Unfortunately, the latter piece of information is not included on the label, which makes it impossible to do your own calculations. The best suggestion we can offer, if you know the percentage of fat in a cheese you select, is to regard it as roughly comparable to a cheese for which you do have information.

Q. Some ice cream appears to be nothing but air. Is there any limit on how much air manufacturers can whip into their products?

A. Yes. Allowable "overrun" as it is technically called, is specified. Ice cream is among the foods for which there is a federal Standard of Identity. That means it must conform to a defined recipe. That recipe specifies the percent increase in volume which occurs as air is whipped into the mixture during the freezing process. Adequate overrun is essential to producing the best-quality ice cream. Too little results in ice cream with a heavy, coarse texture, while too much produces a frothy, foamy texture. While overrun may be as little as 30% to 40%, as is usual in homemade ice creams, it usually ranges anywhere from 70% to 100% in commercial ice creams. A quart of basic mixture with a 100% overrun would therefore produce two quarts of ice cream.

Under the standard, ice cream cannot weigh less than 4½ ounces per gallon, exclusive of microcrystalline cellulose, which is sometimes used as a stabilizer to improve body and texture. While Standards of Identity apply only to ice cream shipped among the states, each state has its own frozen dessert standards. And these generally are similar to the federal regulations.

Q. Are there regulations governing how much meat must be in canned products containing meat, such as chili and beef stew?

A. Yes. All products which contain at least 2% poultry or 3% meat are governed by United States Department of Agriculture (USDA) regulations. Where appropriate, these regulations specify how much meat or poultry must be included in order to feature the word "beef" or "chicken" in the name of the product. (You can recognize these foods by the USDA inspection stamp on the label.) For example, chili con carne must contain 40% beef; beef stew, at least 25% beef; beef with gravy, at least 50% beef. At least 35% of the weight of gravy with beef must be beef. Any less, and a different name must be used. You can get information about other products for which USDA standards exist in a booklet called *Meat and Poultry Products—A Consumer's Guide to Content and Labeling Requirements.* Single copies are available from the Meat and Poultry HOTLINE, USDA-FSIS, Rm. 1165-S, USDA, Wash., D.C., 20250.

Q. How do turkey frankfurters compare nutritionally with beef hot dogs?

A. On the average, turkey frankfurters are lower in fat and calories than frankfurters made from either beef or a mixture of beef and pork. A turkey frankfurter weighing 1½ ounces contains about 8 grams of fat and 100 calories, while a frankfurter of the same size (about 5 inches long and ¾ inches in diameter) made either from beef or beef and pork provides about 13 grams of fat and 145 calories.

The difference in amounts of most other nutrients among the various types of frankfurters is not nutritionally important. However, regular frankfurters are quite high in sodium, and for that reason should be avoided by anyone trying to reduce his or her salt intake. But, on average, turkey franks contain even more sodium. A typical 1½-ounce beef frankfurter contains over 450 milligrams of sodium (as much as you'd get in a pound and a half of fresh, unsalted hamburger). A turkey frank of the same size contains nearly 650 milligrams of sodium, a chicken frank about 615 milligrams. Franks made from beef and pork fall in between, providing about 500 milligrams of sodium.

We should point out that the value for turkey franks was based on a sample of four products and that for chicken franks on just a single sample. You may, therefore, want to check with the manufacturers of the brands available in your area. It may be that some contain less sodium. Also, the recent emphasis on lowering the sodium content of processed foods has convinced some manufacturers to reduce the amounts they were using.

Q. Is it true that pork is now considerably leaner than it once was?

A. Yes. Consumer demand for leaner meat coupled with a declining market for animal fats as vegetable oils have become more plentiful has led farmers to produce leaner, longer hogs. A study by the USDA's Economic Research Service (ERS) shows that, while in 1968 only 8% of the hog carcasses qualified as U.S. Number 1 (the leanest, meatiest grade), by 1980, over 70% made that grade.

Q. Why does the thickness of the skin of navel oranges vary so greatly? It would seem to me that the thickness of a single variety should be fairly constant.

A. The thickness of the skin on citrus fruit depends on seasonal growing conditions. Factors including extremes of temperature, the amount of rainfall, and excess wind all affect skin thickness. Thicker skins apparently are nature's way of protecting the fruit against "the elements."

Q. I understand the Department of Agriculture has changed its designations regarding the quality grading of beef. Could you please provide me with the details?

A. As of November 1987, what was formerly called USDA Good was renamed USDA Select. The name change grew out of concern that consumers did not readily identify "Good" grade as generally lower in fat than the same cut from ahigher grade, and they tended to view it as less desirable than Choice. Ordinarily, the USDA does not allow the use of the quality terms on beef unless they have been officially graded, but because "Select" is a term which has been used by some firms to describe their products, they will be allowed to continue to do so. Just how widespread the use of the term will be is unclear. Consumers should therefore remember when looking for lean meat to make sure they are buying USDA Select.

To give you an idea of the difference in fat and calories between the same cut from two grades, a 3½-ounce portion of Choice top round contains 6.4 grams of fat and 194 calories, while the same amount of Select beef contains 5.4 grams and 184 calories. For blade roast, the difference is a bit bigger. The Choice beef contains 15.8 grams of fat and 275 calories, while the Select meat contains 13.7 grams of fat and 256 calories. It's always a good idea to keep meat portions small. But those who eat larger amounts of meat should take special notice of the difference in grade.

Grade is not the only criterion on which to base your selection if you are looking for the lowest fat options. The amount of fat in a portion of meat may be affected to a great extent by the type of cut you choose. For example, a Select rib steak, which is heavily marbled, or a piece of Select chuck roast will probably have more fat than the same amount of Choice top round or top loin steak.

Q. For some time I have used margarine instead of butter at the table. Now I have read that as oils are developed into a solid mass to create margarine they are saturated. Is that true?

A. It is true that margarine is not as rich in polyunsaturates as the oil from which it was made. That's because in making margarine some of the oil used must be hydrogenated, or hardened. Otherwise it would not hold its shape. So in order to keep polyunsaturated fat intake at the recommended 10% of the total fat you consume, it does make good sense to use liquid oils for cooking whenever possible.

Beyond that, margarines vary in the amount of polyunsaturates they provide. There are two ways to choose those which contain the most generous amounts. If the margarine label includes information about fat and cholesterol, simply select a brand which contains more polyunsaturated than saturated fat. In other words, if the margarine contains 11 grams of fat per tablespoon, a good choice might be one which contains 5 grams of polyunsaturated fat and 2 grams of saturated fat. The other four grams not accounted for are monounsaturates.

If labeling information is not available, check the ingredients list. If the first ingredient list is a liquid oil, such as corn, canola, cottonseed, sunflower, safflower or soybean, it too, is an acceptable choice.

ANATOMY OF A FOOD LABEL

"They ought to call it 'cheese and macaroni,' " says the little girl in the TV commercial, because she finds the packaged macaroni and cheese dinner so "cheesy." In fact, the manufacturer cannot call it "cheese and macaroni." Federal regulations require that when ingredients are used in the product name, they must be listed in descending order by weight. And in this case, there is more macaroni than cheese in the product.

That is just one of the rules food companies must obey when labeling their products. At a minimum, all food labels must provide product name, manufacturer, packer or distributor's name and address, and net weight or contents of the package. The net weight of canned goods includes the liquid in which the food is packed.

Most food labels must furnish a list of ingredients in descending order by weight. This gives the consumer a better idea of exactly what is in the food and allows for comparisons between similar products. A classic example is the position of sugar in the ingredients list for dry cereals. The higher on the list, the more sugar in the cereal.

If you are concerned about fat intake—both type and amount—and there is no nutritional information to guide you, the ingredients list can offer a clue about the relative importance of fat in the product. Regulations governing fat labeling are under review, and it is hoped will soon be revised to better serve consumers. In the meantime, the current law allows manufacturers to be vague about what fats they use. Anyone who reads labels has doubtless seen products that contain "any one or more of the following . . . " fats or oils. Since vegetable oils vary in degree of saturation, exact information is important to consumers who are trying to control their fat intake. Until we have better fat labeling, consumers who want to know what type of oil is being used must contact the manufacturer.

The end of the ingredients list may be vague. Under current regulations, the name of artificial and natural colors and flavorings need not be specified. The only exception is yellow dye Number 5, to which some people are allergic.

Foods that do not require a complete ingredients list are those for which the federal government has established the Standard of Identity or strict recipe formulation. This standard spells out what ingredients a product must contain to warrant being called, for example, "mayonnaise." The more than 300 "standardized" foods include ketchup, peanut butter, jam, soft drinks, orange juice, milk, ice cream, macaroni, and noodles. This standard protects a consumer from buying a product that is not what he or she expects from the name. Peanut butter, for instance, has to contain at least 90% peanuts. A less "peanutty" version, nutritionally inferior to the original, has to be labeled "imitation."

Many food labels also list nutrition information. This information is required when nutrients like vitamins and minerals are added, or when the manufacturer makes a nutrition-related claim on the label, such as "contains more vitamin C than a glass of orange juice." Manufacturers often provide nutrition information voluntarily. Currently, more than half of all food regulated by the FDA bear nutrition labels. They must include, on a per-serving basis, the number of calories, amount of carbohydrate, protein, fat, and sodium, and percentages of the U.S. Recommended Daily Allowances (U.S. RDA) for protein, five vitamins, and two minerals. The amount of cholesterol and fatty acids, both saturated and unsaturated, and the remaining nutrients for which U.S. RDA's exist may also be provided if the manufacturer chooses. To encourage more extensive sodium labeling, the FDA allows information about sodium and potassium without other labeling.

In checking nutrition information, serving size is critical, For some products, it may be listed by weight, 1 ounce in the case of most cereals. Since your serving size is probably influenced by how the cereal fills the bowl, you should also check the volume of that one ounce when comparing prod-

FOOD LABEL INFORMATION
What Does It Really Mean?

	PER SERVING
***Calories**	
Low calorie	40 calories or 0.4 calories per gram
Reduced calorie	One-third fewer calories than unmodified food
***Sodium**	
Sodium Free	Less than 5 mg. of sodium
Very low sodium	Up to 35 mg.
Low sodium	No more than 140 mg.
Reduced sodium	75% less than that of the food as normally prepared
Unsalted	No salt added to foods normally processed with salt, like potato chips
****Light**	
Lite	Lower calories or salt; at least 25% reduction in fat or other ingredients
Lean	At least 25% reduction in fat and less than 10% fat
Extra lean	No more than 5% fat
Low fat	Less than 10% fat

*Applies to foods under FDA jurisdiction.

**Applies to foods under USDA jurisdiction, except raw ground beef, where ground beef contains 30% fat; lean, 22.5%; extra lean, 15%.

ucts. An ounce of cornflakes is about 1 cup, compared to only half a cup of raisin bran, and about a quarter cup for granola. Nutritionally, a cup of one cereal can differ greatly from a cup of another kind.

To complicate matters further, not all manufacturers of similar products use similar serving sizes. A serving of bread may be one slice or two, or in the case of diet bread, a very slim 2–3-ounce slice. And while a manufacturer may consider a can of tuna a single serving, you may not. Beyond that are a whole array of designations manufacturers may use to sell their products.

The information on food labels can be a big help—if you keep in mind what it all means. The following chart is designed to help you with that task.

Questions and Answers

Q. In what situations must a food be designated "imitation?"

A. For over a decade, the term "imitation" has been interpreted by the FDA to mean products that substitute for and resemble a traditional food but which are nutritionally inferior to that food. The FDA defines nutritional inferiority as "any reduction in content of an essential nutrient that is present in a measurable amount but does not include a reduction in the calorie or fat content." The term "measurable amount" is defined as 2% or more of the U.S. RDA for that nutrient.

While this definition does establish certain criteria for deciding whether a fabricated substitute food must be labeled as imitation, it does not tell the whole story. At least 42 nutrients are known to be essential, but U.S. RDA's have been established for just 20 of them. So, over half the essential nutrients are not considered in the comparison. In addition to calories and fat, among those nutrients not considered are carbohydrates, linoleic acid, vitamin K, and nine minerals, including sodium and potassium. This means that a substitute food can be considered nutritionally equivalent and contain none of these nutrients; or it may contain some or all, but in lesser amounts than the traditional food. In some cases, it may contain larger amounts of a mineral like sodium. Finally, it may contain more or fewer calories.

There are questions about the many unexplored and complex interactions which may affect the bioavailability or usefulness of nutrients in these foods to the body. And there are still other questions concerning substitute foods that still need to be answered. So, while fabricated foods can make a positive contribution to the diet, there is no assurance that these foods are consistently equivalent in nutritional value to their conventional counterparts. The extent to which one of them replaces a traditional food as a major component of the diet can certainly be cause for concern.

There are situations in which a substitute or imitation food may be preferable to the traditional food. Margarine, rich in polyunsaturates, is a preferred substitute for butter for those who are trying to limit saturated fat intake. Another example is imitation mayonnaise, which contains less fat and fewer calories than real mayonnaise. As a consumer, it is up to you to use nutrition labeling information to make informed choices about whether an individual imitation or substitute food is the proper choice for your diet.

Q. Are there regulations governing the use of the word "natural" on meat and poultry products?

A. In order to carry the "natural" label, meat and poultry, which fall under USDA jurisdiction, must meet two criteria. First, they cannot contain any artificial flavorings, colors, chemical preservatives, or any artificial or synthetic ingredients. Second, the product and its ingredients cannot have been processed more than minimally.

The USDA Food Safety and Inspection Service (FSIS) policy goes on to define what constitutes "minimal processing." Processes such as roasting, smoking, freezing, drying, or fermenting, all of which make food edible, preserve it, or render it safe are allowed. So, too, are physical processes such as grinding meat, separating eggs, and other procedures which do not really change the raw product.

As long as the character of the product has not been changed to a point where it can no longer be regarded as "natural," the term can still be used even when it contains ingredients such as sugar, which has been processed into the product more than minimally. However, in those cases, the claim must be qualified to clearly and conspicuously identify that ingredient.

In addition to meeting the above criteria, manufacturers who claim that his or her product is "natural" are required to explain on the label just what the term means. Moreover, the right to use the natural label is not in the hands of the manufacturer. FSIS reviews each case and makes judgments on individual products.

Q. How accurate must the nutrient information on a food label be? How sure can I be that the nutrients listed on the package are what I am really getting?

A. Quite sure. Two sets of standards were established at the time that nutrition labeling regulations went into effect. One governs those foods to which nutrients are added for enrichment and fortification. The other covers naturally occurring nutrients.

According to the first set of standards, when nutrients are added, a composite batch of the food must contain amounts at least equal to the value of each nutrient declared on the label. For naturally occurring nutrients, a composite batch of food must contain at least 80% of the nutrient value declared on the label. The second, more liberal standard, acknowledges that a variety of factors can affect the nutritional content of a food.

In fact, studies have shown that some nutrients vary considerably more than others, and in some foods more than in others. For example, in studies of canned fruits and vegetables conducted some time ago, the vitamin A content of spinach varied by almost 150%, and in apricots, by almost 30%, depending on the crop. There was considerable variation in vitamin C content, a function of both natural factors and processing methods. Among the minerals tested, iron values varied to the greatest extent. Calories, probably the most widely used piece of information on the nutrition labeling panel, varied least.

In order to meet compliance standards, manufacturers tend to be conservative in making decisions for food labeling. The result is that what you see is probably what you get at the very least, and perhaps even more.

Q. Sometimes I find it frustrating to try to use nutrition labeling information. Spaghetti is a good example of what I mean. Could you please explain why servings of spaghetti are always described in terms of their dry weight instead of their weight when cooked?

A. While labeling is not perfect, there is a very good reason for what appears to be a needlessly cumbersome presentation of information. The number of calories in a given volume of spaghetti can vary considerably, depending on how long the pasta has been cooked. If cooked for longer periods, it absorbs more water than if it is served "al dente," or until just tender. The former would provide 155 calories and the latter, 190 calories per cup. Depending on how long it has been cooked, 2 ounces of spaghetti, the amount usually listed on the nutrition label, may swell to anywhere from 1 to 1⅓ cups. In order to be sure to comply with labeling regulations, manufacturers choose the safest course, in this case, providing information about the dry product.

Q. I recently bought a microwave oven. Up to that time I had virtually ignored the entrees and dinners in the frozen food section of the supermarket. But I decided it was time to give frozen foods a try. Among the items I purchased was a two-portion enchilada entree. I admit that if I had thought about it more carefully, I would have realized that the exterior packaging might have given an exaggerated impression of what was inside. But I was taken aback by what was supposed to be two portions. They were absurdly small. Isn't there some limit on what manufacturers can call a portion?

A. No. When nutrition labeling first went into effect more than 15 years ago, it was decided that the specification of portion sizes should be left up to the manufacturer. That explains why two brands of an identical food can have different portion sizes. In most cases, portion sizes specified on packaging have been reasonable. The case you point out appears to be an exception. The only real defense for the consumer is to be sure to check labeling information carefully. And perhaps, if you feel strongly enough, a letter to the manufacturer, explaining that you believed you were misguided might be in order.

Q. In buying hot dogs, I have noticed that some packaging lists "beef and pork" while on others the list reads beef, then pork. Is there a difference?

A. There could be. Ordinarily, ingredients are listed in descending order by weight, and that is what you can expect if the ingredients are listed in the second format you describe. If, however, the ingredients are listed as "beef and pork," it is unclear which of the two meats predominate. The USDA's standard allows manufacturers to reformulate their mixed-meat hot dogs within certain defined limits without changing labels. That, of course, permits them to produce the hot dogs as cheaply as possible.

Beyond that, at least 70% of the meat in each hot dog must come from a combination of beef and pork skeletal muscle. The manufacturer may alter the proportion of each, but the combination cannot include less than 30% of either one. Up to 15% of the hot dog may come from poultry and the rest from variety meats and other animal parts. If used, they must be included in the product name and must appear in the ingredients list. A name such as "hot dogs with variety meats" is likely to discourage sales. So such products are rare.

Q. Can you please explain the regulations governing the use of "low calorie" and the term "reduced calorie?"

A. Under FDA regulations which went into effect in July 1980, foods labeled "low calorie" can provide no more than 40 calories per serving and 0.4 calories per gram. The term "low calorie" can only be used to describe foods for which the standard product contains a significantly greater number of calories. For example, a manufacturer of a brand of mushrooms, a food which is naturally low in calories, could not label them "low-calorie" mushrooms since this would imply that his or her mushrooms were substantially lower in calories than another brand. Instead, they could be labeled, "mushrooms, a low-calorie food."

Foods with "reduced-calorie" labeling must contain at least one-third fewer calories than a similar food in which the calories are not reduced. But it must not be nutritionally inferior to the unmodified food. A reduced-calorie food that doesn't smell and taste like the food for which it substitutes must say so on the label. And finally, reduced-calorie foods must back up their label claims with information comparing the number of calories in a serving of the standard food and the reduced-calorie food. All low-calorie and reduced-calorie foods are required to have complete nutrition labeling information.

Q. In reading nutrition labels, I get somewhat confused by the terms "enriched" and "fortified." Can you please explain the difference?

A. Enrichment refers to the restoration of nutrients removed during processing to levels at or not too much greater than those in the original food. The classic example of enrichment is the addition of thiamin, riboflavin, niacin, and iron to white flour. However, many nutrients lost in refining flour, including magnesium, zinc, chromium, vitamin B-6, and folic acid, may not be restored by enrichment. Thus, white bread, although a good food, is not nutritionally equal to whole-grain bread.

Fortification is the addition of nutrients not normally present in a food, or present in amounts too small to be of nutritional significance. Fortification has been dramatically effective in preventing nutritional deficiencies. For example, carotene, which the body converts to vitamin A, was first added to margarine in Denmark during World War II after it was found that switching from butter to margarine was causing blindness in Danish children. Milk, a food which children are likely to consume, was chosen as the vehicle to carry vitamin D for the prevention of rickets. And iodine was added to salt as an effective way of preventing goiter. These were all extremely important public health measures.

In recent years, the rationale for some fortification has been less clear. A statement issued by the American Medical Association several years ago, agreed upon by both the Food and Nutrition Board of the National Research Council and the Expert Panel on Food Safety and Nutrition of the Institute of Food Technologists, points out that some fortification is not defensible. For example, there is no apparent health justification for adding nutrients to cereals intended for older children and adults beyond 25% of the U.S. RDA for vitamins and minerals.

We would emphasize that the regular consumption of these heavily-fortified cereals, or other foods containing as much as 100% of the U.S. RDA for some nutrients, is no substitute for consuming a well-balanced and varied diet.

Q. Could you explain how to interpret the sugar labeling information on cold cereal packages?

A. Sugar is listed as "sucrose and other sugars." Usually this means it is predominantly sucrose, or white table sugar, although many granola-type cereals are made with brown sugar and honey. Some cereals may also contain a small amount of other sweeteners such as corn syrup, and these are included in this category.

To translate grams of sucrose and other sweeteners into the more familiar teaspoons, you need to know that a teaspoon of sugar weighs 4 grams. Thus, for example, a 1-ounce serving of cereal containing 11 grams of "sucrose and other sweeteners" contains nearly 3 teaspoons of sugar. Sugar content varies anywhere from zero to as much as 16 grams, or 4 teaspoons in a 1-ounce serving of cereal.

Q. What is the difference between ice cream labeled as "vanilla flavored" and that labeled only "vanilla?"

A. The difference relates to whether the flavor is all natural or partly artificial. "Vanilla" ice cream contains only pure vanilla, while "vanilla flavored" contains both natural and artificial flavor. But according to the federal Standard of Identity, in order to use the term "vanilla flavored," the natural flavor must predominate. Specifications for a third type of labeling might be something of a surprise. Ice cream labeled as "artificially flavored" may contain either all artificial flavor or a combination of artificial and natural flavors. In this case, the artificial flavor would predominate.

Regulations governing ice cream labeling specify the size of letters to be used and the placement of the words describing the flavoring ingredients. And they clearly define how the predominant flavor is to be measured.

Q. Please explain the guidelines for sodium labeling.

A. The sodium labeling language for foods that fall under FDA jurisdiction uses five terms. First, foods that contain less than 5 milligrams of sodium per serving are called "sodium free." Next, those with 35 milligrams or less per serving are labelled "very low sodium." Third, foods containing 140 milligrams or less per serving are called "low sodium." Fourth, in order for a label to read "reduced sodium," a food must contain 75% less sodium than the same product would, if processed normally. Finally, "unsalted" means no salt has been added to foods that are normally processed with salt.

The FDA will, however, allow manufacturers to use comparative label statements on foods where there is at least a 25% reduction in sodium compared to the food it replaces. The motive is to encourage reducing the sodium content in foods whose level cannot be lowered sufficiently to meet the criteria for "reduced sodium." When this claim is displayed, the manufacturer must also provide the consumer with information about the actual amount of sodium in the product.

In addition, if a manufacturer makes a nutrition claim for a food or puts nutrition labeling information on a package, the label must also disclose the sodium content of the food.

Q. What is "organically grown" produce?

A. The basic definition of "organic" produce is quite straightforward. It applies to fruits and vegetables grown without the use of chemical fertilizers, herbicides, and pesticide, which may be used by conventional farmers. But the translation of that definition to produce labeled "organic" at your local market is far more complex. For one thing, 33 states have no laws governing the use of the term, nor are they currently trying to pass them. Among the states that do, specifications of the law vary considerably. In California, the organic label may be used on produce raised in soil where there had been no chemical treatment of the field for one year prior to the time the food was sold. Several other states, including Kansas, Maine, Minnesota, and North Dakota specify a much longer gap, at least three years. In still others, including both New Hampshire and Oregon, the time lag between the use of chemicals and the use of the term is unspecified. In short, interpreting what is meant by "organic" depends very much on where you live.

FROM RAW MATERIALS TO FINISHED PRODUCTS

As schoolchildren, most of us were warned—under dire threat of punishment—not to "personalize" our books with pen or pencil. That rule made sense in a system where texts got handed down from one class to the next, sometimes over a period of many years. Yet when it comes to producing a diet high in taste, rich in essential nutrients, and at the same time light on fat, salt, and sugar, writing in your books is exactly what we are going to propose.

Once you have returned home from the supermarket with lean meat, low-fat dairy products, and as much fresh produce as your budget and the season allow, the next step in preparing a healthy diet can be summed up in a single word: technique. And for that, cookbooks are the best resources we know. To be sure, a number of excellent volumes written expressly for the purpose provide an array of recipes geared to a healthful diet. However, it is also possible to adapt your own favorite volumes to keep in step with current dietary guidelines. Indeed, we confess a weakness for adding exciting new volumes to our kitchen bookshelves already groaning under an excess load, but several "old friends" personalized with adaptations we have worked out remain the basis of our cookbook library.

In some cases, bringing your favorite recipes into line requires just a few minutes to take a hard look at the ingredients list for obvious targets and make the necessary changes. For other recipes, the process may be slower, and you may need to use the trial and error method to see what works and what fails to meet with family approval. When it comes to cutting back on fat, Chinese stir-fry recipes serve as a model for a generally applicable approach. We find that the amount of fat suggested can be slashed considerably. Far from damaging the quality of the recipe, it actually produces a more agreeable dish. The same is true for many other dishes prepared in a skillet.

A second, very useful ally in cutting back on fat is yogurt, especially the low-fat variety. A salmon mousse recipe is an excellent example of how a minor modification can have a major nutritional effect. Switching from mayonnaise and whipped cream in the original recipe to low-fat yogurt reduced the calories by almost 60%, from 320 to 190 per serving, and the fat by more than 40%, from 26 to 11 grams per serving.

Yogurt is a particularly useful substitute for both sweet and sour cream in many other ways, too. We use it in everything from a topping for haddock baked with white wine, to a mixture with Parmesan cheese for noodles Alfredo, and as a basis for excellent herbed salad dressings. Adding a tablespoon of cornstarch dissolved in a little water will prevent the yogurt from curdling when heated.

We urge caution in altering recipes for baked products, since success can depend on chemical reactions that can be disrupted by radical changes. But in many cases the effect on the product is minimal, while the nutritional difference is considerable. Bran muffins are a case in point. The recipe for 12 standard muffins provided on the cereal box included 1¼ cups whole milk, ½ cup sugar, ¼ cup oil, and ½ teaspoon salt. Each muffin provides 160 calories, 6 grams of fat, 25 milligrams cholesterol, and 300 milligrams sodium.

Switching to skim milk, reducing the sugar to 2 tablespoons, oil to 2 tablespoons, and salt to ¼ teaspoon produces muffins providing 110 calories and 3 grams, or 50% less, fat. Reduction in salt leads to a drop of only 25 milligrams of sodium per muffin because so many of the ingredients, including the bran, milk, baking powder, and egg all contribute to the total. Using an egg substitute would, of course, eliminate all cholesterol from the recipe.

Turning now to salt, Chinese stir-fry dishes also provide a way to slash sodium from a recipe. Begin by switching to reduced-sodium soy sauce, which contains about 200 milligrams per teaspoon compared to as much as 500 milligrams in some regular soy sauces. Among those sauces lower in sodium than soy are oyster sauce (215 to 300 milligrams per teaspoon), sweet bean and hoisin (160 milligrams per teaspoon), and satay sauce (50 to 80 milligrams per tsp.). You may want to rely somewhat more heavily on onions, garlic, and ginger than on some of the very saltiest Oriental condiments.

In general, when it comes to salt and salty condiments, the basic approach is to cut down (or out) and compensate with herbs, spices, and condiments which are lower in sodium than table salt. A virtually salt-free alternative for prepared mustard for roast beef sandwiches is a mixture of dry mustard, marmalade, chives, and freshly ground black pepper. This sandwich always gets rave reviews.

In making the salmon mousse, mentioned earlier, we dilute clam broth, the major source of sodium, with an equal amount of water. By relying more heavily on lemon juice and minced onion than salt, we were able to reduce sodium by 100 milligrams per serving. When served without comment, the response was enthusiastic enough to permit us to assume that taste had not been sacrificed by the changes.

One word of advice about herbs: Whenever possible, buy them fresh. When you must rely on dried ones, try to find a store that specializes in seasonings and sells only the highest quality, and buy them in the smallest quantities possible. Because flavor deteriorates quickly, this is clearly a case where the large economy size is no bargain. A second step to maximizing the flavor from seasonings is to buy whole spices and invest in a small spice grinder. We guarantee you will be suitably impressed with the superior flavor of freshly ground pepper or nutmeg over that which has been sitting on a supermarket shelf for many months.

And finally, here's a word or two about the technique for skimming the fat from your family fare to a bare minimum. Begin by paring away visible fat before you start to prepare meat and poultry. Next, pour off fat as it accumulates during cooking, so that it will not be reabsorbed into the food. And

SALMON MOUSSE

1½ tbsp. plain gelatin
⅓ cup white wine
1 cup scallions, minced
1 tbsp. soft margarine
1½ cups clam broth
3 cups cooked, flaked salmon (or other fish).
salt and pepper
1 tbsp. dried dill weed
3 tbsp. lemon juice (or more, to taste)
⅔ cup part-skim yogurt

1. Soften gelatin in wine, about 5 minutes.
2. Melt margarine, add scallions, and cook until soft.
3. Add clam broth and simmer 5 minutes.
4. Add gelatin and wine and stir until dissolved.
5. Add flaked fish. Puree mixture in blender.
6. Season with salt, pepper, lemon juice, and dill.
7. Fold in yogurt, taste, and correct seasonings.
8. Pour into a single 2-quart mold or into eight individual molds and chill until set.

8 Servings/115 Calories Per Serving

Note: This is the basic recipe for the Salmon mousse. To decrease the sodium content, dilute the clam broth with water, i.e. use ¾ cups of broth and ¾ cups of water.

whenever possible in making soups and stews, refrigerate them so that the grease can be easily lifted from the top of the dish.

There you have our formula for dishes high in taste and nutrition and low in fat and salt. Below are ten general recipe suggestions which illustrate further just how it can be done.

Boneless Chicken Breasts—A Low-Fat Favorite

- When preparing chicken breasts, pound them and season with pepper, thyme, and just a sprinkle of salt. Then sauté quickly in a bit of oil. Squeeze a little lemon juice over the cooked chicken before you bring it to the table, or deglaze the pan with a small amount of Madeira wine.
- Or, when you have sautéed the chicken breasts as above, remove them from the pan to a warm oven and sauté a few chopped shallots and brown mushrooms in the cooking pan. Before adding to the chicken, be sure to drain the fat on paper towels.
- For an Italian-style dish, cut the the chicken breasts into chunks, trimming any visible fat. Heat a small amount of oil, then sauté a little garlic

and minced onion. Add the chicken and toss lightly until done. While the mixture is cooking, season it with oregano and black pepper and just a tablespoon of tomato paste. Remove the meat from the pan, add a little white wine, boil it down quickly, and pour over the chicken.

Luscious Leftovers

- Use leftover roast veal or pork to make an Indian dish. For 4 servings, sauté a medium-sized onion, minced, in a little oil, add ¼ cup raisins, 2 tablespoons slivered almonds, 1 teaspoon ground cumin, and ½ teaspoon turmeric. Add ½ cup low-fat yogurt and heat gently. Serve over rice.
- You can use leftover chicken to make a delicious Middle Eastern dish. Combine shredded chicken with a little fresh ground beef or lamb, sautéed well and drain on paper towels to get rid of excess fat. Sauté a medium-sized onion in a little oil, then add the chicken and meat, along with cooked rice and aromatic spices, like ground cloves, and cinnamon. Heat slowly. The ratio of meat to rice and intensity of seasoning is up to you, but in general, a cup of meat and chicken to 4 of rice seasoned with 1½ teaspoons cinnamon and ½ teaspoon cloves works well.

Pasta Pizazz

- A pasta dish for summer months relies on fresh basil and fresh tomatoes. Simply coat cooked pasta with a little fruity olive oil (about ¼ cup per pound), toss in peeled, seeded, and chopped tomatoes, finely chopped white onion, chopped basil, and Parmesan cheese. Season generously with freshly ground pepper. For a pound of pasta, a cup of fresh tomato, and ½ cup each of onion, chopped basil, and cheese are generally good proportions.
- A second tasty pasta dish is tubular pasta, like penne or ziti, tossed with spinach and low-fat ricotta and Parmesan cheeses. For 6 servings, cook a package of thawed frozen spinach over high heat with 2 tablespoons oil, fresh pepper, and a pinch of salt. Toss with ½ cup each of low-fat ricotta and Parmesan cheeses. For added flavor, toss in some minced green onion.

Sensational Seafood

- A delicious seafood dish is shellfish served on a vegetable puree. For 4 servings, puree a cup of raw green beans or tomatoes in a food processor. Bring the puree to a boil and add a tablespoon of oil. Heat the mixture vigorously for a minute or two. Season with white pepper, a pinch of thyme, and a dash of white wine. Steam a pound of shrimp or scallops until just done and serve over the puree.
- For another seafood dish, equally tasty if made with pieces of whitefish or with shellfish, such as scallops or shrimp, first heat a little oil in a skil-

let. Then, sauté a minced shallot, add the fish, and sauté quickly. As the mixture is cooking, add just 2 teaspoons Dijon mustard, a sprinkling of tarragon, a tablespoon of drained capers, and several grinds of fresh pepper. When the fish is cooked, remove, and quickly deglaze the pan with a little white wine. A pound of fish served over noodles, and prepared in well under ten minutes, serves four.

Stir-fry Classic

■ Basic Chinese stir-fry is hard to beat for speed and versatility. For 4 servings, heat 2 tablespoons oil in a frying pan. Add a clove of minced garlic, a thinly sliced onion, and 3 slices of fresh, minced ginger, and stir fry for a minute or two. Add a pound of lean, thinly sliced beef strips and cook quickly. Season with a teaspoon of soy sauce and a few drops of sesame oil and top with shredded scallion. Drain to eliminate any excess cooking oil or fat from the meat. Accompany with Chinese vegetables quickly sautéed in just a tablespoon of oil and seasoned with a few drops of hot chili oil.

Questions and Answers

Q. What are the differences among skim milk, 1% fat, 2% fat, and whole milk?

A. The differences relate to the amount of butterfat, by weight, that they contain. At one end of the spectrum is skim milk, which contains virtually no fat, while at the other is whole milk, in which about 3.25% of the weight is butterfat.

While fat content is the main marker of caloric differences between the various milks, the addition of protein solids to some of the reduced-fat milks also affects their caloric content. Thus, whole milk contains 150 calories per cup, while 2%-fat milk may contain anywhere from 120 to 135 calories, depending on whether or not protein solids have been added and in what amounts. Similarly, the caloric content of 1%-fat milk ranges from about 100 to 120 calories, and skim milk from a low of 85 to a high of about 100 calories per cup.

Q. Ricotta is often referred to as Italian cottage cheese. It seems creamier than regular cottage cheese. Are the two really nutritionally comparable?

A. No, there are significant differences related to the basic food used to produce the two types of cheese. Whole-milk ricotta, as the name implies, is made from either whole milk or from a mixture of whole milk and whey. It contains 16 grams of fat and 215 calories per half-cup serving. The same amount of part-skim ricotta contains considerably less fat, about 10 grams, and provides 170 calories.

Regular cottage cheese is made from the curd to which a little cream is added. Even the creamed variety contains less fat and fewer calories than the part-skim ricotta. A half-cup serving contains only 110 calories and 5 grams of fat.

If you're interested in controlling the amount of fat, particularly saturated fat, in your diet and/or cutting down on calories, cottage cheese is the better choice. Of course, the lower the fat content of the cottage cheese you buy, the fewer calories you will get.

Q. Can you provide data on the sodium content of various Chinese seasonings?

A. As a basis of comparison, keep in mind that a teaspoon of salt contains 2,100 milligrams of sodium. In analyses of a number of Chinese condiments published several years ago, several seasonings, including sweet bean sauce, hoisin sauce, satay sauce, fermented bean cake, fermented black beans, and dried shrimp all contained less than 200 milligrams, or less than one-tenth the sodium, as a teaspoon of salt. Brown bean sauce contained 425 milligrams of sodium per teaspoon.

For other common seasonings there was considerable variability from one brand to another, and in the absence of labeling information perhaps sensitive taste buds will aid in trying to make the lowest sodium choices. For example, oyster sauce ranged from a low of 215 milligrams per teaspoon in one brand to as much as 330 milligrams in another. And among three light soy sauces tested, values ranged anywhere from 320 to 445 milligrams per teaspoon, while among the dark sauces, five brands ranged anywhere from 310 to as much as 495 milligrams per teaspoon.

Q. In reading pamphlets about controlling sodium intake, monosodium glutamate is often listed among the ingredients to watch. Because it is in so many foods, I would like to know how its sodium content relates to that of salt.

A. Measure for measure, monosodium glutamate, or MSG, contains considerably less sodium than table salt. By weight, salt is 40% sodium, while MSG is only 12% sodium. Thus, while a quarter teaspoon of salt provides about 550 milligrams of sodium, the same amount of MSG would provide only 165 milligrams. However, while the contribution of MSG to the sodium content of a particular food may be small, it is often added commercially to foods which are generously salted. Moreover, salt and MSG may not be the only sources of sodium in a processed food. So to really have an idea of how much sodium a serving of a particular processed food may contain, it's best to check the sodium labeling information now available on an increasing number of processed foods. If it is not available, you have two alternatives: write to the manufacturer and request that information, or buy a comparable product where the information is readily available.

Q. Can you provide some directions for minimizing the greasiness of fried chicken when I do make it?
A. Since fat absorption is related to the amount of time the chicken spends in the oil, it is important to minimize cooking time. To accomplish that, the temperature of the fat should be kept constant, about 350°F. That means cooking just a few pieces at one time. As it is cooked, the chicken should be put in a warm oven, about 300°F, standing on end. Considerable amounts of the absorbed fat will drain to the bottom of the pan, but the chicken will remain crunchy. As a final step, set the fried chicken on paper towels to drain just before serving. But as you point out, even the most careful preparation techniques cannot get around the fact that this remains a fat- and calorie-laden treat best reserved for special occasions.
Q. I really miss putting butter on my vegetables and don't find margarine an acceptable substitute. As an alternative, I use a little sesame oil as a seasoning. I am concerned that it may be highly saturated. Is it?
A. Sesame oil actually contains generous amounts of polyunsaturates, which make it quite an acceptable choice. From the gastronomic point of view, we think it has a certain advantage. Unlike many vegetable oils which are virtually tasteless, sesame oil has a pronounced, and to our taste, pleasant flavor. Thus, a little goes a long way, making it particularly useful for individuals who want to cut down on their intake of fat, calories, or both. Sesame oil, incidentally, is not just a good seasoning for hot vegetables. It is also an excellent dressing for raw vegetables when combined with some white vinegar and a bit of soy sauce.
Q. Can you please tell me how to make a sour cream substitute from yogurt?
A. Yogurt can sometimes be used as is as a sour cream substitute, but for a more dense and creamier alternative, simply dump a container of low-fat yogurt into a funnel lined with a paper filter or cheesecloth. Stand it in a container in the refrigerator for several hours to allow the whey to separate. The resulting "cheese" can be eaten as is, or seasoned with whatever herbs or seasonings you like. Yogurt cheese is especially good as a spread for crackers when blended with some minced garlic. It is a good idea to add the seasonings and then let the cheese sit awhile to give the flavor a chance to permeate. A topping of a small amount of brown sugar and some yogurt cheese over green grapes makes a tasty dessert. Two tablespoons of the cheese itself, if made with low-fat yogurt, contains about 1 gram of fat and 28 calories.
Q. I have heard conflicting reports about whether shellfish are high in cholesterol. Why the confusion and can you straighten me out?
A. The confusion has an historical basis. At the time that restricting dietary

cholesterol was first recommended as one of the measures that could help control blood cholesterol and thereby reduce the risk of heart disease, available laboratory procedures did not distinguish between cholesterol and other sterols present in considerable amounts in shellfish. Consequently, it appeared that shellfish contained more cholesterol than they really did.

Newer procedures indicate that most shellfish are in the same range with chicken, lean beef and veal, and fin fish. That is, 3 ounces of oysters provide 40 milligrams of cholesterol; scallops, 45 milligrams; clams, 55 milligrams; lobster, 75 milligrams; and crab, 85 milligrams Shrimp contains a bit more, about 130 milligrams per 3-ounce serving. By comparison, 3 ounces of lean beef, veal, or chicken provide an average of 80 milligrams, while the same amount of flounder has only 40 milligrams, and tuna, 55 milligrams. In sharp contrast, a large egg—and eggs are, for most people the largest single contributor of cholesterol—contains about 213 milligrams of cholesterol.

Q. What is the evidence regarding a link between a cholesterol-lowering diet and an increased risk of cancer? Is it possible that lowering serum cholesterol is a poor idea?

A. No. Evidence from investigations of a link between serum cholesterol and cancer, now well into the second decade, suggests that in this "chicken and egg" riddle, the cancer comes first and lowered serum cholesterol follows. True, studies in widely different geographic areas ranging from Evans County, Georgia, to the South Pacific have found an increased mortality from cancer in groups with the lowest serum cholesterol levels. However, the level at which this occurs is well below the usual range of cholesterol values in the U.S.

An analysis by the International Collaborative Group of ten years of cancer mortality in over 60,000 men from 11 population studies in eight countries found that cancer precedes lower cholesterol levels. Why any association occurs only at levels below 190 mg./dl. and only in males remains unexplained.

Beyond that, many pieces of evidence suggest that lowering serum cholesterol does not "cause" cancer. For one thing, in a number of worldwide population-based studies, high serum cholesterol and higher consumption of saturated fat have been associated with both increased noncardiovascular mortality and death from cancer, in particular. Second, in studies which have shown a low serum cholesterol and cancer link, there was no attempt, using either diet or drugs, to lower cholesterol levels. Thus, these studies cannot link diet change with cancer. Third, while a study of men in a Los Angeles VA Hospital done in the 1960s reported excess deaths from cancer in men on cholesterol-lowering diets, other studies which compared the results of four independent clinical trials in Oslo, Helsinki, London, and Minneapolis found no increased risk.

The more recent of two international workshops sponsored by the National Heart, Lung, and Blood Institute (NHLBI) in 1981 studied the results of 17 investigations in detail. The panel which analyzed the study findings concluded that there seemed to be a weak and inconsistent relationship between very low cholesterol levels and cancer of the colon in men. However, these studies had been designed to study cardiovascular disease, not cancer. Therefore, other factors of possible importance in relation to cancer had not been examined and could not be considered in the data analysis. Moreover, several inconsistencies in the data tended to weaken the argument for a cancer-cholesterol relationship.

The cancer-cholesterol connection is an issue that researchers will continue to examine. The point here is that there is no evidence to suggest that we should abandon our dietary efforts to lower serum cholesterol.

Q. My cholesterol level was high enough so that my doctor decided to put me on a very-low-fat diet. I have lowered my cholesterol dramatically, but in the process I lost considerable weight. I did need to lose some, but now I am having trouble keeping my weight up. What do you suggest?

A. Rediscover carbohydrates. Over the years, carbohydrate-rich foods have gained the undeserved reputation as "cheap" and "fattening." But gram for gram, they contain less than half as many calories as fat.

Now that you have lost more weight than is desirable, it is time to make a conscious attempt to increase the low-fat foods in your diet. Just how you do it will depend on your own food preferences. You may find that you would enjoy having more bread than you had been accustomed to eating—perhaps a slice or two of a good whole-grain loaf at breakfast, along with some juice and cereal with skim milk; and some more at dinner. Rediscover good thick soups. Many recipes using various dried beans, lentils, and barley, especially those you are likely to find in vegetarian cookbooks, are already or can easily be adapted to fit into a low-fat diet. Enjoy more generous servings of pasta or noodles. Even without much fat, it is quite possible to prepare tasty sauces to season them. Similarly, have larger servings of rice and barley. We suggest you try pilaf, prepared by baking either grain in the oven with chicken broth. If you want to use a bit of the fat allowed on your diet, you can enhance your rice or barley dishes by sautéeing some minced onion and mushrooms in oil to add to the mixture.

Finally, as long as you have not been advised to restrict your intake of simple sugars, there are several desserts you can indulge in from time to time. Among these are angel cake, sorbet, gelatin, and meringues. Even if fat is not a concern, we think that a scoop of good fruit sorbet served on a meringue shell and topped with a raspberry puree is an elegant enough dessert for any festive occasion.

Q. I have a friend who insists that certain foods should never be eaten together, claiming that the digestive system has an entirely different process for breaking down different types of foods. She actually uses a chart to guide her in putting together appropriate food combinations to ensure efficient digestion. Is there any truth to this claim?

A. No. The idea of "ideal" food combinations is hardly new. It has been incorporated into dietary designs for everything from weight-reducing plans to regimens associated with various spiritual beliefs. As long as the end result is a nutritionally well-balanced diet, it is of no harm. But there is not a shred of evidence to suggest that it is of physiological benefit either.

The fact is that the normal, healthy digestive tract is designed to provide the many enzymes we need to break down carbohydrates, proteins, and fats in the foods we eat—regardless of the combinations in which we eat them—and to maintain the internal environment in which they work efficiently.

Q. Are there significant differences in the nutrient values of foods cooked in microwave ovens compared to those prepared by conventional methods?

A. Apparently not. While the number of microwave ovens is multiplying at an enormous rate (it is estimated that at least 75% of American homes have one), there has not been extensive research in recent years on nutrient retention in foods cooked in them. And some of the earlier studies are of limited value for comparison, in part because many important details were omitted from reports of the findings. More recent studies have shown that any differences tend to be of little significance in affecting the overall nutrient content of the diet.

Since ascorbic acid is the most vulnerable to heat, water leaching, and oxidation, it is used as the indicator nutrient in vegetables. And in most cases, ascorbic acid content is higher in vegetables cooked in a microwave oven. Folate destruction in vegetables also appears to be lower.

In evaluating nutrient retention in meats, thiamin, which is sensitive to both heat and oxidation, is commonly used as an index of vitamin loss. In this case, overall decreases in the thiamin content of a serving of microwave and conventionally cooked meats appear comparable. So, too, were levels of riboflavin and niacin, both of which are more stable when heated.

Finally, comparisons of nutrient losses in foods reheated by the two methods appear to be similar. On the other hand, and not surprisingly, most nutrient losses are lower in microwave reheated meats, entrees, and vegetables, than in foods held on a steam table for up to three hours.

DINING OUT, DINING SMART

In an earlier era, dining out for most people was reserved for special occasions. What we ate away from home had little bearing on our nutritional well-being.

Today, the tables are turned. If you're a typical American, you now eat one out of every three meals and snacks out of your house or ordered from take-out restaurants. The options are endless, from fast-food shops to traditional restaurants, lunch counters, packaged food sold in machines, pizza pavillions, croissant cafes, supermarket salad bars, and so on. What it boils down to is that one-third of all your meals are selected from a menu devised by someone you probably don't know, cooked by someone you'll probably never meet, prepared in a kitchen you'll probably never see, and made with ingredients of which you are not quite certain.

As we see it, prudent restaurant eating is a responsibility to be shared by those who provide the choices and those who select among them. It is unrealistic to suggest that every item on every menu be compatible with a prudent diet. On the other hand, we can reasonably expect restaurants to offer some healthful menu alternatives and to provide nutrition information that allows consumers to make wise choices.

In fact, many restaurateurs have responded to changes in consumer demand by creating dishes lower in fat, sauces of fresh vegetable purees rather than of richer ingredients, or, for example, making a vegetable fish chowder as delicious as the sea of cream and butter for which New England is famous. They are offering salad dressing on the side and low-calorie dressing or lemon as a regular option, and they are providing a choice of butter or polyunsaturated margarine for rolls and potatoes. Some are learning, at long last, to prepare fish without encrusting it in a layer of breading that transforms it beyond recognition. Attractive dishes of fresh fruit have sprung up on menus, and fat free sorbets are becoming increasingly common.

Also responding to consumer demand are some fast-food chains, which have found that there may even be profit in such formerly alien items as salads. And while it may not be the biggest seller, low-fat milk is making an appearance on restaurant menus. Among the more innovative landmarks is Pawtucket, Rhode Island, where as part of a cardiovascular risk reduction program, participating restaurants designate "heart healthy" menu choices with a little red heart.

Some restaurants have hired professional dietitians to analyze their dishes and provide customers concerned about salt, fat, and calories with nutrition information on menu items. Now that computers are widely available to make such calculations quickly and cheaply, we wish more restaurants would follow suit. Fast-food restaurants, whose receipts account for more than 30% of all away-from-home sales, have a special responsibility to supply customers with in-store data about nutrient content. Given the limited scope of the menu (and the fact that many major chains already have the information anyway) the task should be relatively easy, and would be a boon to consumers seeking to make informed choices.

But while there are measures restaurants can take to facilitate prudent eating for their clientele, the thickest slice of responsibility belongs to the individual. Step one is to use discretion in choosing the restaurant. If "deep-fried" is the dominant mode of cooking, the chances of finding food that both tastes good and is good for you are slim.

The second step is to plan ahead to choose the appropriate options and to resist the temptation to be lured by Reuben sandwiches, oversized cheeseburgers gilded with bacon and Russian dressing, deep-fried veal cutlets, and myriad other fat-rich dishes. Also, you should decide what proportion of your daily quota of calories you plan to consume at this meal. You may want to tell the waiter to leave the french fries off your plate, even if there is no price difference. If they're not there, you can't possibly eat them!

Apart from steaks and lobsters, which are commonly priced by size, there are few restaurants which offer small portions for less money. But it's certainly possible to request a smaller portion, especially if you find yourself in a restaurant notorious for Gargantuan servings. When ordering meat or poultry with a sauce, inquire about the ingredients. If you think the dish might be high in fat but want to order it anyway, ask to have the sauce served on the side. Request that vegetables be served unbuttered. Order your potato plain, either boiled or baked, perhaps garnished with a lemon wedge, or ask for rice with a tomato sauce. Ask that butter not be served with your bread. Finally, if you are among the millions of Americans who frequent fast-food restaurants and are concerned about your diet, request nutrition information about the menu items for your favorites and become familiar with them.

Birthdays, anniversaries, and other milestones may still be occasions to toss dietary discretion to the wind, but routine eating out demands a more prudent approach—that is, if you are committed to a healthy lifestyle.

DINING OUT, DINING SMART II: CHOOSING FAST FOODS WITH CARE

In case you had any doubts about just how much food is being consumed in that special type of eatery born in America about 40 years ago, consider this: Nearly one out of every two dollars spent in restaurants is spent in a fast-food outlet. Skyrocketing business has boosted sales to four times the level of 1954, making these chains the fastest-growing restaurants of all. The lure of convenience and the consistent quality of the products reel in millions of Americans to the quickie counter over and over again. In many cases, meals away from home represent a significant slice of our overall diet.

But is fast food good food? Back in the days when quickie meals usually meant a burger, fries, and a shake, the nutritional picture left room for improvement. Though not generally short on protein, overreliance on typical convenience menus could lead to inadequate intake of calcium, magnesium, copper, and vitamins A, B_6, C, and folic acid. Moreover, many of these fast foods were high in fat, saturated fat, and cholesterol.

Gradually, the fast-food concept has been successfully applied to different types of foods, allowing for wider variety and balance. Far from just lunchtime fare, fast food is now eaten for dinner and even breakfast. The choices can range from traditional American to Mexican, Chinese, and others—a rainbow of ethnic menus. Fresh fruits and vegetables are available, too, as well as whole-grain dishes like tabbouleh and whole-wheat pocket sandwiches.

The increase in choices means more than just new taste adventures. Greater variety makes it possible for the consumer who, for whatever reason, relies heavily on fast foods to eat well. The key point is that an adequate diet depends on wise selections wherever you are eating. Your food choices when eating in fast-food restaurants are just as important as the ones you make in the supermarket.

How can you enjoy the speedy service of meals on the go and still maintain a healthy diet? Follow the same guidelines as you would at home. Take advantage of the salad bar or choose the vegetable soup. Try the frozen yogurt instead of the ice cream, and replace the Danish with a whole-grain roll. When making selections, take into account how food is prepared, in light of your own nutritional needs. For instance, most of the fish at convenience chains is served deep-fried, adding so many calories to an otherwise lean protein source that the fish may wind up more calorie-laden than the beef. A fish sandwich would thus be a poor choice for someone trying to cut calories.

While many individuals who eat out often do have adequate diets, some members of the population may not. These are people with higher needs for particular nutrients. One example was provided by a Cornell University study which analyzed data from the nationwide food-consumption survey. Findings suggested that the intake of some nutrients—vitamins A and C, as well as calcium and iron—tends to decrease as the proportion of calories eaten away from home goes up. This trend could be especially important for teenagers and for women in their childbearing years, many of whom fail to get enough iron. This same group also tends to take in less than the recommended amount of calcium. For these individuals, careful choices in fast-food restaurants can make the difference between a satisfactory diet and the short end of the stick. Take the typical fast-food shake. One serving may supply over one-fourth of a woman's recommended daily allowance for calcium, but most also contain 50% more calories than a glass of whole milk and may add substantial sodium to the meal as well. Too many shakes can add up to an overload of calories in relation to other essential nutrients.

If you visit fast-food restaurants regularly, the best advice is to select a variety of foods from several types of eating places. Learn to combine foods and to scan the menu for items that will add up to a nutritionally balanced meal. A meal out of the house shouldn't mean a meal out of step with good nutrition. It is the wisdom of your choices, not the speed with which the food is prepared, that makes the nutritional difference.

Because major fast-food chains provide such a large proportion of the calories for so many people, we think they ought to provide nutrition information right in the restaurant. A few do. To help you make your choices, we have put together the latest nutritional information provided to us by the fast-food companies. That information can be found in Appendix, p. 299.

HIDDEN DEMONS
Preventing Food Poisoning

The party's over, the guests have gone. It was a successful affair highlighted by a well-planned, creative menu. But the next day: disaster. Two-thirds of the guests become ill, and the blame is laid on your food. Was the chicken underdone? Could it have been the artichoke dip that stayed out a long time, or maybe the ceviche?

Whether for you, your family, or a house full of guests, gastronomic delights need never be the source of illness. A few simple precautions in handling and storing food can virtually eliminate the risk of food poisoning. But before we review the guidelines for preventing foodborne illness, let's examine some of the more common causes.

The greatly increasing number of salmonella infections in the past decade has made this microorganism a regular household word. Studies have implicated chicken and other poultry as major sources of contamination. Recently, infections have also been traced to beef, improperly pasteurized milk, and grade A eggs. Evidence indicates that just a small number of salmonella bacteria is enough to cause a fleet of flulike symptoms including diarrhea, nausea, fever, headache, abdominal cramps, and sometimes vomiting. Symptoms usually appear within 12 to 24 hours after eating a contaminated food. The bacteria are killed by high temperatures, so infection can be prevented by cooking.

Staphylococcus (staph) infection is more difficult to control because, unlike salmonella, these bacteria produce a heat-resistant toxin in food that sits too long at room temperature. It is the toxin, rather than the bacteria themselves, that makes us sick. For this reason, cooking a food already containing the toxin will usually not render it safe. Meats, egg products, macaroni and potato salad, and other prepared foods that have been left at room temperature, or kept warm for an extended period, are frequent sources of staph infection. Symptoms of staph poisoning also mimic the flu and include diarrhea, vomiting, nausea, and abdominal cramps. These symptoms occur 1 to 8 hours after eating and usually last for 12 to 24 hours.

While less familiar to the public, *Campylobacter jejuni* is one of the most common causes of bacterial diarrhea in the United States. Raw or undercooked meat and poultry and unpasteurized milk are recognized sources of these bacteria, but recent studies have pointed to chicken as the chief source of contamination. Diarrhea, fever, and abdominal cramps usually occur two to five days after eating a contaminated food. Botulism, a very serious foodborne illness, is caused by the bacteria *Clostridium botulinum.* These bacteria grow under anaerobic (no oxygen) conditions and produce a potentially fatal toxin. In comparison with other foodborne illnesses, botulism is relatively rare, but when it does occur, it can be deadly. According to the Centers for Disease Control in Atlanta, 124 outbreaks of botulism, involving 308 people, were identified between 1976 and 1984. Of these, 23 were known to be fatal.

Because an anaerobic environment is necessary for the bacteria to produce the toxin, home-canned foods, especially low-acid foods such as green beans, are the most common sources of botulism. However, in recent years, such unexpected foods as baked potatoes, commercial pot pies, and sautéed onions were among the unlikely sources of the illness. In each case, anaerobic conditions were created by peculiar preparation and storage of the foods. The potatoes, for example, were left tightly wrapped in foil in a warm environment for several days before they were used.

The symptoms of botulism include double vision and other visual disturbances, generalized muscle weakness, inability to swallow, dry mouth, and constipation. These symptons occur 8 to 36 hours after the spoiled food is eaten.

If all of this sounds grim, keep in mind that the best prevention is proper handling and storage of food beginning at the time of purchase. While we tend to associate the warm weather of spring and summer with an increase in foodborne illness, the risk also rises right after holidays, when leftovers abound. Whatever the season, follow these ten sensible guidelines and you can reduce the risk of foodborne infection to zero.

1. First, check your refrigerator temperature. Proper storage calls for temperatures below 40ºF.
2. Keep fresh meat and poultry in the refrigerator for no more than a couple of days. And be sure not to let juices drip on other foods. Unwrap poultry and cover loosely; in tightly sealed packages, anaerobic bacteria will multiply and release offensive gases.
3. If you want to keep meats more than a couple of days, wrap them tightly, date, and freeze them at or below 0ºF. Frozen ground meat keeps up to three months at this temperature, other meats up to a year.
4. Thaw meats gradually, and only in the refrigerator. Thawing at room temperature is dangerous because the inside of the meat may remain frozen for hours, while the bacteria multiply on the warm outer surface.
5. Scour cutting boards and utensils which have been used for raw meat, fish, or poultry with plenty of soap and hot water to prevent contamination of cooked foods or those which will be eaten raw.
6. Keep food at room temperature for no more than two hours. Temperatures between 45º and 115ºF provide a danger zone where the bacterial population can double every 15-20 minutes. Cool leftovers quickly by transferring them from the cooking pot to a shallow pan on a cooking rack. When storing warm foods in the refrigerator, allow air to circulate around the container. Freeze leftovers if you are not going to eat them within four to five days. Despite common belief, even thawed foods can be refrozen.
7. Wash raw fruits and vegetables thoroughly before using. Occasionally, they can be contaminated with bacteria from the soil or from human handling.
8. Store canned foods in a cool, dry place, preferably for not more than a year. Canned foods stay edible as long as the container remains airtight, but storage at high temperatures can downgrade flavor and nutritional value. Date cans when purchased and use the oldest first. Dented cans are acceptable as long as the ends are flat and the seams don't leak, but use them soon. Discard, without opening, any can which bulges or has a swollen lid.
9. Avoid eating raw eggs, raw meat, and raw fish. Dishes like steak tartarè (raw ground beef) and sushi (raw seafood) can contain parasitic larvae. These larvae, which are destroyed by cooking, can go undetected in raw foods, even under careful inspection.
10. Cook beef to an internal temperature of 160ºF and poultry to 180ºF. Raw or undercooked pork may cause trichinosis. It should be cooked to

an internal temperature of 170ºF to kill any trichina larvae which might be present.

At a minimum, foodborne illness can bring uncomfortable, flulike symptoms. At the extreme, it is fatal. Luckily, with proper storage and preparation, the problem is entirely preventable. So play it safe. Remember that menacing organisms often do not change the appearance, taste, or odor of food. So, don't let looks fool you—when in doubt, throw it out.

Questions and Answers

Q. Can you please explain the dangers of eating raw fish?

A. Expanding interest in cuisines from other parts of the world has led to a surge of enthusiasm for raw fish dishes such as sushi (a traditional Japanese dish containing thin slices of raw fish) and ceviche (marinated raw fish). Unfortunately, the enjoyment of these foods is not without risk.

Certain popular varieties of fish available in the U.S., including herring, cod, squid, mackerel, pollock, and salmon, are commonly infected with *anisakiasis* larvae, a type of roundworm. *Anisakiasis,* or herring worm disease, is a recognized public health problem in Japan, the Netherlands, and other countries where people frequently eat raw or poorly cooked fish. Reported cases in the U.S. have been few (and restricted to the West Coast and Alaska) but it is believed that *anisakiasis* infection is more common than the reports suggest. Moreover, *anisakiasis* is not the only threat. Periodically, other types of worms from fish are identified as the source of severe symptoms, some of which even require surgery.

Since most fish have larvae in their muscles, as well as in their viscera (internal organs), prompt cleaning is not an effective preventive measure. These larvae survive marinating, inadequate smoking, and salting, but they do not survive temperatures over 140ºF for ten minutes or freezing at very low temperatures. In short, the only way to be absolutely sure of avoiding infection from fish is to deep freeze it (a practice which adversely effects the flavor and texture) or to cook it thoroughly before you eat it.

These cautions also apply to shellfish. For over 50 years, consumption of raw shellfish has been linked with outbreaks of serious gastrointestinal diseases such as typhoid, cholera, and hepatitis A. As a result of careful monitoring, these illnesses no longer pose a widespread health threat in the United States. The National Shellfish Sanitation Program, administered by the FDA, currently works with state agencies to insure that shellfish are taken only from clean waters.

However, every year restrictions on harvesting areas increase, causing financial hardship for the harvesters. And some unscrupulous individuals market shellfish taken from restricted areas. Bouts of diarrhea, abdominal pain, nausea, and vomiting, the result of microbiologic contamination, are still associated with eating raw oysters and clams. Periodic outbreaks of hepatitis are also traced to shellfish. Our advice is not to take the risk—cook all fish (and shellfish) thoroughly before eating it.

Q. Does a bulging lid on a can always signify the presence of botulism toxin?

A. No. A bulging lid may be an indication of botulism poisoning but it can also have other causes. A bulge could be caused by denting, or it could also be the result of a chemical reaction between certain foods, in which hydrogen is liberated. However, it is impossible for the consumer to determine the cause of a bulge. Since botulism poisoning is extremely dangerous and even potentially fatal, suspicious cans or jars should be returned, unopened, to the store where they were purchased. If, for any reason, this is not possible, the cans should be discarded in such a way that they are inaccessible to children or pets.

Q. Is it possible to get botulism poisoning from frozen food?

A. No. In order for botulism spores to grow and produce their toxin, they require a rather narrow range of temperatures. Some will not grow in an environment that is colder than 50°F, while others are able to grow slowly at temperatures as low as 38°F. Obviously, your freezer is considerably colder than that.

We should caution that freezing does not kill botulism spores. It is possible that if frozen food was thawed and left in a sealed container in a warm environment, spores could begin to grow and produce toxin.

Q. Is it safe to cook a turkey in a microwave oven?

A. According to experts at the USDA's Food Safety and Inspection Service it is safe as long as you follow directions carefully. First, the bird should not be stuffed, since the heat may not penetrate thoroughly enough to kill potentially harmful microorganisms. Second, it should be cooked covered for at least part of the time, since steaming in a closed environment promotes good heat conduction and is therefore effective in killing bacteria. Microwaveable cooking bags are well suited to the task. Third, turn the dish in which the turkey is cooking to help insure that heat penetrates to all parts of the bird. Finally, use a thermometer to insure that the internal temperature reaches 180°F.

Q. If you suspect you have food poisoning, what should you do?

A. The USDA's Food Safety and Inspection Service recommends treating mild symptoms of diarrhea and vomiting by taking plenty of fluids. Contact your physician or local emergency room if symptoms are severe or if the victim is very young, elderly, or chronically ill. Report the incident to your local board of health or other public health officials if you suspect it involves food eaten at a large gathering, restaurant, or purchased prepared food. When you call, have on hand the container or information about the restaurant. Wrap the product in plastic and label "danger" in case officials want to examine it.

For more answers to questions about food safety of meat and poultry products, contact the USDA's Meat and Poultry Hotline (800-535-4555) between 10 A.M. and 4 P.M. EDT, weekdays. For other food safety questions, contact your local county extension service.

Q. Are canned foods that have accidentally been frozen still safe?

A. They may be, although it is important to exercise caution in using them. The Canned Food Information Council advises that if a canned food is accidentally frozen, check the container carefully after it thaws to make sure that ends that bulged during freezing are once again flat and that there are no signs of leakage. In addition, it is important to watch for the several signs of spoilage—food spurting when the can is opened, off odors, and mold. Discard any food that is at all questionable. Once thawed, containers should be wiped dry to prevent rust. While some foods show a breakdown in texture, their nutrient content is not affected by freezing.

We should add that the USDA's Food Safety and Inspection Service recommends stricter precautions for accidentally frozen canned meat and poultry. Even if a can does not appear to have burst—an indication for discarding the contents without tasting—there is a real danger that there may be microscopic openings in the seams as a result of the stress. The USDA recommends that when canned foods have been frozen they be used immediately, boiling them first for 15 minutes to eliminate any possibility of food poisoning bacteria.

Q. I always thought that once foods have been thawed they should not be refrozen. Recently, I have heard that such a drastic measure is not always necessary. Is that true?

A. Refreezing is not a procedure of choice, but is a safe and acceptable alternative under certain conditions, and when it is necessary in order to avoid wasting food. The admonition not to refreeze thawed food apparently originated with Clarence Birdseye, the father of the frozen food industry, who was concerned with the negative effects of refreezing on the quality of his products. This was especially important during the early days of the industry, before commercially frozen food had gained widespread consumer acceptance.

The fact is that while thawing and refreezing may result in vitamin losses and usually affects the quality of the food adversely, as a general rule, foods that still contain ice crystals or have been held no longer than a day or two after thawing in the refrigerator are probably safe to refreeze. The likelihood that the food you are refreezing is safe will be much greater if it has been thawed in the refrigerator. When you do find it necessary to refreeze food, do it as quickly as possible, by placing it directly on a rack so that air can circulate around it, hastening the removal of heat.

Q. What is known about the safety of aspartame?

A. Quite a bit. Probably because of the considerable notoriety that has attended its predecessors, aspartame received more testing before it was approved than any other additive in the history of the FDA. So far, it has come up with a clean bill of health for safety, However, in a statement a couple of years ago, the FDA commented that given the limitations of existing data, it is impossible to state whether aspartame is associated with any clinical syndrome.

Aspartame is made up of two amino acids, phenylalanine and aspartic acid, both commonly found in food. The amounts of these amino acids contributed by artificial sweeteners are quite small compared with the amounts provided by other foods.

Specific concerns have focused in several areas. Questions have been raised about the fact that when aspartame is digested, or, to a lesser extent, as it sits on the shelf in an artificially sweetened liquid at warm temperatures for an extended time, some methanol is formed. In fact, fruit and vegetable juices naturally contain two or three times as much methanol as that provided by the same amount of soft drink. Moreover, studies in which doses were as much as four times the maximum level advised by the FDA failed to raise blood methanol beyond normal levels, nor did these high doses increase blood levels of its toxic breakdown product.

Another concern centers on the hazards of phenylalanine to a particular group of individuals who lack the enzyme to break it down. The condition, called phenylketonuria, or PKU, is rare, only about 1 in 15,000 live births. However, in these children, unrestricted amounts of phenylalanine can result in serious damage to the nervous system and permanent mental retardation. It is because of these individuals that products contain the label warning: "Phenylketonurics: Contains Phenylalanine."

While PKU is usually identified at birth, and a strict diet instituted at once, concern has been raised about the possible harm to a fetus in a pregnant woman who does not know that she is a carrier of the gene. Scientific evidence does not seem to support that concern, however. Similarly, reports linking seizures to aspartame ingestion in experimental animals have not been substantiated. A recent, carefully controlled study conducted by researchers from Duke University was unable to demonstrate that aspartame, even when administered in amounts far larger than anyone would normally consume, causes headaches. There was no difference in the incidence of headaches, or of other clinical symptoms as the result of a number of laboratory tests using either aspartame or a placebo.

In short, except for those who have phenylketonuria or who may need to limit their intake of phenylalanine for other reasons, there seems to be no evidence that aspartame, if used in moderation, should pose a threat to health. Nonetheless, with an eye to the wisdom of moderation, the FDA has set an acceptable daily intake at 50 milligrams per kilogram of body weight. Translated into actual consumption, a 132-pound adult would need to drink over 18 cans a day of artificially sweetened soft drink to obtain that amount. Clearly, that is well beyond the amount even the biggest consumers are likely to get.

Q. A friend of mine told me that vinegar is sometimes used commercially to retard mold development in bread. Does it work?

A. Vinegar is one of several alternatives (others include concentrated raisin juice, fermented flour, and fermented dairy solids) that some bakers now use to replace artificial preservatives which act as mold antagonists. The idea is that by using these alternatives, it is possible to make a label claim that the bread product is "additive free" or contains all "natural" ingredients.

These substitutes are not, however, as effective as the commercially available mold antagonists. It is estimated that bread baked without additives will mold within five to seven days. If baked with vinegar or one of the other "natural" products, shelf life is extended by about a day. When commercial mold antagonists, including propionates and sorbic acid are used, bread can be expected to remain on the shelf mold free for 10 to 12 days.

Q. I have read that you should discard any can with a swollen or bulging lid in such a way that not even pets could get at it. But shouldn't consumers who discover a problem of that type report it to some type of agency concerned with food safety?

A. Indeed they should. Should you find that you have a can with a swollen or bulging lid, the U.S. Food and Drug Administration would like you to let them know about it at once so that they can determine whether your problem is an isolated incident or the result of some processing defect necessitating a recall of a product line. Each telephone book in the U.S. has the number of the FDA office nearest you. An official will probably want to come and pick up the product in question in order to determine right away whether there is a problem. In the meantime, however, do not open the can.

PESTICIDES AND OUR FOOD SUPPLY

 Since the end of World War II, our food supply has become more abundant, more varied, and less expensive than ever before. These changes have helped Americans lead longer, healthier lives. Ironically, one of the forces behind this improved picture is pesticides.

Ironic, we say, because pesticides are often associated with images of illness and death. The word conjures up contaminated farmers languishing with cancer, food tainted with poisonous chemicals that no amount of scrubbing can wash away, and the ravaging of our nation's breadbasket through dire ecological imbalance. It's certainly true that some pesticides have been linked to an increased risk of cancer. That is why the government stopped the use of the cancer-causing agent EDB several years ago and why manufacturers no longer make apple juice and apple sauce from apples treated with a potentially harmful chemical known as daminozide (trade name, Alar).

Despite these moves, consumer advocacy groups argue that mistakes are corrected too slowly. In many cases, their concerns are legitimate. Even the former commissioner of the Food and Drug Administration, Frank Young, M.D., acknowledges that there are "gaps that need to be addressed." One such gap is that although as much as 25% of our fresh fruits and large amounts of our winter vegetables are imported from countries whose allowances for pesticides are less strict than our own, hardly any of that produce is tested before it enters the U.S. And of foods grown here, only about 14,000 samples were analyzed in 1987, which Commissioner Young admited is insufficient.

But here's the other side of the coin: fully half of those domestic samples had no pesticide residues at all, and less than 1% had levels exceeding established tolerances. Even more to the point, environmental experts at FDA maintain that while pesticides loom large in people's minds as an immediate and particularly onerous threat to health, a more significant problem, one that poses a far greater risk to consumers' well-being, is foodborne contamination from bacteria like salmonella.

Still, the government is attempting to limits hazards related to pesticides. One step is to allow new and safer pesticides to replace older, more dangerous types without the red tape that had been required in the past. Pesticides developed since 1972 (which have automatically gone through rigorous analysis) and found to carry fewer health risks than older compounds, are allowed to take their place on raw and processed foods immediately. Until 1972, any pesticide already on the market, even if suspect, was allowed to remain there until it had undergone a lengthy testing process. Now, a nine-year deadline has been set for completing tests on all older pesticides. Before that deadline was established, the analysis of the pre-1972 chemicals—some 600 in all—could conceivably have stretched into the next century.

The Environmental Protection Agency has also been relieved of having to reimburse a manufacturer when it bans one of its pesticides. In the past, if the EPA deemed that a pesticide was unsafe and should no longer be sold to farmers, it had to compensate the maker of that pesticide at fair market value for as-yet unused supplies. Freed of that financial burden, the agency can now take action more easily.

As these regulations are slid into place, the government is simultaneously studying the use of biological alternatives to pesticides. An example is exploring whether insects and other small animals that do not hurt food can be used to prey on animals that do harm crops as a partial solution for cutting back on pesticides.

Of course, these several measures will not eradicate all concerns completely. It is impossible for the government to insure the safety of every bite of food that goes into our mouths. But a perfect food supply has never been a reality, even before the era of pesticides. Foods have their own built-in toxicants, in fact. Mushrooms contain potent animal carcinogens, and alfalfa sprouts harbor a poison that can cause illness in laboratory animals. But since it would be difficult to eat enough of these foods to create problems in humans, no one would argue that we should avoid them. The same thinking can be applied to pesticides. Technologists can now detect pesticide residues in foods in concentrations as low as one part per trillion. But the presence of these chemicals in minute amounts does not automatically signify a heightened threat to the health of people who eat foods that contain them.

To sum up, risk from pesticides is technically present, and certainly we need to continue exploring both safe compounds and appropriate alternate forms of pest control. We also need to beef up our monitoring system, especially of imported foods. But when you mesh all these factors together, and weigh the risks and benefits, a general outcry against pesticides is unwarranted.

2 THE NUTS AND BOLTS OF NUTRITION

The curtain rose on the scientific study of nutrition in a laboratory in France in the 1770s with Antoine Lavoisier's ingenious method for measuring energy expenditure. His identification of the calorie as a unit of heat was the source from which all further discovery flowed. Lavoisier's studies, later extended by scientists through the centuries and across the world, led to the establishment of tables giving the caloric equivalent of common foods and the caloric cost of various forms of exercise.

One might roughly divide the history of nutrition into three great eras. Between 1770 and 1905, attention focused on calories and the energy nutrients: carbohydrate, protein, and fat. Cholesterol was also discovered during that period, and the role of some key minerals present in the body in large quantities, like calcium, iron, sodium, and potassium, was examined.

Toward the end of the nineteenth century, the French physiologist Magendie showed that the body was not a perfect chemist, and that to support life, some as yet undefined chemical entities had to be supplied by food. This realization opened the door to the second period in the history of nutrition, between 1905 and 1945, the time of the great discoveries of the relationship between micronutrients, vitamins and minerals, and nutritional deficiencies. The concept of "essential" amino acids, constituents of proteins which the body could not manufacture and which had to be present in the diet, emerged. In the 1920s, a major breakthrough occurred when scientists discovered that a collection of complex compounds—called "vitamins"—was necessary in tiny amounts to keep the body running smoothly. Scientists also recognized the serious consequences of the lack of particular vitamins in the body and pinpointed the effects of mineral deficiencies. Goiter, commonplace in inland regions in the U.S., was successfully combatted with iodine. Zinc deficiency, the cause of dwarfism in some Middle East areas, was identified.

Since World War II, it has become increasingly evident that what is in the diet can, over time, be as important as what is missing from it. This knowledge marks the third period in nutrition's history. The links between tooth decay and sugar consumption, high cholesterol and the intake of saturated fat, and heavy salt intake and hypertension are all examples. Further, a correlation was shown between obesity and conditions like diabetes, atherosclerosis, and liver and kidney disease. It was also demonstrated that when people don't exercise, their mechanism for regulating appetite may suffer.

Today, growing evidence links certain types of cancer to diet; for instance, high fat levels are associated with breast cancer. There is much left to learn along these lines, as well as about other dietary factors such as fiber and the role of genetics in shaping health. As research breaks new ground, understanding the basics of nutrition, the energy nutrients, vitamins, minerals, water, and fiber, is crucial to interpreting the millions of messages we receive on everything from the morning cereal box to the latest meal-in-a-bar snack food.

THE SUPPLY AND DEMAND CURVE IN HUMAN NUTRITION

What's the difference between a nutritional requirement and a dietary allowance? The same difference as between a necessity and a safety net, which allows a margin for error. For many consumers, the failure to make that distinction in thinking about nutrients churns up a whirlpool of confusion.

The concept of a minimum nutritional requirement is pretty clear. It is the smallest amount a person needs in order to avoid gross deficiency disease. When nutritionists first met to create a table of nutritional recommendations, their focus was more on economics than on health. It was the time of the Great Depression and millions were unemployed. The International Labor Organization got the idea that if they could define a family's minimum nutrient needs, they could estimate the cost of a satisfactory diet. If a family spent no more than one-third to one-half its income on food, it was possible to estimate the minimum amount of money necessary to live. Such nutritional brinksmanship, just enough to stay out of trouble, is not a lofty goal. Clearly more is better—at least up to a point. Therein lies the distinction between minimum requirements and the Recommended Dietary Allowances, or RDA's, as they are commonly called.

First established in 1943, the RDA's were intended as a guide to wartime planning and stockpiling of nutritious food supplies for national defense. Today, the board of scientists which sets the standards still focuses on the question of what the nutrient does, and who needs how much of it.

For example, size makes a difference. Usually the bigger you are the more nutrients you need. Women during their childbearing years need more iron than men of comparable age because they lose blood through menstruation each month. Pregnant women and those who are breast-feeding need more iron because of the needs of the unborn or nursing baby. Children generally need more nutrients per pound to meet the demands of rapid growth and because they "burn up" nutrients slightly faster than adults.

Then comes the extra margin for safety. Here, the experts take into account the varying amounts of food consumed every day and whether a nutrient is available in many common foods or in only a few. They weigh whether or not the vitamin is widely found in low-calorie foods and whether the best sources are too expensive for many people. They also worry about the safety of the margin itself. For example, you can consume fairly large amounts of vitamin C without harm. Beyond a certain point, the body just gets rid of what it can't use. Thus, the allowance level is set fairly high, six times the minimum needed to prevent scurvy, but no higher, because any excess above that would be wasteful. In contrast, the RDA for vitamin D is much closer to the bare minimum because too much can be harmful.

The end result is that if people get 100% of the Recommended Dietary Allowances of the basic nutrients every day, some people will be getting more than they need—but no healthy person will be getting too little. Despite the endless onslaught of advertising suggesting otherwise, there is no valid reason for climbing far beyond the RDA's. Two-hundred percent of the RDA for a nutrient is not twice as good for you. The minimum plus the margin of safety standard is true for just about every nutrient covered by the RDA's.

In all there are RDA's for eleven vitamins, seven minerals, and protein. The recommendations are divided into ten categories by age and sex, with extra slots for pregnant and nursing women. A separate set of "safe and adequate dietary intakes" covers 12 nutrients for which we still lack sufficient data to set RDA's. All this information would never fit on a tuna fish can, so when nutrition labeling went into effect something more compact was needed. To fill the bill, the U.S. Recommended Daily Allowances (U.S. RDA's) were adapted from the parent RDA's. There are special categories for pregnant and nursing women, as well as for children under four, but the one most commonly used for nutrition labeling is that for children four years and older through adulthood. The standards in that table are generally the highest level for adults, and therefore, in some cases provide even more generous margins. To complicate the explanation a bit further, the U.S. RDA for iron, 18 milligrams, exceeds any value in the current revision of the FDA tables. It was the value for women taken from an earlier version. In the 1989 edition, the RDA for iron for adult women has been dropped from 18 to 15 milligrams.

Meeting the RDA's for essential nutrients is an important goal, but it does not guarantee a nutritionally adequate diet. Implicit in the concept of the Recommended Dietary Allowances is that they be met by a diet containing a wide range of foods, not by taking a nutritional supplement.

Questions and Answers

Q. A friend of mine has just had a hair analysis. Based on the findings of that analysis, she was told to take a supplement containing several minerals. I had not heard of this procedure before and wondered about its validity. What is your opinion?

A. In recent years, hair analysis has become just one more weapon in the arsenal of self-styled nutritionists. Yet hair analysis is thought to be useless for assessing vitamin status and of limited value for assessing mineral status.

Hair analysis as a research tool does have some value. For example, it has been used to detect high levels of heavy metals, such as mercury or lead, in a particular population. However, the usefulness of data resulting from the hair analysis of individuals remains unclear, with unanswered questions about both analytical procedures and about the interpretation of the results of these procedures. Indeed, the relationship between the concentration of a vitamin or mineral in hair and the concentration in other body tissues has not been established.

Despite the fact that researchers are unsure about its role in evaluating nutritional status, the results of commercial hair analysis are used to sell supplements. In some instances, the significance of low levels of heavy metals is exaggerated. In others, "deficiencies" are detected and megadoses of vitamins and trace minerals are prescribed to correct so-called "metabolic imbalances." This is just one more form of nutritional quackery that in some cases may be costly but harmless and in others downright dangerous.

Q. What is "megavitamin therapy." How much more than a normal amount is considered a megadose?

A. Megavitamin therapy is simply the use of vitamins at several times the Recommended Dietary Allowance (RDA). It has been suggested that a general description might be ten times the RDA for each vitamin. There is, however, a serious flaw in that definition. While it is true that ten times the RDA is the lowest level at which symptoms of toxicity may begin to appear, vitamin D toxicity can develop in infants at substantially lower doses—just five to seven times the RDA (between 2,000 and 3,000 International Units a day) normally, but as little as 2½ times in certain extremely susceptible infants.

In view of the serious side effects of taking too much vitamin D, giving infants anything above what is recommended by the pediatrician is courting disaster. As for normal, healthy adults, while many people like to take a single multivitamin as a bit of nutritional insurance, there is no reason for an individual to dose him- or herself with any single vitamin or take two or three times beyond what is needed. Groups for which it is a good idea to take a single multivitamin daily are the elderly, pregnant and lactating women, and young children.

Q. I have heard that supplements of individual minerals can create "mineral imbalances." Could you please explain why this happens?

A. While we have a very long way to go in understanding the complexities of mineral interactions in the body, we do know that there is considerable potential for undesirable effects as a result of unsupervised self-dosing with supplements of individual minerals. High intakes of one mineral, such as you might get by taking a supplement, can affect the way the body handles a second mineral not necessarily even consumed at the same time. The intestine may respond to high, chronic doses of a specific mineral with an adaptive mechanism which limits the uptake of that mineral into the body. At the same time, however, transport of a chemically similar mineral which occurs at a low concentration in the diet may be reduced. While the body's supply of the supplemented mineral thus remains adequate, a deficiency of the minor mineral could eventually develop. Another potentially hazardous situation could result from the adverse effects of one mineral on the mechanism by which the body absorbs and regulates another.

The best and safest way to make sure you get all the minerals you need is not to take supplements but to eat a varied diet containing lots of fresh and lightly-processed foods which supply these essential nutrients.

Q. A young man I know is suddenly losing his hair quite rapidly. He has been evaluated and found medically healthy. He is now considering going to a "nutritionist" who claims to be able to treat the problem. It means a lot more expensive tests, and I suspect it will be a waste of money. Are my suspicions correct?

A. Yes. We would urge anyone seeking the services of a "nutritionist" who claims nutritional cures for baldness to reconsider. Baldness, especially a patchy form of hair loss known as alopecia, as well as other hair changes, including color loss and changes in texture are associated with true nutrient deficiencies in both humans and animals. Loss of body hair has been associated with the consumption of excessive amounts of vitamin A in people. But these are extreme situations. Having ruled out a medical cause for the problem, the most likely explanation lies in heredity. That, of course, is beyond control.

PROFILE ON PROTEIN

A common image of early man shows a brawny fellow with a huge club dressed in animal skins gnawing on a bone. While it's true that our ancient ancestors did engage in hunting, researchers have shown that meat was not their main source of food. Roots, berries, leaves, nuts, eggs, and fruits were staples of their diet, and even such game as they did catch was far leaner than the choice, farm-grown meats we eat today. Yet the view persists that meat, rich in protein, connotes strength and survival. Eating large quantities is linked in many people's minds to surging growth, bulging muscles, and athletic prowess.

Protein is indeed a vital nutrient that plays a spectrum of roles in our bodies. Carbohydrates, fats, and proteins can all provide us with energy, but only protein has the capacity to build, repair, and maintain the body's tissues, including those in the kidneys, liver, and skin. Proteins are components of enzymes and certain hormones, and are needed to make blood cells and infection-fighting antibodies, as well as for hair and nails. Proteins are part of the carpentry that helps keep the body erect and the glue that holds the cells together.

Like other constituents of the body, proteins eventually get used up and must be replaced. The body assembles its own proteins from those in the foods we eat. Every different type of animal, vegetable, or microbe has its own special types of protein, so there are countless kinds, all designed to meet the needs of particular organisms. These millions of proteins are all formed from only 20 different building blocks—amino acids—put together in different ways, just as words are made from the alphabet or structures from a Lego set.

Our body's task is to take the proteins of other organisms and transform them into types we can use to repair and maintain our cells. By breaking down foods into their component amino acids, and then rebuilding them to suit our needs, we can manufacture some of the amino acids and hence, some of the proteins, ourselves. These amino acids are called "nonessential" because we do not have to get them ready-made in foods. However, there are eight amino acids that we cannot make, and which must be included in our diets. Referred to as the "essential amino acids," they must be present in the foods we eat or we will be placed in nutritional jeopardy.

Here's where meat comes in. Animal foods most closely resemble the proteins in our bodies. They contain all the amino acids in the right proportions, which makes them of highest biologic value. This is to say that a smaller, overall amount of protein of high biological value will give us the same amount of amino acids (and thus, overall usable protein) as a large amount of a poor protein, such as a plant source.

Does that mean we should all don cave-man clothes and go out with clubs in search of meat? Absolutely not. While we certainly need to include animal foods in our diets, the truth is that it is not necessary to depend exclusively on high-quality proteins—some of which are high in fat and/or cholesterol and expensive to boot—to meet our needs for amino acids. Habitually, we eat a variety of foods containing proteins of differing qualities. The daily Recommended Dietary Allowance is 56 grams (or 2 ounces) of pure protein for a man and 46 grams (1.6 ounces) for a nonpregnant, nonnursing woman.

These quotas are not all that hard to meet. One cup of milk, for instance, has 9 grams of protein. An ounce of ground beef has 7, an egg has 6, and one tablespoon of peanut butter, 4. A woman, then, can get nearly 40% of her daily protein requirement from 2 cups of milk. Add an egg and 3 ounces of meat, fish, or poultry, and she will have all the protein she needs for the day. Many other foods are also good protein sources. A half-cup of oatmeal has 3 grams, as does one slice of whole-wheat bread. A cup of spinach has 5 grams, a stalk of broccoli, 6, one medium baked potato, 3.

A very small amount of protein of high quality, contributing the missing essential amino acids, can be mixed in to upgrade the quality of "poor" proteins. For instance, cereals are generally low in the amino acid, lysine, whereas milk contains ample amounts. When we pour milk on breakfast cereal, we create a complete protein. A Chinese meal that supplements rice with beans or combines the two with small portions of fish, poultry, or other meat is a particularly good model of this mutual supplementation of protein.

To include protein in a healthy diet we don't need to become hunters, but we do need to chose wisely which foods we eat—and in what combinations.

Questions and Answers

Q. Is yeast a good protein supplement?

A. We would be hard put to recommend it for several reasons. An ounce of yeast does provide about 11 grams of protein, roughly equivalent to the amount in an 1½ ounces of meat. However, that is about ¼ cup, rather a formidable amount to consume, unless you happen to like the taste. Second, the protein in yeast, a plant food, does not contain all of the essential amino acids necessary for growth and repair of body tissue. In this case, the sulfur-containing amino acids are lacking. So in order for the body to use it efficiently, it should be taken with a variety of other protein foods. Third, yeast tends to be an expensive source of protein. Finally, there is a basic question about the advantages of protein supplements. Most people in the U.S. get far more protein than the body needs. Any extra is either burned for energy or stored as fat. So why take supplements?

Q. Is there any truth to the claim that the amino acid, lysine, is a useful supplement for treating genital herpes infections?

A. Lysine has been promoted for the treatment of herpes in the popular press. However, there is no good evidence to support its effectiveness. The origin of the claim dates back to laboratory observations first published in 1964. Research conducted to determine amino acid requirements of the virus found that lysine exerts a partially inhibitory effect on the growth of the virus, while another amino acid, arginine, seems to promote replication. However, several clinical trials, conducted over a period of ten years, provided inconclusive results. Moreover, these studies suffered from design flaws which limit their value. Unfortunately, the amount of lysine study subjects consumed in their diets was not reported, nor was there any attempt to control the amount of lysine or arginine in their diets.

Q. I have read that a medium-sized stalk of broccoli contains a respectable amount of protein. I had always thought that the calories in vegetables came from starches and sugar. What other vegetables are good sources of protein?

A. Quite a number of them. Starting at the top of the list, a cup of black-eyed peas provides 15 grams of protein and a cup of baby lima beans, about 13. The same amount of peas or brussels sprouts will give you 7 or 8 grams, and spinach will contribute 6. You can get 5 grams of protein from a cup of asparagus, collard greens, or corn, and about 4 from the same amount of kale, potato, bean sprouts, or winter squash. Other vegetables provide smaller amounts.

By themselves these vegetables do not contain all of the essential amino acids and therefore cannot be used to build and repair body tissue. Eaten as part of a meal containing other proteins which supply the missing amino acids, they can however, contribute significantly to your protein intake.

FAT FACTS

With the emergence of the links between fat intake and both cardiovascular disease and certain cancers, terms such as "cholesterol," "saturated," and "polyunsaturated" have become household words—almost. A vast number of Americans are trying to cut down on fat. Yet, despite the intense focus on fat in recent years, and the widespread use of these terms everywhere from TV sitcoms to commercials for peanut butter, there remains a wealth of misunderstanding about what the terms actually mean and how they relate to health. But in the enthusiasm to cut back on fat, almost to regarding it as a dirty word, we forget that it actually plays a crucial role in the diet. So let us turn for a moment to why we need fat and then straighten out some of the often confused terminology crucial to understanding the role of fat in disease, especially cardiovascular disease.

We need fat because it provides energy, and, after all, we need fuel to function. Several essential vitamins, including A, D, E, and K are soluble in fat. Fatty foods, therefore, act as carriers of these vitamins. They also provide essential fatty acids that the body needs and cannot make. They slow the rate at which food leaves the stomach, thereby contributing to a feeling of fullness. Finally, they absorb and hold flavors and, in combination with other nutrients, provide textures that increase palatability. In plain English, their major contribution to making foods smell and taste good is the very reason that people find it so difficult to reduce their fat intake. But that is exactly what we are being asked to do in order to insure that we will lead longer, healthier lives.

In order to understand the "down side" of the fat story it is essential to understand the relationship between serum and dietary cholesterol and dietary fat. Cholesterol, both dietary and serum, is a waxlike compound that is one of a group of complex molecules called sterols. Sterols are present in one form or another, in both plant and animal tissues. Dietary cholesterol is the cholesterol in the foods you eat. Serum cholesterol is the measure of cholesterol in your blood.

Cholesterol itself, however, is not found in plants. That is why one brand or another of potato chips, peanut butter, corn oil, or any number of other foods is advertised as containing "no cholesterol." By virtue of the fact that they are plant foods, none of them would contain cholesterol. While the claim often causes no end of confusion for consumers, it is true and it has been proven absolutely to be effective in selling products.

Cholesterol, found only in animal foods, is part of every animal cell. It is especially high in eggs, liver, and organ meats, and is found in varying amounts in shellfish. Unlike the plant sterols, dietary cholesterol is absorbed by the body, which also manufactures it for a number of important functions. It is necessary for the formation of bile acids and steroid hormones, and it reacts in the skin with ultraviolet light to produce vitamin D.

When, for reasons which are not yet understood, atherosclerotic plaques slowly begin to form on the inner walls of arteries, waxy cholesterol is their major component. The deposits gradually grow tough and fibrous, and may eventually harden and become chalklike. They narrow the passage through which blood can flow, and make the artery wall inelastic, so that it cannot expand to allow for greater blood flow when you run to catch a bus or suddenly decide to do ten push-ups in the morning. But while dietary cholesterol does seem to contribute to atherosclerosis, it appears to have a far less important effect on serum cholesterol than dietary fats, and particularly saturated fats.

Dietary fats are mainly compounds called triglycerides. Ninety-eight percent of the fat in our foods and 90% of the storage fat in our bodies is triglyceride. Triglycerides are made up of three molecules of fatty acids, attached, like the tines of a fork, to one molecule of glycerol, like a short handle. The fatty acids, which are strings of carbon atoms with hydrogen atoms attached to them, may be all the same kind, there may be two of one and one of another, or all three may be different. Some are saturated with hydrogen. That is, they contain all the hydrogen atoms their molecule will hold. They are solid at room temperature. Other fatty acids, called monounsaturates, have two less hydrogen atoms than their structure allows. Still others, the polyunsaturates, have more "vacancies" along the carbon chain. These differences in structure have important effects on serum cholesterol. Saturated fats, found mainly in animal fats, dairy products, and in coconut and palm kernel oil, tend to raise cholesterol levels. Many shortenings contain vegetable fats which have been "hydrogenated," or saturated, by chemically forcing hydrogen into the fat. This makes them harder, or more solid at room temperature, and improves their storage life. Polyunsaturated fats, found chiefly in vegetable oils, such as corn, cottonseed, soybean, canola, sunflower, and safflower oil, and monosaturates found mainly in canola and olive oil help lower serum cholesterol.

Cholesterol and fatty acids travel in the blood in different protein-coated "packages." Two types are of particular importance in relation to heart disease. Low-density lipoproteins, or LDL's, which have a thin protein coating and large amounts of cholesterol have come to be known as "bad cholesterol." They carry most of the cholesterol in the blood and if not cleared from the blood, cholesterol and fat can deposit in the arteries, contributing to atherosclerosis. When it comes to lowering LDL cholesterol, the emphasis is clearly on diet, and particularly on getting less saturated fat, more polyunsaturated fat, and less cholesterol.

High-density lipoproteins, or HDL's, which have a thicker protein packaging, carry cholesterol back to the liver for processing or for removal from the body. They are commonly referred to as "good" cholesterol. Several factors, including losing weight, if necessary, quitting smoking, and increasing physical activity all may raise HDL levels. Diet has not been identified as an important factor in raising HDL's.

In terms of reducing the risk of cardiovascular disease, the message quite simply is this: Cut way down on saturated fat to no more than 10% of total calories, replace some of it, up to no more than 30% of total calories, with mono- and polyunsaturated fat, and reduce cholesterol intake. The evidence for reducing the risk of certain cancers, especially cancer of the breast in women and cancer of the bowel in both men and women, suggests the need for a reduction in total fat intake. Ditto for controlling weight. So while fat has much to offer, the message is clear—eat less and enjoy it more.

Questions and Answers

Q. Why do fats smoke when they get too hot?

A. Triglycerides, composed of fatty acids and glycerol, begin to break apart at very high temperatures. Gradually, the glycerol becomes dehydrated into a compound called acrolein, which is responsible for the unpleasant odor and irritating effect on the eyes and mucus membranes.

Some fats, like butter and lard, reach their "smoke point" quite rapidly, while liquid oils, such as corn, sunflower, soybean, and peanut oil can withstand much higher temperatures before they begin to break down. That naturally makes them better choices for deep frying. In addition, in this country, oils are processed to keep their so-called "smoke points" as high as possible to make them suitable for cooking at high temperatures.

Q. How are liquid oils hydrogenated?

A. To understand hydrogenation it is first necessary to understand just a bit about the chemical makeup of fats. Nearly all fats are made up of compounds called triglycerides, which contain three chains of fatty acids attached to an alcohol called glycerol. The fatty acid chains are strings of carbon atoms to which hydrogen atoms are attached. When the carbon chain holds all the hydrogen it can possibly take on, it is said to be saturated. In that case each carbon is attached to the next by a single bond. When there is a "vacancy" along the chain, two carbons are attached to each other by a so-called "double bond." It is at these double bonds that hydrogen is added to the fatty acid.

The hydrogenation process actually involves several steps. First the oil is mixed with a catalyst (usually nickel) to speed up the reaction; then it is heated to a fairly high temperature; and finally it is exposed to hydrogen under pressure. During this last step, the oil must be agitated to help dissolve the hydrogen, insure thorough mixing of the catalyst, and get rid of the heat generated by the reaction. When the desired degree of hydrogenation is achieved, the oil is cooled and the catalyst is filtered out.

Q. We frequently hear suggestions for cutting down on dietary fat intake. But is it possible to consume a diet containing too little fat?

A. It is quite unlikely since the amount we need is really quite small. Besides providing calories to meet our energy needs, fat has two major physiological functions in the body. Fats are essential for the absorption of fat-soluble vitamins and they are a source of essential fatty acids the body uses for a variety of purposes. Essential fatty acids are important components of cell membranes; they are used as raw material in producing prostaglandins, a group of hormonelike compounds which perform a wide range of tasks in the body; and they are involved in the metabolism of cholesterol.

The Food and Nutrition Board of the National Research Council estimates that to meet these needs, it takes 25 grams (just 225 calories-worth) of fat a day or in terms of "visible" fat, 5 teaspoonfuls. And as you know, much of the fat we consume is hidden in foods so we really don't see it. Consider, for example, that a cup of regular cottage cheese, a food we tend to think of as relatively low in fat, contains about 5 grams, a 6-ounce piece of a very lean fish, like halibut, contains a little over 2 grams, and even a typical slice of bread provides about a gram. So it's easy to see how, over a day's time, it is possible to get to 25 grams of fat and more without realizing it.

Looked at another way, even those of us trying to limit our fat intake to no more than 30% of the total calories are probably getting more than that amount. For example, on a 1,200 calorie diet, 30% of the calories would total 40 grams; on 2,000 calories, 67 grams; and on 2,500 calories, 83 grams.

While the available evidence seems to indicate that it is a good idea to limit fat to no more than 30% of the total calories, it is important to remember that fats do have other positive attributes. They absorb and hold flavors in foods, and in combination with other nutrients, provide texture that increases palatability. And they slow the rate at which food leaves the stomach, thereby contributing to a feeling of fullness.

Q. For some time I have used margarine instead of butter at the table. Now I have read that when oils are developed into a solid mass to create margarine they are saturated. Doesn't this offset the benefits of using margarine?

A. No. It is true that margarine is not as rich in polyunsaturates as the oil from which it was made. That's because in making margarine some of the oil used must be hydrogenated, or hardened. Otherwise it would not hold its shape. So in order to maintain your polyunsaturated fat intake at the recommended level of at least 10% of the total fat you consume, it does make good sense to use liquid oils for cooking whenever possible. When using a table spread, however, margarines are preferable.

Q. If butter, margarine, and oil are all "pure fats," it would seem that they should all contain the same number of calories. According to my calorie chart, oil contains 125 calories per tablespoon, while the same amount of either of the solid fats contains only 100. Why?

A. True, the only source of calories in all three is fat, but there is a difference. Oils contain nothing but fat, while 15% of the weight of both butter and margarine is water. That caloric difference should not play a major role in your decision about which type of fat to use for two reasons. For one thing, if you are concerned about trying to keep your serum cholesterol in check, it is a good idea to use the more unsaturated liquid oils wherever possible. Second, when substituting oil for margarine in recipes for baked products, the amount of oil is reduced by about 2 tablespoons per cup. That virtually wipes out any caloric difference between the two types of fats.

Q. With the discovery that fish oils might provide some protection against heart disease, the term omega-3 fatty acids seems to have crept into the language of food supplements. Can you provide an explanation of where that name comes from and tell me whether they are of benefit?

A. Fatty acids, the building blocks of triglycerides, are the main type of fat in food and the type stored in adipose tissue. Chemically, they are made up of chains of carbon atoms with varying numbers of hydrogen atoms attached. Fatty acids differ in the number of carbon atoms in the chain, the number of double bonds they contain, and the position of the first of these double bonds. "Omega," the last letter in the Greek alphabet refers to one of the carbon chain, specifically the left end, and the "3" to the number of carbon atoms in from the end at which the double bond appears.

The possible link between omega-3 oils, found mainly in oily fish, and the prevention of heart disease began with the observation that Eskimos who eat a diet quite different than ours, and one which contains large amounts of fish, rarely die of heart disease.

Subsequent studies examined the link between fish consumption and cardiovascular disease in other groups. Some found it to be of benefit, with as little as two fish dishes a week offering cardiovascular protection. Others found no effect. These observations were the beginning of a long process of identifying and understanding the possible relationships. That process is far from complete.

Omega-3's do prolong bleeding, inhibit blood platelets from sticking together, and decrease produciton of a compound associated with the constriction of blood vessels. Other studies suggest that they may promote changes in blood cells that increase the supply of oxygen to the tissues, and that they may help lower blood pressure. Another area of research focuses on possible links between fish oils and inflammatory and autoimmune disease. And a few studies suggest a role in treating psoriasis and some types of dermatitis.

In many studies in which fish oils were found to be of benefit, however, the amount used was large enough to be considered a pharmacologic dose. And often forgotten is the fact that, beyond their cost, they are calorically potent. Doses used in many studies provided nearly 300 calories a day. It has been suggested that large doses may not be without hazard.

In short, the wisest course for normal individuals is to get their fish oils not from capsules but by eating fish two or three times a week, within the context of a cholesterol-lowering diet. In fact, the lack of agreement that omega-3's are the "active ingredient" where fish consumption has shown to be of benefit in reducing cardiovascular risk suggests that you choose a variety of fish, rather than only those rich in omega-3's.

Q. Does heating oil cause it to become more saturated?

A. No. In a study conducted a number of years ago, a group of British researchers heated corn oil to temperatures 50 degrees above that normally used for deep frying. After seven heatings, the proportion of linoleic acid, the predominant polyunsaturated fatty acid in the oil, dropped minimally. Similarly, in tests of several batches of cooking oil which had been used many times for deep frying, linoleic acid levels were quite similar to those in fresh oil.

Q. Do lecithin capsules prevent blood cholesterol from rising?

A. The claim that lecithin cannot only lower blood cholesterol but also prevent and cure heart disease has been around a long time. It is based on the fact that lecithin, a "phospholipid," acts as an emulsifier and functions in the transport of fats. Unfortunately, oral lecithin supplements don't seem to have any effect on the way the body handles fat or cholesterol. This may be explained by the fact that the body doesn't absorb lecithin intact, but breaks it down during the digestive process.

Lecithin should not be thought of primarily as a nutritional supplement to be purchased in the health food store. It is widespread in the food supply, and is found in largest amounts in egg yolk, organ meats, whole grains, and legumes. Moreover, if you look at the ingredients lists on food packages, you will find that is a rather commonly-used additive.

FRIENDLY CARBOHYDRATES

When it comes to trends in nutrition, carbohydrates have been through the mill, both literally and figuratively. The literal part has been the refining process that strips whole grains of essential nutrients and creates overly processed, often bland, foods, to which sugar, fat, and salt may be added. On the figurative side, carbohydrates have been reviled by dieters as starchy villains, hailed as saviors for athletes, shunted aside in favor of protein, and gobbled down as sources of "quick energy."

Although the subject of carbohydrates has often fueled heated discussion, many of those who enter the debate still do not understand exactly what they are. Carbohydrates are chemicals ranging from very simple molecules in sugars like glucose (the sugar in blood), fructose (the sugar in fruit), sucrose (ordinary beet or cane sugar), and lactose (milk sugar), to much more complex molecular structures such as starches or cellulose, composed of hundreds of glucose units.

Carbohydrates can be generally classified into three groups: monosaccharides, disaccharides, and polysaccharides. All derive from the Greek word for sugar. Monosaccharides are the simple sugars such as fructose, glucose, and the much rarer mannose, found in Biblical manna, the dried sap of a species of ash trees growing in the Sinai desert. Disaccharides are pairs of simple sugars. They include sucrose, lactose, and maltose, a breakdown product of starches found in corn syrup, malted milk, beer, and malted breakfast foods. Polysaccharides, the starches, are long chains of simpler carbohydrates. Most, like glycogen, contain glucose molecules, anywhere from 3,000 to 60,000 of them. But they may be made from other monosaccharides, too. Inulin, a polysaccharide in artichokes, contains 40 fructose units. And agar, a polysaccharide in seaweed, is a string of units of another monosaccharide, galactose.

In terms of bulk, polysaccharides are far and away the most important carbohydrates. In grains (especially if not stripped of nutrients by milling), dried legumes, potatoes and other vegetables, and some fruits, they come hand in hand with essential vitamins and minerals, particularly the important trace minerals. Without fruits and vegetables we would not get our fair share of ascorbic acid, alias vitamin C. Carbohydrate-rich foods also provide fiber, which is increasingly recognized as a key player in promoting long-term health.

Carbohydrates are available in a lot of different varieties of foods, many of them very high in nutritional value. In fact, the only carbohydrate that might be considered a nutritional enemy is sucrose. The large sackful of average American consumes each year provides nothing but calories and certainly contributes to tooth decay.

Apart from sucrose, we can view most carbohydrates as friends. Most are synthesized by green plants under the influence of sunshine. Part of the synthesis goes into building the stiff skeleton and plant cell walls. The rest the plant stores for its own energy as starch in tubers like potatoes, in roots like carrots, in seeds like wheat and corn, or as sugars in fruits and some vegetables. Thus, such diverse foods as milk, grapefruit, baked beans, and broccoli all contribute carbohydrates. The milk provides lactose, the grapefruit both fructose and glucose, and the baked beans and broccoli, complex carbohydrate.

The moment we bite into foods containing a carbohydrate we start digesting it, as enzymes split the starch into smaller fragments. Then, in the small intestine, enzymes cleave them into even tinier parts, splitting both starches and sugars into the very simple sugars, glucose, fructose, and galactose. These are absorbed through the intestinal wall into the blood. The fate of the carbohydrate from that point follows one of three routes.

Most of this sugar is burned for energy. Like other animals, we store a small portion, in the liver, muscle, and heart as glycogen. When blood glucose is low, liver glycogen is converted to glucose to prevent hypoglycemia. With physical stress, during a vigorous tennis game, for example, muscle glycogen is used as a backup. Carbohydrates not needed immediately for either purpose are converted to fat and stored in our fat cells, just like excess dietary fat or protein.

According to current recommendations aimed at reducing the risk of both cardiovascular disease and certain types of cancer, we should be striving to get as many as 55% to 60% of our allotted calories from carbohydrates. Recent evidence suggesting that it takes considerably more calories to store carbohydrates than fats makes them particularly desirable for weight control, as well. With all these points in their favor, it is time to recast the role of dietary carbohydrates (with the exception of sugar and sweets) not as dietary adversaries, but as allies to good health.

Questions and Answers

Q. If the body stores starch as glycogen in both the liver and the muscles, it would seem that meat should provide some carbohydrate. However, I have always read that the calories in meat come from protein and fat. Could you please straighten me out?

A. Your logic is correct. Your confusion stems from a missing fact. Animals and humans do store starch, as glycogen, in both the liver and muscles. However, at the time of slaughter, most animals are in the fasting state, and thus their muscles have been largely depleted of glycogen. Liver, on the other hand, still contains some glycogen, though certainly not in amounts great enough to make a significant contribution to the day's carbohydrate intake. A three-ounce piece of beef liver, for example, contains roughly 5 grams or 20 calories'-worth of carbohydrate.

Q. I have read that substances called raffinose and stachyose are responsible for the gas problem associated with eating dried beans. Can you explain what these substances are?

A. Both raffinose and stachyose are classified as oligosaccharides, compounds made up of several simple sugars. Raffinose is a trisaccharide, containing a single molecule each of galactose, glucose, and fructose, while stachyose is a tetrasaccharide made up of two molecules of galactose, and one each of glucose and fructose. The body lacks the enzymes necessary to break these compounds into the simple sugars which can be absorbed. So they move on to the intestine where bacteria digest them, producing the gas associated with dried beans.

It is possible to reduce the flatulence problem associated with dried beans by soaking each cup of beans in 2 quarts of water for four or five hours before cooking. Drain and add fresh water for cooking. If more cooking is necessary after 30 minutes, drain and add fresh water once more. There is some loss of B vitamins and protein, but the procedure seems to be effective in significantly reducing the gas problem. Moreover, people who begin to eat beans regularly gradually develop some adaptive mechanism and the problem seems to diminish.

Q. What is the nutritional difference between sugar and honey?

A. Despite the claims of honey lovers and health food enthusiasts, there is simply no scientific basis for the idea that honey is nutritionally superior to table sugar. Like sugar, it contains no nutrients except calories.

Claims for honey really make little sense when we consider the facts. For example, the sweetener in the nectar that bees use to produce honey is actually sucrose in a dilute solution. By a chemical process called "inversion" the bees simply convert this "raw material" to the simple sugars glucose and fructose. Neither vitamins nor minerals are added along the way.

It is similarly difficult to defend the idea that honey is better than sucrose because it is a "natural" food. That much overused term, which implies but really carries no guarantee of better nutritional value, can be applied to both sweeteners. While it is true that the "natural" source of honey is nectar from flowers, sucrose comes from the equally "natural" plants, sugar cane or sugar beets.

Because it contains a greater percentage of fructose, the sweetest of the sugars, honey is somewhat sweeter than table sugar. Therefore, some people find that they can get by with less of it. However, in order to realize a significant caloric saving, you really must cut back considerably on the amount you use. The reason is that honey contains 65 calories per tablespoon while the same measure of sucrose provides only 45 calories.

Q. Does activated charcoal prevent gas formation after eating dried beans?

A. A carefully conducted study reported several years ago by researchers from the University of Minnesota failed to demonstrate any benefits of activated charcoal claimed in an earlier study. Researchers began their effort with a series of laboratory experiments designed to uncover which of three possible mechanisms explained why charcoal reduced the volume of bacterial gases after eating beans. Instead, their experiments failed to demonstrate that activated charcoal had any effect at all on bacterial fermentation.

As a result, the investigators decided to repeat the earlier studies which had claimed that activated charcoal was of value.

The gas-producing properties of beans are believed to be due to their high concentration of so-called oligosaccharides, carbohydrates which the body cannot digest or absorb. These carbohydrates are fermented by bacteria in the colon, releasing carbon dioxide and hydrogen which may be excreted in flatus, metabolized to other compounds by bacteria in the colon, or absorbed into the bloodstream and excreted through the lungs. A rise in breath hydrogen, therefore, is a useful and easily obtained indicator of bacterial fermentation.

After an overnight fast, subjects were given 8 ounces of canned baked beans. Over the next nine hours they were allowed to consume nothing but water or black coffee. On two occasions they were given four capsules containing activated charcoal with the beans and four more every 30 minutes for the next hour and a half. On two other trials, they were given placebos, identical in appearance to the charcoal. Neither the investigators nor the subjects knew which was which. Breath hydrogen was measured at the beginning of each test and every hour for nine hours. In addition, subjects were asked to record hourly the number of times they passed flatus. There was no difference in either measure, regardless of whether activated charcoal or the placebo was used.

WHAT IS A VITAMIN?

If you stopped a passerby on the street and asked him or her to define vitamins, you would probably get a vague answer on the order of "something we need" or "pills we take with our food." Chances are that hardly anybody would describe them as organic compounds, essential catalysts for thousands of body reactions. Yet, every day, a multitude of Americans religiously downs a daily multivitamin, multivitamin and mineral supplement, or individual vitamin pills—and most have only the cloudiest notion of why they do.

Some of us fall victim to the vitamin advertising with which we are continuously inundated, much of which is outrageous. Vitamins have been touted as miracle cures for everything from cancer to baldness. Others choose to take supplements because they think "if a little is good, a lot must be much better." Unfortunately this simply isn't true.

How can we make sense of advertisements which hold out false hopes and of the maze of conflicting scientific evidence, and tell for ourselves which nutritional messages are valid? To begin with, it is essential to understand what vitamins are, what they do, and why we need them.

Vitamins are organic compounds necessary for reproduction, to maintain life, and to promote growth. They are usually grouped according to their solubility. The water-soluble vitamins include the B vitamins and vitamin C. These cannot be stored in the body for long. They are either utilized soon after they are ingested or else eliminated, mostly in the urine. Vitamins A, D, E, and K are all fat-soluble and can therefore be stored in the body's fatty tissues for future use.

Although certain vitamins are involved in the metabolism of energy-yielding nutrients, they themselves do not provide us with energy. They are nutrients the body needs in minute amounts but cannot make itself. Vitamins must be obtained from the diet. Several vitamins are partial exceptions to this rule. Given certain conditions, the body does have the capability of manufacturing vitamin A, D, K, biotin, and niacin. If there is sufficient tryptophan (an amino acid) available, the body can use it to manufacture niacin; so-called "provitamin A," carotenes which are found in plant foods, can be converted by the body to vitamin A; the action of ultraviolet light can convert cholesterol in the skin to vitamin D; and both biotin and vitamin K are among the essential nutrients which can be manufactured by a friendly population of bacteria which inhabit our intestines.

Because vitamins are required for normal metabolic functions, their absence from the diet results in characteristic deficiency diseases. Deficiencies result when a person is not getting a vitamin in his/her diet because a variety of foods have been excluded, the absorption of the vitamin is inhibited due to a metabolic disorder, or if a special condition has increased the need for a vitamin above what is normally required. Deficiencies can be corrected by feeding sufficient amounts of the particular vitamin.

If you eat a well-balanced diet, with plenty of fruits and vegetables, whole-grain or enriched grain products, vitamin D-enriched milk, and other animal products, it is highly unlikely that you will be deficient in any vitamin and won't need to take a supplement.

The "if" however, is a big if. If your food habits are irregular, if you eat snacks on the run rather than meals, or if you don't eat whole groups of food (such as vegetables), then you may be quite short in one or more vitamins and minerals. If that's the case, you may choose to take a supplement. Just remember that vitamin and mineral supplements are no excuse for a poor diet. Too often people fool themselves into thinking that if they take a vitamin pill they don't need to worry about what they eat. A vitamin C pill may give more than the RDA for C but it won't provide you with all the nutrients that an orange will. Obtaining all the essential nutrients from food is the best guarantee that you're getting everything you need in balanced amounts.

If you do choose to take a supplement, stick to a multivitamin and mineral preparation which provides nutrients at the level of the RDA's and not above. You should certainly stay clear of megadoses, a term commonly used to describe amounts greater than ten times the RDA. Such high doses are also frequently referred to as "therapeutic doses" and are used in an attempt to cure a variety of symptoms.

Vitamin supplements are only effective in treating symptoms that are caused by a deficiency of that vitamin. They are ineffective in treating conditions whose causes are totally unrelated to vitamin intake. So don't buy any preparation that gives you doses much in excess of the RDA's. At best, you would only be wasting your money. At worst, especially with fat-soluble vitamins such as A and D, you could be risking toxicity. In these amounts, vitamins are no longer nutrients but drugs and should be treated as such.

Questions and Answers

Q. Is there anything wrong with preparing vegetables in the morning to serve for that evening's dinner?

A. Ideally, to maximize nutrient retention, it is better to prepare vegetables just before they are to be cooked or eaten raw. But the reality is that for many people such last-minute preparation is incompatible with other demands on their time. An alternative is to wash the vegetables, shake off excess moisture, and store them in plastic bags in the refrigerator for that night's meal. This helps to keep them fresh and preserve the nutrients they provide.

It is best to leave the vegetables in large pieces. That minimizes the amount of cut surface exposed to air, and limits vitamin C losses. Finally, with exception of vegetables like potatoes, which turn an unattractive brown color if not kept in water, avoid extended soaking. That leaches out both the vitamins and minerals.

KNOW YOUR B's AND C's

There seems to be a prevailing misconception that large doses of water-soluble vitamins are not harmful because the body will just eliminate them. Recently, however, it has been observed that excessive supplementation with vitamin B_6 can lead to loss of muscle coordination and impaired sensations of touch and temperature. It is suspected that high doses of B_6 (2 or more grams) can cause irreversible nerve damage and doses as low as 200 milligrams per day, taken over a period of time, can cause a sensation of "pins and needles," numbness of the hands, difficulty walking, and other symptoms.

Routine self-medication with large doses of vitamin C can alter your body's utilization of the vitamin. Your body adjusts to large doses of C over a period of time by limiting absorption and excreting or destroying the vitamin in amounts greater than usual. If you suddenly stop supplementation and your body doesn't adjust to the lower intake rapidly enough, you can develop deficiency symptoms.

Although vitamin C and all of the B vitamins are extremely important in maintaining our health, the new evidence should offer a word of caution to those who insist on taking excessive amounts of various nutrients. With this in mind, let's have a closer look at the water-soluble vitamins and why we need them.

The B Vitamins

The biological importance of the B vitamins stems from their presence in coenzymes—molecules which facilitate the function of enzymes. Of the many vital roles which they have in the body, B-complex vitamins are involved in the metabolism of fats, carbohydrates, and proteins, in the production of DNA (which carries the genetic code) and thus, in the replication of cells. Just as excessive amounts can cause physical complications in the body, inadequate supplies of the B vitamins can lead to serious disorders.

Thiamin

Since World War II, thiamin, also known as vitamin B_1, has become one of the vitamins added to white flour, corn and rice as part of this country's standard enrichment program. Thiamin is also found in whole grains, organ meat, pork, dried beans, and fruits and vegetables. In fact, its presence in food today is so widespread that nobody needs to worry about not getting enough.

One of the most well-known vitamin deficiency diseases, beriberi, results from a lack of thiamin. The disease is characterized by a loss of appetite, decreased muscle tone, depression, and neurological disorders. It is still seen occasionally in the Orient among poor people living on highly restricted diets of mostly polished rice. It's also found among severe alcoholics, but that's about the extent of it these days.

Niacin

In the late 1930s it was found that the disease, pellagra, whose symptoms are referred to as the four D's—dermatitis, diarrhea, dementia, and finally death—resulted from a lack of niacin. It was later discovered that if niacin is lacking from the diet, the amino acid tryptophan can be used by the body to manufacture it. Therefore, three conditions must exist for a niacin deficiency to develop: (1) There must be too little niacin in the diet; (2) too little dietary tryptophan; (3) a relatively large amount of other amino acids, so that what tryptophan the food does contain cannot be spared to manufacture niacin.

Fortunately pellagra is rarely seen today. Whole wheat, rice, fruits, and vegetables are good sources of niacin, while milk and other animal products provide us with tryptophan.

Folacin

In recent years, folacin and vitamin B_{12} have received increasing attention due to their link with different types of anemia. Folacin, necessary in the metabolism of certain amino acids, is also involved in providing components for the synthesis of DNA and RNA. A deficiency affects both the production of proteins and cell division, especially of red blood cells which multiply rapidly. Without sufficient folacin, cells "get stuck" as they attempt to double their DNA before dividing and become enlarged. As a result, new red blood cell production is impaired and anemia soon follows.

Megaloblastic anemia, which is caused by a deficiency of folacin, is often seen among pregnant women. It occurs most commonly during the third trimester when fetal blood supply is increasing rapidly. For this reason, many obstetricians prescribe prenatal vitamins containing additional folacin, usually 0.8 milligrams, twice the usual adult level.

The best sources of folacin are liver and other organ meats, green leafy vegetables, and dried peas and beans. Since large amounts of folacin can be destroyed by heat or exposure to air, it's best to eat raw or slightly cooked fresh vegetables and to store them covered in the refrigerator.

Vitamin B_{12}

Vitamin B_{12} functions as a coenzyme in a reaction that permits the absorption of folacin. Without B_{12}, folacin cannot be absorbed and becomes trapped inside the cells of the intestinal wall. This is why a deficiency of B_{12} produces the same symptoms as a folacin deficiency. In addition to the megaloblastic anemia, a B_{12} deficiency also causes nerve damage and paralysis which, if not detected and treated early on, is irreversible.

Even when the amount of B_{12} we eat in out diet is adequate, a deficiency can result if it is not absorbed properly in the body. In order to be absorbed from the intestines to the bloodstream, B_{12} must bind with an intrinsic factor (a compound produced in the stomach). If the intrinsic factor is not present, B_{12} is not absorbed and pernicious anemia develops. Persons who have had their stomachs removed or injured are at risk of not having enough intrinsic factor. Fortunately, as this is not a common situation, for most of us this is not a concern.

Animal products are rich sources of B_{12}. If a person places himself or herself on a diet completely devoid of any animal product, he/she would have no source of vitamin B_{12} and would be at risk of a deficiency. Therefore, vegetarians who do not include eggs, cheese, or other dairy products in their diets should take a B_{12} supplement.

Riboflavin

Although riboflavin deficiency still remains a problem in much of the world, it is rare in the United States. Milk is the most important source of riboflavin (also called Vitamin B_2) in the American diet. An 8-ounce glass supplies 0.84 milligrams, or about half the daily requirement for the adult. Meat, fish, poultry, and eggs are other excellent sources of riboflavin. Leafy vegetables, broccoli, asparagus, and enriched or whole-grain cereals and breads also contain appreciable amounts. Because direct sunlight can destroy up to three-quarters of the riboflavin, it is best to buy milk in opaque paper cartons.

Biotin

Biotin is found in a wide variety of foods, especially liver, kidney, legumes, nuts, egg yolk, and some vegetables. Bacteria in our intestines also synthesize significant amounts which we then absorb and use, so deficiencies of this nutrient are generally not a concern.

Vitamin B_6

A deficiency of vitamin B_6 (also known as pyridoxine) can lead to dermatitis around the mouth and nose, ulcers in the mouth, depression, and irritability. This probably accounts for the increasing attention that B_6 has received as a possible cure for PMS, oral lesions, and other illnesses. To date, evidence indicates that B_6 is effective in curing such disorders only if they are caused by a B_6 deficiency.

Vitamin B_6 deficiencies are observed in alcoholics because alcohol causes the breakdown of the coenzyme with which it is associated and also because the B_6 intake of alcoholics is often inadequate. But, if you eat a well-balanced diet, chances are you are getting enough of this nutrient. Poultry, fish, liver, whole grains, beans, and brewer's yeast are all good sources of B_6.

Vitamin C

What most of us know about vitamin C can be summed up in two points: it's found in large quantities in citrus fruits, and it is frequently espoused as a miracle cure for the common cold. The first point is correct, but evidence supporting the second is sketchy, at best.

Although vitamin C wasn't discovered until the 1890s, history's greatest seafarers were well acquainted with scurvy, a disease now known to be caused by a deficiency of this nutrient. Ocean voyages usually began in the early spring after the seamen had been through a long winter without fresh fruits or vegetables. Invariably, many of the seamen developed bleeding gums, loose teeth, hemorrhages, sore joints, lethargy, and wounds that would not heal—all signs of scurvy.

The widespread tissue damage and hemorrhages caused by scurvy make it obvious that vitamin C plays a vital part in maintaining the health of tissues, cells, and blood vessels. In addition, it plays a part in the absorption of iron from the intestines and in its storage in the liver.

But what about the claims that it can protect against the common cold? Although vitamin C may act like an antihistamine and help alleviate cold symptoms in some people, thus far there is no conclusive evidence that would warrant the use of supplements for cold prevention or treatment. Many manufacturers add it to foods, but the fact is that most people get all the vitamin C they need, and then some, just by eating a variety of fruits and vegetables.

Clearly, the water-soluble vitamins are essential for many of the body's vital functions, and it is important to eat a varied diet to ensure that we are getting enough of each. Yet, one must be wary of the endless claims that are made about the curative properties of vitamins—save your money and avoid buying supplements which will provide you with excessive doses.

Questions and Answers

Q. Recently my son began taking large doses of niacin for reasons which are not clear to me. He assures me that niacin is not toxic. Is that true?

A. No. There are actually two forms of the vitamin, both of which are capable of preventing niacin deficiency. One, niacinamide, which is used to treat deficiencies, produces no reaction and has not been associated with toxic symptoms. The other, nicotinic acid, has been shown to reduce blood levels of fat and cholesterol and is used as part of the treatment for elevated serum cholesterol in some cases. This is done only under medical supervision, however, and it is associated with a number of problems.

Nicotinic acid causes the release of histamine, leading to dilation of the blood vessels and flushing, which can occur within 15 minutes after taking as little as five times the Recommended Dietary Allowance. The Coronary Drug Project Research Group (CDPRG), which evaluated nicotinic acid as a cholesterol-lowering agent several years ago, found flushing in 92% of patients taking 3 grams a day. Eventually, about half developed a tolerance.

Proponents of nicotinic acid therapy for a variety of conditions, who argue that flushing is "only a symptom," might be slowed by reports of other side effects. High nicotinic acid intake has been associated with liver toxicity, and niacin-related jaundice has led to needless surgical procedures. Nicotinic acid can also elevate blood uric acid levels, and at high levels competes with uric acid for excretion. This can be a particular problem for individuals predisposed to gout. Indeed, the CDRPG found an increased incidence of acute gouty arthritis in patients taking niacin.

Nicotinic acid has also been associated with irregular heartbeat, with a variety of dermatologic problems, and with elevated blood sugar levels both in the fasting state and after taking large "test" doses of glucose. Gastrointestinal symptoms including stomach pain, nausea, and diarrhea have been associated with nicotinic acid taken in pharmacologic doses. Because of the release of histamine, there is particular concern about the potential hazard to individuals with peptic ulcers and asthma.

The risks associated with taking niacin in large doses led the CDPRG to conclude several years ago that "great care and caution must be exercised for the treatment of persons with coronary heart disease." Taking it as a self-help measure is unwise.

Q. I know that taking megadoses of vitamins can be dangerous, but I have read that there are individuals who do need many times the normal requirement of a particular vitamin. Is this true?

A. Yes, although cases are extremely rare. Nearly 40 years ago, in 1954, an individual infant with convulsions was found to respond to pharmacologic doses of pyridoxine, or vitamin B_6. That case marked the beginning of the concept of vitamin-responsive inborn errors of metabolism. Since that time, at least 25 genetically-determined disorders have been described, involving eight of the nine water-soluble and one of the four fat-soluble vitamins. These disorders may be related to a defect in the body's ability to absorb, transport, or use a vitamin. Pharmacologic doses required to treat these cases can vary anywhere from 10 to 1,000 times the Recommended Dietary Allowance. The fact that these cases exist and are effectively treated with enormous doses of vitamins should never be used as a rationale for self-medicating with pharmacologic doses of any vitamin for any reason.

Q. While browsing around the shelves of vitamin supplements, I noted a vi-

tamin B_{12} preparation which contained 8,333% of the Recommended Dietary Allowance. Is there a reason for taking B_{12} in such massive amounts?
A. No. The amount we need on a daily basis is minute, only 3 micrograms a day. Moreover, the body has a remarkable capacity to store the vitamin. The liver can store enough to take care of our B_{12} needs for anywhere from three to five years. And that still adds up to only between 2,000 and 5,000 micrograms. So why anyone would want to take 25,000 micrograms or as much as 12 times that amount every day is a mystery to us.
Q. How is folate related to folic acid?
A. The terminology for this B vitamin is rather complex. "Folate" is used interchangeably with "folacin" to describe a group of compounds having nutritional properties and chemical structures similar to the parent compound, folic acid. These terms come from *folium,* the Latin word for leaf, and reflect the fact that dark green leafy vegetables are prime sources of the vitamin.

Folic acid actually includes three compounds: pteridine, a yellow, phosphorescent pigment similar to that found in butterfly wings; para-aminobenzoic acid, an essential growth factor for bacteria and a raw material that some animals can use to produce their own folacin; and glutamic acid, an amino acid. Thus, the true chemical name, taking these components into account, is pteroylglutamic acid, or PGA.
Q. After taking a B-complex vitamin supplement, I noticed that my urine turned a bright yellow color. Why?
A. In all likelihood, what you observed, if you will pardon the irresistible pun, was a most colorful demonstration of the physiological effects of an overdose of riboflavin. It was a clear message that you're taking in more than you need.

Riboflavin is an orange-yellow solid, which when dissolved in liquid, gives off a yellow-green fluorescence. When large amounts pass through the body unused, they turn the urine a color sometimes described as canary yellow. Like the other B vitamins, riboflavin is water-soluble, which means that the body lacks the capacity to store any excess. If you took a urine specimen to the laboratory, we'd bet an analysis would find large amounts of other B vitamins that were in your capsules, too.
Q. Is it true that when orange juice is processed and frozen into concentrate, most of the vitamin C is lost?
A. No. If you are among the millions of people who depend on their morning glass of frozen reconstituted orange juice as a reliable source of vitamin C, rest assured. Modern processing methods are designed to protect the vitamin from the tree to the supermarket. The rest is up to you.

Frozen concentrate is made in batches using ripe oranges with peak amounts of vitamin C. A closed vacuum process that returns all vapor to the concentrate results in minimal nutrient loss. Once frozen, it is stored and shipped at temperatures well below 0°F. If kept thoroughly frozen at the supermarket and in your home freezer, reconstituted orange juice supplies between 90 and 100 milligrams of vitamin C per 8-ounce cup. This is just 20 milligram less than the amount in freshly squeezed juice, and perhaps more importantly, more than one-and-a-half times the U.S. RDA for the vitamin.

How does frozen concentrate compare to orange juice in the refrigerator dairy case? Any differences are considered too small to be of practical importance. So taste and cost, rather than nutrient differences, should dictate your choice.

Regardless of which type of orange juice you buy, the economy size makes sense only if your family consumes it quickly. While deterioration in the first two or three days is minimal, if stored properly, over time all juices lose both flavor and substantial amounts of vitamin C.

"FAT-SOLUBLE" ISN'T FATTENING

Do fat-soluble vitamins have more calories than other vitamins? No. In an age when dieting has become a common preoccupation, people see "fat" and immediately think "calories." The truth is that vitamins, whether fat-soluble or water-soluble, contain no calories. Only protein, fat, carbohydrate, and alcohol contain calories. And contrary to popular belief, vitamins do not make us hungrier, either.

So, what does "fat-soluble" mean? Exactly what it says—that these vitamins (A, D, E, and K) are soluble in fat, not in water. In biological terms, this means that excess amounts are not readily excreted in urine, but are stored in the body's fatty tissues. That explains why megadoses of fat-soluble vitamins, especially A and D, can be toxic.

The Fat-Soluble Vitamins

Vitamin A

There are two forms of vitamin A. First are the so-called provitamins or carotenes which come exclusively from plants. They are water-soluble and can be broken down into the active form of vitamin A in the intestine. Of the carotenes, beta carotene is the most abundant form with potential for vitamin A activity. Then there is fat-soluble vitamin A itself, also known as retinol or preformed vitamin A. It is found only in animal products.

Vitamin A is necessary for growth and the development of bones and teeth, and it is vital to the health of epithelial tissues. These tissues includes not just skin but all the membranes that line passages leading to the outside of the body, as well as glands and their ducts. Insufficient vitamin A causes epithelial cells to become dry and to deteriorate.

Vitamin A is also part of a pigment in the retina which transmits visual images to the brain through the optic nerve. This accounts for a well-known symptom of vitamin A deficiency—night blindness. This symptom, in which a flash of light at night causes a period of blindness, is easily detected in adults and is one of the first signs of vitamin A deficiency.

To make sure you have enough vitamin A in your diet, include dark green leafy vegetables and deep yellow fruits and vegetables. Liver and whole milk are also good sources of the vitamin. Nowadays, low fat and skim milk usually have vitamin A added. Since high doses lead to toxicity, it is obviously unwise to self-prescribe vitamin A supplements for any reason.

Vitamin D

Vitamin D has long been called the "sunshine vitamin" because sunlight, rather than food, is our major natural source of the vitamin. Ultraviolet rays act on a form of cholesterol present in our skin and convert it to vitamin D.

However, 50 years after its discovery, there are still many things nutritionists do not know about the ways in which vitamin D acts in the body. But we do know that the vitamin is essential for calcium utilization, and that either a deficiency or an excess can cause serious physical disorders.

Vitamin D must undergo two transformations, one in the liver and one in the kidneys, before it can be used in the body. Once activated, it plays a crucial role in maintaining blood calcium levels and in the mineralization of bones, including the deposition of calcium. When blood calcium falls below a safe level, vitamin D signals for more to be absorbed from the intestines. If that is not enough, vitamin D stimulates calcium release from bones.

A lack of vitamin D, either as a result of too little sunshine or not enough in the diet, means the bones cannot mineralize properly. Natural vitamin D production can be hampered by tall buildings which block the sun's rays, air pollution, and long hours spent inside during the winter months. Vitamin D deficiency results in rickets among children and osteomalacia (softening of the bones) in adults. Rickets, an epidemic in many parts of the world during the Industrial Revolution, was essentially wiped out in this country when milk was fortified with vitamin D.

Fortunately, most milk is fortified with vitamin D today. It is especially important that growing children, pregnant women, and the elderly consume only D-fortified milk. The few other good sources include fatty fish, such as sardines, and egg yolk. For reasons which are quite unclear, dry cereals are commonly D-fortified, too. Vitamin D is extremely toxic in large doses and should be taken as a supplement only when prescribed by, and under the supervision of, a physician.

Vitamin E

Touted for decades as improving everything from one's libido to slowing the aging process, vitamin E has remained a best-selling supplement in pharmacies and health food stores. Unfortunately, research has failed to provide support for any of these claims. While marketers continue to reap profits from supplement sales, scientists are still trying to determine the exact roles that vitamin E plays in the body.

It is known to act as an antioxidant, by combining with and deactivating certain potentially harmful breakdown products called free radicals. It prevents them from reacting with and damaging cellular components, especially the polyunsaturated fatty acids in cell membranes. In this way, vitamin E protects and maintains the walls of red blood cells and other cells from oxidative damage. Vitamin E has also been shown to help maintain normal muscle function, possibly acting as a coenzyme.

Even though vitamin E is essential for these processes, humans need very little. Because it is fat-soluble, the vitamin is readily stored in the body, and it is excreted slowly. The small amounts that are used can be regenerated, even after it has been oxidized. Furthermore, the body has other antioxidants that, in some instances, can substitute for vitamin E.

Vitamin E occurs in a wide variety of foods including vegetable oils, nuts, seeds, grains, vegetables, and to a lesser extent, meats. For all these reasons, deficiencies are rare in humans and occur only under very unusual circumstances. It is not surprising then, that an exasperated scientist once referred to vitamin E as "a vitamin in search of a deficiency." In fact, it was not until some 40 years after its discovery that a vitamin E deficiency in humans was identified. In the mid-1960s, inadequate vitamin E was recognized as the cause of a particular type of anemia in infants. Since then, a deficiency has also been shown to occur in diseases such as cystic fibrosis, where absorption is impaired. But these conditions are, happily, uncommon. Given the lack of data supporting the benefits of large supplements and the absence of evidence that dietary intakes are inadequate, there is little reason why vitamin E should remain among the fastest moving items in the health food store.

Vitamin K

We all go through life suffering minor cuts, scratches, lacerations, and a variety of bumps and bruises. We may suffer a moment's pain, but our blood promptly clots and within minutes of a small injury, the flow of blood is stemmed. After that, we are already on the road to recovery. For a small number of people, however, this is not the case. Almost everybody is familiar with the problem of the hemophiliac. What most people don't know is that a small number of other people also suffer from impairment of coagulation. But unlike the hemophiliac, their disorder is not genetic; it is nutritional.

Vitamin K plays a crucial role in the clotting process. Without it, our blood would not coagulate, and a small cut could be a life-threatening occurrence. Fortunately, most of us have no problem getting enough vitamin K. It is widely found in liver, egg yolk, soybean oil, and green leafy vegetables such as lettuce, spinach, kale, and cabbage. In addition, bacteria that live in our intestines manufacture considerable amounts. With vitamin K so readily available, few of us ever need any additional supplies.

There are, however, three groups of people who may be easily treated with vitamin K supplements because they suffer from coagulation impairment. These include some newborn infants, people who don't properly absorb fats and, therefore, vitamins that are soluble in fats, and patients who are taking anticoagulant medication for heart disease.

It's clear that although vitamins A, D, E, and K are usually grouped together because of their solubility, they are very distinct compounds. Each has a different function in the body, all vital to our well-being. Getting enough—but not too much—of each them is the key to good health.

Questions and Answers

Q. If milk provides vitamin D, why is there none in yogurt?
A. Neither milk nor yogurt, which is made from milk, are naturally good sources of vitamin D. The amount that milk actually contains as it comes from the cow is small and variable, depending on both her diet and her exposure to sunlight. Moreover, since it is fat-soluble, vitamin D is removed along with the butterfat in producing skim or low-fat milks. Consequently, the vitamin D content of most milk sold in this country is increased in one of two ways. It can be exposed to ultraviolet light, which converts a sterol in the milk to vitamin D. The amount that can be produced in this way is somewhat limited. So it is more practical to add vitamin D concentrate to a level where milk contains 400 International Units per quart. Yogurt, however, is not fortified.
Q. Several months ago I began losing hair from a particular spot on the back of my head. On the advice of a friend, I began rubbing vitamin E cream on it, but to no avail. In fact, the spot appears to be getting larger. Do you think the vitamin E may actually be doing more harm than good?
A. It is probably not making the condition any worse, but there is no reason to believe that it will help either. Our advice is that you seek the service of a professionally-qualified dermatologist.

Vitamin E has been an enormously popular ingredient in countless skin and hair preparations for years. This is rather curious considering the complete lack of evidence to justify its use. A review of the scientific literature regarding deficiency in both man and animals reveals only the most remote basis for any dermatologic claims for vitamin E.

A varied diet should insure that you will get all the vitamin E you need. The only people who benefit from adding vitamin E to cosmetics are the manufacturers who charge premium prices for their vitamin E-enriched products.

Q. I have heard that eating too many carrots can turn the skin a bright orange color. Is this not a form of vitamin A toxicity?

A. No. Hypercarotenemia, as it is called, does occur in individuals who consume an excess of carotene, the precursor of vitamin A found in fruits and vegetables. It has been estimated that a daily intake of a pound of carrots will cause the characteristic color changes after several weeks. That, of course, is a large amount of carrots to munch down on a daily basis. And, indeed, the problem is usually traced not to eating large amounts of carrots and other produce, but to the consumption of large amount of carotene-rich vegetable juices produced in vegetable juice extractors often sold in health food stores. The yellow-orange skin color results from the excess amounts of carotene stored in the fatty tissue immediately below the skin. The color, though not especially attractive, gradually disappears when dietary carotene intake is reduced.

Q. I realize that it is a poor idea to overexpose one's skin to the sun for several reasons, not the least of which is increased risk of skin cancer. But I have often wondered why no one mentions the potential risk of vitamin D toxicity as a hazard. Isn't it true that substances in the skin are converted to vitamin D, which is toxic?

A. Ultraviolet rays do convert a particular type of cholesterol, known as 7-dehydrocholesterol, into vitamin D. Happily, however the body has regulatory defenses against overproduction. Vitamin D can be stored in the skin in an inactive, nontoxic form and released gradually as needed. When the stores are filled, the raw material simply travels along different metabolic pathways.

Q. I have read that vitamin E has been found effective in treating children with neurological problems. I have a child with some neurologic problems and would like to know more about this.

A. Vitamin E has been used successfully to help alleviate neurological problems in a small number of children who apparently developed a secondary deficiency of the vitamin—that is, a deficiency brought about by another disease.

The children who have shown some improvement in neuromuscular disease after receiving supplements of vitamin E had congenital liver disease characterized by cholestasis, or a blockage in bile flow. These children were also shown to have low serum vitamin E levels and muscle cramps similar to those seen in E-deficient animals.

While the details of the mechanism of vitamin E absorption are unknown, a crucial role for bile acids has been recognized. Thus, oral supplements of vitamin E routinely given along with other vitamins to children with disorders of this type could not be adequately absorbed. Consequently, neurological symptoms of vitamin E deficiency gradually appeared and grew steadily worse. Some children can absorb adquate amounts if larger doses are given. In most cases, however, the vitamin must be given in an injectable form.

It is exciting to be able to explain and to successfully treat a severe constellation of symptoms. However, this is a very specific situation. The results must not be extrapolated to suggest that vitamin E will answer all the heretofore unexplained and as yet untreatable neurological conditions.

Q. Despite my warnings, my sister takes large doses of vitamin A, saying that until you get up to dosages of 50,000 units (she takes about half that amount) there is no danger. Is that true?

A. Absolutely not. There is no absolute black-and-white distinction between toxic and nontoxic intakes of vitamin A. A number of factors can affect the level which is toxic for a particular individual. Second, it is important to remember that what one gets in a supplement represents only part of the story. Diet can also contribute significant amounts. Finally, symptoms of toxicity can be precipitated by the onset of other medical problems. Several examples from the medical literature illustrate how it happens.

In one case, liver damage developed in a 63-year-old man who had followed a restricted diet for seven years and had taken several vitamin supplements, including 25,000 IU's of vitamin A a day. He was also getting between 15,000 and 30,000 IU's from foods. A second case was unmasked in a 42-year-old man who had been healthy. Symptoms appeared when he developed viral hepatitis. He had taken 25,000 IU's a day for ten years and an additional dose occasionally when he felt stressed. Dietary sources had also supplied 25,000 additional IU's.

Q. What is carotene and how does it relate to carotenoids?

A. Carotene is one of the carotenoids, a family of several hundred naturally occurring compounds responsible for the color of everything from apricots to watermelon, and even for many of the bright colors in autumn leaves and birds.

Only about 20 of the carotenoids have vitamin A activity. And three of the most common of those contain different types of carotene. Beta carotene is probably the one you have heard most about because of studies suggesting that generous intakes over a long time may be associated with a lower incidence of certain types of cancer. It was first isolated from carrots more than 150 years ago and is available in large amounts in yellow and orange vegetables and fruits, as well as in a number of dark green vegetables, where the chlorophyll masks the yellow or orange color. Two other forms of carotene, alpha and gamma, differ a bit in their chemical structure, and have only half the vitamin A activity of beta carotene.

Q. I know that the two most reliable ways to get vitamin D are from sunlight or from vitamin D-fortified milk. But what other foods contribute to vitamin D intake?

A. Few foods naturally contain significant amounts of vitamin D, and most are foods we do not eat frequently enough or in large enough amounts to make a difference. Moreover, the amount of vitamin D in some of these foods can vary widely, depending on both the animal's diet and the extent to which it was exposed to sunlight.

To put the potential contribution of these foods into perspective, it is helpful to use a cup of vitamin D-fortified milk as the standard. It provides 100 International Units (IU's) of vitamin D, or half the adult Recommended Dietary Allowance. Three-and-a-half ounces of one of the fatty fish, like herring or salmon would provide over 300 IU's of vitamin D, or 150% of the RDA, while the same amount of tuna (a rather generous portion) would provide between 200 and 300 IU's. In sharp contrast, a piece of liver weighing 3½ ounces before cooking would contain anywhere from 15 to 40 IU's, a medium egg only about 25 IU's, and a tablespoon of butter 15 IU's.

In short, except for those of us who consistently eat significant amounts of the fattier fish, fortified milk remains the most dependable dietary source of vitamin D.

MINERALS: GOOD THINGS COME IN SMALL AMOUNTS

Over 96% of our body weight is made up of just four elements: carbon, hydrogen, oxygen, and nitrogen. By contrast, the remaining 4% includes some 60 minerals. Among these minerals, concentrations vary greatly. For example, calcium makes up almost 2% of your body weight, whereas some of the trace minerals are present only in fractions of a thousandth of an ounce.

But just because minerals are present in such minute amounts doesn't mean that they are any less vital to life than other nutrients. A perfect illustration of this is zinc. This mineral was first recognized as a nutritional necessity over 50 years ago. Today, we know that it takes part in over 100 different enzymatic reactions. Zinc is vital for the health of the skin, the healing of wounds, and for maintaining a normal sense of taste. It is essential for the formation of the nucleic acids RNA and DNA, which are the basic materials of genes. It enhances the action of a number of hormones, including insulin. It is necessary for fertility in adults and must be present for the normal growth and development of the embryo and the newborn.

Given all of its crucial functions, it is not surprising that a deficiency of zinc can have serious consequences. Zinc deficiency has been associated with a variety of symptoms, including retarded growth, poor appetite, taste abnormalities, and slowed healing of wounds.

Not all problems of poor zinc nutrition can be traced to inadequate dietary intake. Other factors, such as gastrointestinal disease, cirrhosis of the liver, excessive alcohol consumption, tuberculosis, and chronic infections can deplete the body's supply of zinc. In addition, laxatives can impair the absorption and utilization of zinc and other trace minerals. Large quantities of vegetable fiber can also interfere with its absorption.

This is not to say that you should run out and buy zinc supplements. Large doses of zinc have been found to interfere with the absorption of copper, another essential trace mineral, and may eventually result in copper-deficiency anemia. As with all nutrients, it makes far better sense to satisfy your body's needs by eating a wide variety of foods. Good sources of zinc include seafood (Atlantic oysters, in particular), poultry (especially the dark meat), organ meats, eggs, dried beans, legumes, and whole grains.

About 50 years ago, fluoride, another trace mineral, was also receiving a good deal of attention. It was at this time that studies first showed a relationship between fluoride in water supplies and a reduction in the incidence of tooth decay. Flouride's principal effect is to help form a stronger and more acid-resistant enamel when the teeth are being formed in the jaw. Although the effect isless dramatic, it appears that adult teeth can also benefit from the topical application of fluoride (i.e., from flouride-containing water, toothpaste, or mouthwash). As it washes over the teeth, it becomes incorporated into the crystals that make up the structure of tooth enamel.

There may be other benefits from flouride as well. Because it is rapidly taken up by bone and known to stimulate bone growth, there has been increasing interest in flouride as a possible treatment for osteoporosis. Therapeutic doses must be monitored carefully because it can have undesirable side effects at high levels, but we are apt to hear more in the next few years about its relationship to bone health.

Like flouride in water, iodine is another trace mineral which is provided in our diet through fortification; we ingest it through iodized salt. Iodine is an important component of the thyroid hormone which regulates body temperature, controls protein synthesis, and promotes physical and mental growth before birth and during childhood. Without enough dietary iodine, the thyroid gland enlarges as it tries to trap what little amount of the mineral is available—a condition known as goiter. In the United States, iodine deficiency was once widespread in the so-called goiter belt that runs through the Ohio Valley and the Great Lakes region (where the soil does not contain much iodine). What once had been a serious health problem rapidly disappeared when iodine was added to salt.

Today, we no longer worry about iodine shortages. It is found naturally in seafood and increasing amounts have been creeping into our diets through food processing. Some additives, such as dough conditioners, contain substantial amounts of iodine. In addition, appreciable amounts have found their way into milk from the animal feeds and salt licks which are given to dairy cows. Several years ago, because of the potential hazards associated with excess iodine, the government began to take steps to reduce the amounts that were getting into the food supply. They also began monitoring the iodine content of the American diet. At present there is thought to be little cause for concern.

Until fairly recently, magnesium received comparatively less attention than other essential minerals such as sodium, potassium, and calcium. Today, we have an increased awareness of its physiological importance. Magnesium is a component of about 300 different enzymes; included are those that supply energy to cells, cause muscles to contract, send electrical impulses between nerve cells, and metabolize protein, fat, and carbohydrate.

A deficiency of magnesium rarely occurs alone. It is usually seen as a result of other pathological conditions such as alcoholism, intestinal malabsorption, kidney disease, or as a consequence of food deprivation. However, current research is focusing on the effects of long-term borderline magnesium intake and its relationship to hypertension. Evidence is still lacking, but in the meantime, we can ensure that our intake is adequate by eating whole-grain cereals (especially oats), nuts, soybeans, green leafy vegetables, fruits, milk, and fish.

Selenium is yet another mineral that has been in the news these days. This mineral is part of an enzyme that protects cell walls, and the genetic material within, from damage caused by the breakdown products of fat metabolism. Various claims have been made about selenium's role in health, ranging from its ability to prevent cancer to prolonging life. As is the case with most outrageous assertions, there is just no evidence to support these claims. Because too much selenium can be toxic, it is best to avoid the supplements currently on the market and depend on a varied diet to meet your needs. Good sources of the mineral include seafood, kidney, liver, meat, and grain products.

The list of minerals certainly does not end here. Chromium, nickel, tin, manganese, aluminum, sulfur, cobalt, and phosphorous are just some of the many other minerals which are present in our bodies. For some, we know specifically what role they play and how much is needed in the diet each day. For others, we are not so sure. In years to come, advancing technology may lead us to discover their precise roles and our daily requirements for each. Meanwhile, all we can do to ensure a health-giving supply of the wide array of minerals is to eat a balanced diet.

Questions and Answers

Q. Sea salt is considerably more expensive than regular iodized salt and I would like to know if it's worth it?
A. No. Sea salt is one of the numerous items which owes its rise in popularity to the emphasis on "natural" foods. The implication is that salt from the sea sold in small bottles at considerably higher prices than ordinary salt is somehow superior. In truth, the minute amount of trace minerals sea salt provides is of little consequence and hardly justifies its additional cost. Moreover, contrary to popular belief, sea salt is not a good source of iodine.
Q. Is zinc toxic in large amounts?
A. No. Zinc is one of the less toxic minerals, and poisoning has rarely occurred. The inhalation of zinc-containing fumes has poisoned metal workers, and zinc poisoning has also occurred in individuals who consumed an acid fruit drink that had been stored in a galvanized container. And a few cases have apparently resulted from the ingestion of massive amounts of the mineral itself. But fortunately, one of the early symptoms of zinc toxicity is vomiting and this affords natural protection against more serious symptoms.

The reason it is a poor idea to take zinc supplements relates primarily to the fact that the body does not use individual nutrients in a vacuum. Indeed, much current research is directed toward expanding our knowledge and understanding of how the availability of one nutrient affects the absorption and utilization of other nutrients. So while we know that zinc is not particularly toxic, we really do not have sufficient evidence to predict what effects the regular consumption of large doses of zinc might have over an extended period.

While it is certainly important to get enough zinc in your diet, you should depend on foods such as meat, fish, eggs, milk, nuts, legumes, and whole grains as your source of supply. They'll not only provide you with all the zinc you need, but with generous amounts of many other trace minerals your body also needs.
Q. In a gourmet cookbook of mine, the author recommends whipping egg whites in a copper bowl to get the best volume. Isn't copper toxic?

A. Not in the amounts you'd be likely to get from the exposure of the egg whites to the copper bowl. While we really don't know at what levels copper is toxic, it is estimated that people can tolerate at least 20 times the normal intake over a prolonged period before toxicity develops.

We tend to think of copper as an industrial metal, but it has numerous essential functions in the human body. For example, ceruloplasmin, a copper-containing protein in the blood, is involved in various stages of iron metabolism. Copper also enhances iron absorption from the intestine and helps mobilize the iron stored in the liver and other tissues. Enzymes containing copper are involved in the synthesis of hemoglobin, in the metabolism of glucose and the release of energy, and in the formation of both connective tissue and vital substances in the nerve wall. Copper itself also activates certain enzymes.

Even with all of these important roles in metabolism, the need for copper is quite small, only about 2 milligrams a day. To give you a graphic picture of just how much that is, a single penny would provide enough to meet the body's demands for four years.

Fortunately, copper is found in many foods, and therefore, a varied diet should provide all you need. The richest sources include organ meats, shellfish, nuts, dried beans, and cocoa. Copper may also find its way into the food supply from other routes. For example, if milk, which is itself a poor source, is passed over copper rollers during pasteurization, it may take on some copper. And in similar fashion, water traveling through copper pipes can carry considerable amounts of the mineral.

Q. Is it true that selenium supplements are associated with some severe toxic symptoms?

A. Yes. A case report from medical literature provides a graphic example of selenium toxicity. A woman in New York began taking a selenium supplement, which according to the label, contained 150 micrograms, an amount within the safe and recommended 50 to 200 micrograms. She should have been fine.

Within 11 days, however, she began to notice marked hair loss on her scalp, which grew progressively worse. Two weeks later she observed white, horizontal streaking on one fingernail. Next, the woman experienced swelling and tenderness of the fingertips and a discharge around the nail bed. Over the next three weeks the condition spread to all her fingernails, and she finally lost the nail that had been affected first. She also suffered periodic nausea and vomiting, sour-milk breath odor, and fatigue.

Not surprisingly, the first doctor this woman visited did not identify the problem. Human toxicity had never been documented in this country. (It has been found in a large number of villages in the People's Republic of China.) Fortunately, the woman heard on a radio program that some selenium supplements had been recalled when it was discovered that they contained excessive amounts of the mineral. This time she consulted her internist, who found that her blood selenium level was four times what is considered normal in this country. Ironically, the woman would have been even more severely affected if not for other megadosing. With each selenium tablet she also took 1000 milligrams of vitamin C (the Recommended Dietary Allowance is 60 milligrams). Vitamin C changes the chemical nature of the selenium into a form which is poorly absorbed.

The selenium supplements were found to contain 182 times the amount declared on the package. In round figures each tablet provided 31 milligrams rather than the stated level of 150 micrograms. They were recalled by the distributor, but not in time to prevent seven other cases of apparent selenium toxicity.

The point is that there was no reason for her to take a selenium supplement in the first place. Supplements of individual minerals should be used only on the advice of a qualified physician.

CALCIUM: NO BONES WITHOUT IT!

Most of us know at least one elderly woman whose bones became so thin and brittle that a simple fall resulted in a broken hip. We are also aware of the cause of such easily broken bones: osteoporosis, a progressive disease that afflicts one out of every four American women over the age of 60.

Although weak bones were once thought of as a problem confined to the elderly, we now know this is not the case. Studies have shown that many American women are beginning to display evidence of bone loss as young as age 25. Several factors contribute to this disturbing trend.

One cause appears to be a shortage of calcium in the typical adult diet. We all know that children need lots of calcium for strong teeth and growing bones, and that pregnant and nursing mothers require additional amounts to provide for the fetus and the infant. But many people have the mistaken notion that adults outgrow their need for calcium. On the contrary, this mineral remains essential throughout life.

Ninety-nine percent of the calcium in our body is found in bones and teeth. The other one percent is in a "free" form in the blood and soft tissues, where it serves a number of vital functions. Free calcium must be present for the blood to clot, the heart to pump, the muscles to contract and relax, and the nerves to transmit impulses.

Life itself would be in jeopardy if the supply of free calcium were to be exhausted. Because of its importance in bodily functions, the amount of calcium in the blood is allowed to vary only slightly, no matter how much is taken in from foods. Fortunately, the bones act as a reservoir from which the body can draw more calcium whenever blood levels are low. When the blood level is sufficient, dietary calcium is redeposited in the skeleton. Calcium must therefore be replenished by the foods we eat, or the body will gradually deplete its reserves.

Unfortunately, most adults do not get the Recommended Dietary Allowance for calcium, which is 800 milligrams a day (the equivalent of 3 cups of milk or 3 ounces of Swiss cheese). In the face of deficient intake the body draws upon its bone reserves. Over the years that contributes to loss of bone density. Bones become porous and brittle, and they fracture easily.

Women are at greater risk of developing osteoporosis than men for a number of reasons. Men have a heavier bone structure than women. On average, they have a 25% greater bone density at age 25. Pregnancy and breast-feeding raise the calcium requirement of women dramatically. Women are also more likely to go on reducing diets, often eliminating good sources of calcium.

The absence of exercise has also been linked to osteoporosis. It is well known that people who are bedridden or paralyzed lose bone strength. The same thing happens to astronauts who spend several days in a weightless environment. Research indicates that this occurs even with adequate calcium intake. So, frequent exercise, whether it is walking or weightlifting, is essential to maintaining healthy bones.

Several other factors appear to be linked to the incidence of osteoporosis. High-protein diets increase the rate at which calcium is excreted from the body. With age, the small intestine absorbs the mineral less efficiently, so more must be taken in to maintain the same level. And after menopause, women are at greater risk because lower estrogen levels accelerate the rate of bone loss.

Evidence indicates that an increased intake of calcium during young adulthood and middle age can help prevent osteoporosis from developing later in life. The National Institutes of Health recently recommended that women increase their intake to 1,000 milligrams per day and 1,500 milligrams per day after menopause. Given these recommendations, it is sobering to realize that despite all the publicity, many younger women don't even come close to meeting the 800-milligram RDA.

How can you get more calcium? Dairy products are the richest sources. An 8-ounce glass of milk (whole, low-fat, or skim) contains 290 milligrams—almost one-third the RDA for adults. For anyone who is lactose intolerant, the problem can be surmounted by drinking enzyme-treated milk or taking enzyme tablets with milk or other dairy products. Alternatively, most people with lactose intolerance can eat hard cheese and yogurt without ill effects. One cup of yogurt contains as much calcium as in a glass of milk. Small fish (such as sardines) eaten with their soft bones are excellent sources of calcium. Dark green vegetables such as broccoli, kale, and collards, and tofu made with calcium sulfate also provide considerable amounts. Vegetables like spinach, rhubarb, and beet greens have a fair share of calcium, but they contain oxalates which may interfere with calcium absorption.

As experts continue to review the possible benefits of increasing calcium intake, we should be concentrating on getting our intake at least up to the RDA. Although large doses of calcium are unlikely to reverse the disease once it has become established, it appears that a combination of adequate calcium intake, avoiding excessively high protein diets, and regular exercise is the best recipe for prevention of osteoporosis. Supplements may be indicated in some situations, in some children with milk allergies, or in individuals with severe lactose intolerance. But supplements as a source of calcium should be used only on the advice of your doctor.

Questions and Answers

Q. While eating a peanut butter sandwich on whole-wheat bread and drinking a glass of fat-free milk and thinking I was consuming a nutritionally impeccable combination, I read an article that said that bran and whole grains were among the foods that inhibit calcium absorption. If this article was correct, it doesn't seem to make sense that there is so much emphasis on whole grains. Can you straighten out the apparent contradiction for me?

A. Your faith in peanut butter on whole-wheat bread washed down with fat-free milk should not be shaken. It remains an excellent meal, one which provides generous amounts of many essential nutrients.

Phytates, found in whole grains, are among the substances that can interfere with the availability of calcium. However, the extent of the binding that makes calcium unabsorbable is considered insignificant as long as calcium intake is adequate.

On the other hand, it is known that very large amounts of fiber, as one might consume by taking generous amounts of bran, can tie up appreciable amounts of minerals: not just calcium but essential trace minerals as well. The long-term effects of large fiber supplements on mineral absorption have not been fully evaluated. To get more fiber without hurting mineral absorption, the wisest course is to eat plenty of whole-grain breads and cereals, raw and dried fruits, dried peas, beans, nuts and seeds, and lots of vegetables.

Q. I have trouble getting all the calcium I need and still consuming few enough calories to maintain my weight. The problem is compounded by the fact that while I can drink low-fat milk, I do not like skim milk. Do protein-fortified low-fat milks contribute significantly more calcium?

A. Some do. A cup of 2% low-fat milk provides about 120 calories and almost 300 milligrams of calcium. However, if you choose low-fat milk labeled "protein fortified," which contains at least 10% nonfat milk solids, you would get about 137 calories, but the calcium level would be up to 350 milligrams per cup.

Similarly, a cup of 1% fat milk without added milk solids contains 102 calories and 300 milligrams of calcium. If nonfat milk solids are added at levels below 10%, neither the calories nor the calcium climb appreciably. However, milks labeled as "protein fortified" provide 119 calories per cup and, like the 2%-fat, protein-fortified milk, 350 milligrams of calcium.

Q. Could you provide me with information on the differences among calcium supplements?

A. The most common oral preparations are several calcium salts: carbonate, gluconate, lactate, and phosphate. All but one are sold strictly as calcium supplements. The exception, calcium carbonate, is also used as an antacid. The most well known, of course, is Tums.

Be aware that the actual amount of calcium in a calcium salt varies. Calcium carbonate and tricalcium phosphate both contain about 40%, but lactate contains only 18%, and gluconate, just 9%. This could mean the difference between taking one or two tablets, or downing as many as ten or twelve to get the same amount of calcium. Remember, too, that while Tums, and other chemically similar products are an inexpensive source of calcium, many popular antacids contain *none.*

Recently, several manufacturers have started to add more calcium to multivitamin and mineral preparations. Check the label. Some contain as much as 450 milligrams, an amount comparable to that in 1½ cups of milk.

While amounts of calcium in various supplements may differ, with one exception, they are believed to be equally useful. Calcium carbonate may be poorly absorbed by the elderly. Although bone meal and dolomite also provide calcium, we do not recommend taking these because they may be contaminated with toxic metals such as mercury or lead. When choosing a supplement, it is wise to compare prices. Generic brands can cost as little as 50% less than nationally advertised equivalents.

Q. My doctor has said that I should try to get even more than the Recommended Dietary Allowance of 800 milligrams of calcium a day, as much as 1,200 to 1,400 milligrams a day, in fact. Before I begin taking a supplement, I would like to have an idea of how much I am getting in my diet. Can you give me an idea of the amounts in some of the better food sources?

A. Dairy products are the major sources of calcium in the diet. Without them it is difficult to consume as much as 800 milligrams a day, unless you consistently eat reasonably large servings of a few other foods. A cup of milk provides 300 milligrams, a cup of plain, low-fat yogurt somewhat more, about 415 milligrams. Hard cheeses contain between 150 and 270 milligrams per ounce. Part-skim ricotta, at 335 milligrams per half-cup is a particularly good source. At the other extreme, the same amount of low-fat cottage cheese contains only about 75 milligrams. A number of leafy vegetables supply appreciable amounts. A half-cup serving of kale provides 90 milligrams of calcium, turnip greens, 110 milligrams, bok choy, 125 milligrams, and collards, 165 milligrams. A cup of cooked, dried beans provides 90 milligrams, and if prepared with molasses, somewhat more. Canned salmon and canned sardines can be quite good sources, but only if you eat the bones. Three ounces of canned salmon provides 165 milligrams. The same amount of sardines contributes 370 milligrams. And if tofu is prepared with calcium sulfate, 4 ounces will contain 145 milligrams.

These few figures may be adequate to provide you with a ballpark estimate of your intake. However, to do a more detailed estimate, you will need to keep a record of everything you eat for at least three typical days and then use a food composition table to calculate how much you consumed.

IRON'S DIETARY SHORTFALL

Like the five-cent candy bar and the Model T, the black iron kettle has faded from our lives. The gleaming stainless steel which replaced it is lighter to handle and easier to clean, but there is a trade-off: loss of iron in our diets. In days past, food cooked in iron pots and pans contributed to our needed supply of the mineral. Now, recent surveys show that many Americans fall short of their quota. Women of childbearing years take in an average of almost 40% less than the Recommended Dietary Allowance.

The RDA for schoolchildren and men 19 and over is 10 milligrams. For women who have not yet reached menopause it is set at 18 milligrams, to minimize iron loss from menstruation. The American diet averages only 6 milligrams of iron per 1,000 calories, and most women eat between 1,000 and 2,000 calories a day. This leaves them understocked in the iron department.

Premenopausal women are not the only group at risk. People who lose blood through hemorrhage or trauma need to make up the deficit. And during periods of rapid growth in adolescence, the demand goes up. As for the elderly, their tendency to eat less food means that they have to be especially careful to eat a balanced diet which includes sufficient iron.

Iron is not a luxury item; it's a nutritional necessity. Our red blood cells need it to make hemoglobin, a protein which transports oxygen throughout the body. The body contains 100 trillion red blood cells. Every second of our lives, 900 trillion molecules of hemoglobin have to be synthesized. When too little iron is taken in over a long period, stores are depleted. The oxygen transport system slows, and muscle function falters. If the deficiency grows severe, anemia develops, accompanied by symptoms of "iron poor blood," among them fatigue, irritability, and headaches. Luckily, most of us do not suffer from anemia. But we still may be deficient in iron and would do well to boost our supplies through a nutritious diet. This means paying close attention to what we eat—and in what combinations.

Dietary iron comes in two forms: so-called heme and non-heme iron. The main type found in animal forms (except dairy products) is heme iron, which the body uses far more efficiently than non-heme iron. Ironically, two of the best sources of heme iron—liver and oysters—are not exactly staples of the American diet. A more accessible source to most people are red meats. Ounce for ounce they contain more of the mineral than most other foods. Lean beef has over 3 milligrams in a 3½-ounce serving. Non-red meats also provide us with heme iron.

Green leafy vegetables, enriched and fortified breads and cereals, legumes, dried beans, and dried fruits contain non-heme iron Although not absorbed as efficiently as heme iron (only 10% as compared to 40%), it is an important dietary contributor of the mineral.

If you are making a special effort to add iron to your diet, use the mix-and-match method. Eating a food containing non-heme iron together with one that contains heme iron will increase the amount absorbed from the plant food. For instance, you will get more iron mileage out of peas if they are served at the same meal as, say, roast beef, turkey, or flounder.

Foods that supply vitamin C (citrus fruits, tomatoes, potatoes, green peppers, and cabbage, to name but a few) also enhance iron absorption. Drinking orange juice at a breakfast that includes an iron-enriched cereal, or mixing vitamin C-rich cantaloupe into a fruit salad made with raisins, are good iron-absorbing practices.

Even if you no longer use grandmother's iron cookware, following these guidelines will help put your iron account in the black—and keep red blood cells healthy. As for iron supplements, before you take them make sure they are necessary. During your next routine physical, your physician can check your blood and give you the answer.

Questions and Answers

Q. Should women athletes take iron supplements to protect themselves against "sports anemia."

A. Sports anemia, or a low blood hemoglobin level, does develop among some women who exercise vigorously. It tends to appear during the early stages of training, for reasons which are not understood. Poor intake, decreased absorption, and increased loss of iron, as well as expanded blood volume, decreased production or greater destruction of red blood cells, and inadequate dietary protein have all been suggested as contributors. All women athletes need not take iron supplements to prevent anemia. Indeed, whether supplements are of value even to women who have the condition is unclear. The best hedge against iron deficiency anemia, in general, is to make sure to get plenty of iron in your diet.

Q. I cook with iron pans and wondered whether my family might be getting an excess. Is that possible?

A. No. In this country iron overload, or hemochromatosis, a condition in which excessive amounts of the mineral build up in nearly all body tissues, occurs most often as a result of a metabolic error. Individuals who have hemochromatosis are unable to limit the amount of iron absorbed. Iron overload is also associated with other conditions, including alcoholism. The iron content of some wines is quite high, and alcohol apparently increases both the efficiency with which it is absorbed and adversely affects the liver's normal defense mechanisms.

However, iron intake at levels so high that the body absorbs it in toxic amounts from dietary sources has been identified only among the African Bantus, who both cook in iron pots and brew beer in iron drums. The net effect of these practices is that they consume as much as 20 times the normal iron intake, an amount which can overwhelm the body's ability to limit absorption to safe levels.

Q. Do iron pills cause gastrointestinal problems?

A. They can. Some individuals taking iron supplements complain of nausea, heartburn, and abdominal distension, as well as diarrhea or constipation. This association between iron supplements and GI symptoms has also been confirmed by objective observation. In a double-blind study conducted in Sweden a number of years ago, twice as many subjects given 200 mg. doses of iron reported side effects as those given a placebo. When the dose was increased, the percentage of subjects experiencing side effects increased proportionately.

However, some studies have indicated that at least in some individuals the effect can be psychological. For example, in one study reported over 30 years ago, 14 of the 16 patients experienced symptoms when given green, but not white, ferrous sulfate pills. In another study, placebos labeled as iron pills produced symptoms in the same percent of patients as did accurately labeled iron. However, placebos labeled as controls did not.

The important point is that any real effects appear to be dose-related.

One approach to treating mild anemia when an individual complains of GI symptoms is to reduce the dosage of the supplement. A slower but satisfactory increase in blood cell production can occur on a single dose providing anywhere from 36 to 74 mg. of iron a day. An iron supplement should, of course, be used only after the doctor determines that it is necessary.

Q. Are some iron supplements better than others?

A. Several iron preparations are absorbed about equally. They include ferrous sulfate, gluconate, succinate, glutamate, and lactate. Of those, ferrous sulfate tends to be the least expensive. Advertising for iron supplements sometimes suggests that the likelihood of developing gastrointestinal symptoms is reduced by selecting one preparation over others. In fact, symptoms are believed to be related to both the amount of soluble iron in the dose and to individual physiological differences.

WATER: THE MIRACULOUS MOLECULE

If asked to name the single most important nutrient, most people would probably say "protein" or "vitamins." Yet they would be wrong. Sometimes it takes an extreme of nature like a drought or a heat wave to remind us that the most vital nutrient—and food—in our diet is water.

Water is second only to oxygen in its importance in maintaining life. While we can live for around five weeks without a source of carbohydrates, protein, or fats, deprived of water we can survive just five days in a temperate climate, and an even briefer span in the dry, hot desert. The loss of only 10% of body water can cause severe symptoms of dehydration. The loss of 20% is deadly.

The Bible speaks of a "river of water of life," and indeed it is impossible to imagine anything happening in living systems without water. Although flesh at times seems all too solid, in reality more than half the weight of an adult body is water. This "internal sea" of fluids bathes every cell and actually represents the major component of the cells themselves.

Water transports nutrients and removes waste products. Acting as a lubricant, it ensures that organs and joints move smoothly. In saliva it makes chewing and swallowing a comfortable process.

At birth, an infant starts out containing about 77% water. As adults, depending on age and sex (men tend to have more water than women) our bodies are between 45% and 65% water. Beyond that, more than 90% of the remaining dry material is made up of three types of large molecules. These substances—proteins, nucleic acids, and polysaccharides—are composed of small, repeating units linked together by the elimination of water. When the units are broken down, the long chains are split apart by the addition of water to the molecule.

It is no accident that water provides the primary internal environment for the body. Several extraordinary features make it ideally suited for living systems. A single water molecule has an oxygen atom at one end with two hydrogen atoms sticking out as arms to form a triangular structure. Since oxygen attracts electric charges, one end of the molecule has a partial negative charge and the other a partial positive charge. This separation of electric charges gives water one of its most important properties: polarity. Polarity allows water to carry many dissolved substances and helps the molecules in body fluids interact easily. It works to stabilize the membranes that partition cells into compartments.

Water also makes a perfect fluid for the body's natural air conditioning. Because water molecules do tend to stick together, they can hold a great deal of heat. This means that it takes a relatively large amount of heat to raise the temperature of water. As a result, it is a good insulator, minimizing the effects of body heat production and loss. Perspiration thus makes an efficient cooling process because a lot of heat is given off when only a small amount of water evaporates from the body.

Our internal conservation system recycles body water over and over, but some loss of fluid is inevitable. Since the outer layers of skin must be kept moist, nearly 2 cups of water leave the skin surface daily, even without sweating. Still more is lost from the moist surface lining the respiratory tract. Each time we exhale, the expired air contains water vapor. Although ordinarily we do not release much water through the lungs, losses increase with exercise. At high altitudes, where the air is thinner, we respire (inhale and exhale) more often to meet the body's need for oxygen. In a day of mountain climbing, several quarts of water may escape through the lungs alone.

Normally there is no significant fluctuation in body fluid levels, even though about 2½ quarts are lost and replaced each day in the average adult. While we lose water through several sites, including the skin, lungs, and in feces, the primary regulatory organ for water balance are the kidneys. They adjusts urinary excretion so that water loss exactly equals water gain.

Because fluid needs vary, it is impossible to set a precise daily requirement for water. Individual needs depend on factors like body size, basal metabolic rate, physical activity, and climate.

Can you drink too much water? It's not likely. The kidneys are very efficient at disposing of the excess, and "water intoxication" is rarely seen in healthy people. If you find that you've become abnormally thirsty or are passing large amounts of urine, you may have a condition known as diabetes insipidus. On the other hand, edema (water retention), if not related to the menstrual cycle, may be a sign of impaired liver or kidney function. See your doctor in either case.

Under normal circumstances, we should consume about 2 to 3 quarts of water a day. That sounds like a lot, but it does not all come from drinking liquids. As much as a pint is provided by the last step in the breakdown of proteins, fats, and carbohydrates for energy. Called oxidation, this process produces carbon dioxide, which we exhale, and water. And our food contributes about half the fluid we need. Vegetables, fruits, and most milk products are more than 75% water; meat and fish are 50% to 65% water. Even breads and dry cereals may contain between 5% and 35% water. To make up the rest, we should try to drink about 6 to 8 cups a day of fluids like milk, fruit juice, and, of course, just plain water itself.

We might add that, while soft water may taste better than hard, hard water offers the bonus of a higher mineral content. If you enjoy bottled water, the nutrition label on some brands will show you what you're getting.

And, as a real bonus, water is absolutely calorie free. It also tastes good, quenches thirst—and it is vital to your life.

Questions and Answers

Q. Is it true that some vegetables have a diuretic effect?
A. No. The myth that some vegetables are "natural diuretics" has been around a long time, but is just that, a myth. The only dietary substances we normally consume that have a diuretic effect are coffee, tea, and alcohol. In the case of coffee and tea, caffeine and chemically similar substances increase the blood flow through the kidneys, thereby altering the transport of salts and water by the kidney's tubules and increasing urinary output.

The ethanol in alcoholic beverages works somewhat differently. It depresses the production of ADH, the antidiuretic hormone. ADH is secreted by the pituitary gland and is essential for maintaining normal fluid balance. When secretion of the hormone is suppressed, as it is by ethanol, fluids are not reabsorbed. Instead they are excreted. The thirst and other symptoms often described as the "morning after" feeling are the body's signal that it needs liquid to restore fluid balance.

Q. What exactly defines water as "mineral water?"
A. The definition of mineral water in this country is really quite broad. It is simply water obtained from government-approved and regulated natural springs or underground sources. The mineral content is not modified by the bottler.

Since nearly all water contains some minerals, in most states almost any bottled water can legally be called mineral water. One exception is California, where mineral water must contain 500 parts per million of dissolved solids.

While there are no federal standards regarding mineral content, the FDA does have standards to ensure the safety and purity of mineral water and requires domestic producers to adhere to good manufacturing practices. Imported waters must meet similar standards. They must be obtained from pollution-free sources, be bottled under sanitary conditions, and be of good sanitary quality as judged by bacteriologic and chemical analysis.

WHAT'S NEW WITH FIBER?

For more than a decade we have witnessed an avalanche of research aimed at identifying the role of dietary fiber in health and disease. Seizing on the purported benefits, food manufacturers have exhorted us, albeit often prematurely, to eat fiber-rich cereals and oat bran bagels, and to bake bran into our meat loaf. The jury is still out on many counts, but there is no doubt that we know a lot more today than we did ten years ago. Most importantly, we recognize that the varied benefits of a high-fiber diet are such that we should all be making an effort to boost our intake.

Fiber is generally defined as the portion of the diet that cannot be broken down by digestive juices. It includes the tough structural portion of vegetable foods our grandmothers called "roughage." Four-stomached animals, like cows and sheep, have a multitude of microbes in their rumen which can break down fiber. We have no such obliging bacteria or protozoa. Once separated from the digestible components of our food, fiber passes, more or less unchanged, through our intestines.

Although we usually speak of fiber as if it were one compound, we now know that there are two different types, each with unique properties. One type includes cellulose, hemicellulose, and lignin, the insoluble components of plant walls. The second type includes the pectins and gums, water-soluble nonstructural components of plants.

An important characteristic of the insoluble fibers is their ability to hold large amounts of water. In the intestine, insoluble fiber fractions tend to increase the size of the stool, making it softer and allowing it to pass more easily and quickly through the gastrointestinal tract. Insoluble fibers are found in greatest amounts in cereal brans and vegetables. Wheat bran is an excellent source of insoluble fibers.

Pectins and gums absorb water and characteristically form a bulky gel which slows the rate at which food empties from the stomach. The fleshy parts of an apple and the white portion of citrus fruits are common dietary sources of pectins and gums. Oat bran, which has become so popular recently, provides us with soluble fibers.

When compared to less industrialized countries, the fiber content of the American diet is quite small. Since the turn of the century, our fiber intake from whole grains and fresh fruits and vegetables has steadily declined. Although estimates vary, it is thought that we consume only one-third to one-half as much fiber as people in less industrialized countries. Decreased fiber intake has been associated with a number of health problems. Currently, the spotlight is focused on the links between fiber and atherosclerosis, diabetes, colon cancer, diverticular disease and constipation.

Fiber has long been recognized as an effective antidote to constipation. But gastrointestinal benefits may extend well beyond preventing this common affliction. For one thing, studies suggest a relationshp between a low fiber intake and the development of diverticulosis. In this disease, small, hard stools containing little water pass through the gastrointestinal tract with difficulty. This can strain muscles and increase the pressure. Over time, weak areas herniate into pouches called diverticula. A high-fiber diet is thought to play a role in preventing the disease from developing in the first place, and nowadays it is commonly used to treat the condition.

Population studies also indicate an inverse relationship between fiber intake and colon cancer. The results of these studies are difficult to interpret. Many factors other than fiber content of the diet vary from one population to another. Other lifestyle differences may also influence the incidence of colon cancer.

It has been suggested that dietary fiber may reduce the risk of colon cancer by decreasing the production of carcinogens (cancer-causing agents) in the feces, and by lowering the concentration of bile salts which seem to play a role in tumor development. Animal studies suggest that the type of fiber may be an important factor. Wheat bran seems to have more of an effect than other fiber sources. Further studies are needed, however, to fully understand the role of fiber in colon cancer.

High-fiber diets also appear to be of benefit to diabetics. Large amounts of soluble fibers seem to help control the rise in blood sugar after a meal. And the soluble fibers, including pectins and gums, can lower the amount of insulin needed to control the disease.

Finally, oat bran, which contains soluble fiber, has recently been the focus of enormous attention. Studies have shown that the soluble fibers it contains lower LDL cholesterol levels, the type associated with an increased risk of atherosclerosis and coronary heart disease, without affecting HDL cholesterol, the type associated with decreased risk. The reason for the effect is unclear. Bile acids are the major raw materials from which we make cholesterol. Fiber, especially soluble fiber, binds to bile acids, and prevents them from being absorbed into the bloodstream. This may be one way in which fiber acts to lower blood cholesterol levels, but that is not the whole story. Other possible mechanisms under current study include the effects of fiber on enzymes which regulate cholesterol and bile acid production.

Contrary to what many food manufacturers would like you to believe, oat bran is not the only source of soluble fiber in our diet. Legumes and vegetables also have large amounts and are also effective in reducing blood cholesterol levels.

In short, fiber is beneficial, with different types of fibers having different effects. Processing and refining generally remove fiber. So, the best way to reap all the potential benefits of the several components of fiber is to include more whole grains, dried beans, fruits, and vegetables in the diet. Increasing fiber intake of all types is not a nutritional quick fix. It is one crucial element of a well-planned diet.

Questions and Answers

Q. In checking the ingredients in a loaf of pumpernickel, I was suprised to learn it contained only white flour, and that the deep color came from caramel coloring. Are some pumpernickels a better source of fiber than others?
A. Yes. In most supermarket brands the first ingredient is refined flour. However, the types and amounts of other flours, some of which are whole grains and others not, vary from one bread to another. Lacking fiber information, you can check the ingredients list on the package; or, if you are buying bread at a local bakery, ask the baker. The higher up on the list the whole grains are listed, the more fiber the bread is likely to contain.

Perhaps the rather loose definition of pumpernickel, "a sour bread made of 'dark rye' " explains the fact that darkness is about the only thing that one can expect. We checked recipes in several cookbooks, and found no less variety there. One loaf, relatively high in fiber, was to be baked from 100% whole wheat, dark rye, and unbolted cornmeal. At the other extreme, there was a recipe for pumpernickel baked from light rye and degermed cornmeal. While it may come as a surprise, mashed potatoes were a common ingredient, and chocolate and cocoa were used in several recipes.
Q. In checking bread labels, I was puzzled by one for a dark diet bread which weighed .66 ounce per slice. The label said that it contained 1,350 milligram of fiber per slice. The label on a second, where the slice weighed .75 ounce, said that the bread contained 10% total dietary fiber. The fiber in the second bread appeared to be mainly cellulose, with some bran flakes. Can you interpret this information for me?
A. Yes. The lack of a standard labeling format for fiber allows for a variety of approaches, which, understandably can confuse consumers. In both cases, deciphering the information requires the use of the metric system. In the first case, it appears that the manufacturer believes that larger numbers are more impressive. Moving the decimal point three places to the left provides you with more intelligible information. The bread contains 1.3 milligrams

of fiber per slice. This is smaller than a typical slice, but when compared as if they were of equal weight, this slice contains as much fiber as a slice of 100% whole wheat bread.

As for the second, simply multiply the metric weight of the slice by 10% to determine the amount of fiber in the bread. In metric weight, an ounce is 28.35 grams. Since this slice is .75 ounce, it weighs about 21 grams and contains 2 grams of fiber. Finely ground cellulose does make it possible to provide white bread with a high fiber content, but the fiber is not of the same composition as that in whole-wheat bread.

Q. Often included in lists of fiber fractions is a substance called lignin. What is it?

A. Fiber is made up mostly of a group of substances sometimes classified as nonstarch polysaccharides. These include such things as cellulose, hemicellulose, inulin, guar, plant gums, and mucilage. Lignin, however, is not a carbohydrate-like substance. It belongs to a group of compounds called polyphenols.

Lignin is one of the substances which contribute to the rigidity of the plant cell wall. It apparently is not digested in humans and is known to inhibit the digestion of cell-wall carbohydrate by intestinal bacteria. The exact way this works has not yet been identified, however.

A basic problem which limits our understanding of the role of lignin in human nutrition is the fact that it is extremely difficult to develop laboratory methods which accurately analyze the lignin content of the diet or the feces. It is known, though, that lignin contributes significantly toward making wheat bran one of the most poorly-digested fiber sources.

Q. How much fiber should one get on a daily basis?

A. It has been suggested that healthy adults should consume about 10 to 13 grams of fiber per 1,000 calories: this means about 27 to 35 grams per day for men (with an average intake of 2,700 calories/day) and 21 to 27 grams per day for women eating 2,100 calories/day. To put this into perspective, a slice of whole-wheat bread contains 2.4 grams of fiber, an apple provides 2 to 3 grams (depending on the size), and a cup of cooked broccoli provides 6.3 grams.

The important thing to remember is to get your fiber from a variety of sources. Daily consumption of whole grains, legumes, fruits, and vegetables is best.

Q. I use bran cereal regularly to avoid constipation. I am concerned that the bran is "locking up" trace minerals and preventing my body from absorbing the minerals it needs. I wondered whether I should begin taking a mineral supplement?

A. While there is no harm in taking a multivitamin and mineral supplement containing levels at the Recommended Dietary Allowance as a bit of nutritional insurance, you need not be concerned that fiber, in moderate amounts, will affect mineral absorption significantly. Whole-grain breads and cereals are excellent foods and contribute many essential nutrients as well as fiber.

However, with the "rediscovery" of fiber several years ago, an enormous number of publications appeared in the popular press proclaiming fiber as the nutritional panacea. At that time people began taking bran three times a day, sprinkling it on salads, adding it to soups, and baking it into everything from meat loaf to custard pudding. Not only is there no good evidence to warrant the consumption of excessive amounts of fiber, but we simply don't know what adverse effects it might have. Bran contains phytates which tie up minerals and make them unabsorbable. What long-term effect consumption of huge amounts might have on mineral nutrition is an unanswered question.

Q. The current nutrition "message" includes the advice to consume more "complex carbohydrates," but I don't understand exactly what the term means. Please explain.

A. Complex carbohydrate is really a synonym for polysaccharide, a term which means "many sugars." Occasionally an acid may be included in the structure. For example, inulin, the polysaccharide in Jerusalem artichokes, is made up of units of the simple sugar, fructose. And pectins are polysaccharides made up of galacturonic acid, as well as two simple sugars, glucose and arabinose.

The way the sugars are linked together determines the character of the carbohydrate formed, and consequently its chemical and physical properties. For example, amylose, a starch contained in common foods, including wheat and corn, is made up of the same glucose units as cellulose. But a difference in the way the glucose units are attached to each other means that while humans can digest the former completely, they are quite unable to break down the latter.

Whole grains and lightly milled cereals, rich in complex carbohydrates, also provide generous amounts of vitamins and minerals, especially trace minerals and fiber.

Q. Is there any evidence that fiber supplements or a high-fiber diet is advantageous to individuals on weight-reducing diets?

A. The results of studies conducted to date produce evidence which can, at best, be called equivocal. A recent review examined the findings from more than two dozen studies to see whether any generalizations emerged. Dietary fiber was associated with changes in either caloric intake or bodyweight in two-thirds of them. Unfortunately, however, many of the experiments had seriously flawed designs, limiting the usefulness of the conclusions that can be drawn. For example, in over half of those experiments in which fiber was associated with decreased caloric intake, there was no provision for examining the "placebo" effect. So the question of whether the observed difference is psychological or whether it was explained by a real benefit from fiber remains unanswered.

Other investigators observed the effects of fiber on caloric intake for just a single meal, hardly a basis for drawing conclusions about the long-term benefits of fiber in regulating weight. None of the studies were of sufficient length to make judgments about long-term benefits.

Thus, while there are good reasons to eat plenty of fiber from a variety of sources, at present there is little scientific support for taking fiber supplements to help you to eat fewer calories or to lose weight.

Q. I thought that cooking reduced fiber content, but recently I read that cooking can actually increase the fiber in some foods. Is that true?

A. It is possible that cooking can increase the fiber content of foods. The browning process, or so-called Maillard reaction, is a chemical reaction between a carbohydrate and an amino acid that results in changes in both color and texture, creating molecules which closely resemble lignin, an insoluble component of fiber naturally found in food. Thus, toast and bread crusts have more of this fiber fraction than either untoasted bread or the center of the loaf. However, while cooking can increase the amount of lignin in food, it can also result in the loss of some of the other fractions of fiber, both gums and pectins. While all this is interesting, from a practical point of view, it is more important to depend on a variety of dietary sources of fiber.

Q. Please describe what is known about the benefits of oat fiber.

A. Oat bran, either plain, in oatmeal, or in cold oat cereal, appears to help lower serum cholesterol, but it should be viewed as only one small part of dietary efforts in that direction. The hefty amounts of oat bran used in earlier studies are not appropriate as steady fare. When taken in reasonable amounts, some studies have shown a drop in cholesterol of only about 5%. A drop of 5% in an individual whose cholesterol was 253 milligrams per deciliter of blood would keep that person in the high risk range for coronary heart disease, over 240 milligrams. So adding oats is no license for shedding a diet low in saturated fat and cholesterol.

When buying oats, you will want to check labels carefully. Some oat cereals which contain considerable oat bran also contain considerable fat. In oatmeal bread, oats may be far down the ingredients list, which indicates that the bread contains very little bran. Similarly, on a package of oat bran cookies, oat bran was listed after juice concentrate, a clear indication that the amount was insignificant.

VEGETARIANISM AND HEALTH

"Is my teenage daughter harming herself by becoming a vegetarian?" asks a concerned mother. To fully respond we would need more details about the young woman's diet. But the general answer, for this and other worried parents, is reassuring: a vegetarian diet, if sensibly planned, is nutritionally sound.

The 1960s saw a surge of interest in meatless meals. Yet vegetarianism actually dates from early times, and through the centuries millions of our ancestors survived perfectly well without eating flesh. Vegetarianism was practiced by Utopian groups whose members included the authors Henry David Thoreau and Louisa May Alcott, and such early entrepreneurs of the cereal industry as C.W. Post and John Harvey Kellogg. Certain religious groups, among them the Seventh Day Adventists—a group in extremely good health—have practiced vegetarianism for years. Today the vast majority of the world's population follows traditional vegetarian or semivegetarian diets.

The real key to nutritional well-being is that the more broadly based the diet, the better the chances of getting enough of all the essential nutrients, as well as the other beneficial components of food such as fiber. This is as true for vegetarians as for nonvegetarians.

In expressing concern about the adequacy of a vegetarian diet, both young people and parents usually mention protein first. In fact, protein needs can be met easily. Many plant foods, like dried peas, beans, and other legumes as well as nuts, seeds, and cereal grains are rich in high-quality protein. Some vegetables, including lima beans, potatoes, and green peas also provide some. When two or more of these foods are eaten in a meal, the proteins complement each other and are nearly equivalent to a serving of meat. The easiest way to match proteins is with a combination of some animal foods and some plant foods, as in a lacto-ovo vegetarian diet. It might be dry cereal with milk, cheese with pasta, or a glass of milk along with a bowl of bean soup.

In contrast to worries about getting sufficient protein, some people fear that their vegetarian diet will be too high in carbohydrate and will lead to weight gain. In truth, too many calories cause weight gain, and ounce for ounce, high-fat meat contains more calories than does carbohydrate. Thus, many people report that they actually lose weight on a vegetarian diet.

Another plus is that vegetarian eating can be low in both total and saturated fat, especially if the diet emphasizes low-fat dairy products. Using vegetable oils for salads and in cooking raises the proportion of fats rich in polyunsaturates. For people interested in controlling cholesterol consumption, acceptable egg substitutes are available. These measures add up to a diet directed toward lowering cholesterol.

When it comes to vitamins and minerals, the picture is fuzzier, especially for vegetarians who eat no animal foods. Vitamins B_{12} and D, and at least two minerals, calcium and iron, are lacking or in short supply in pure vegetarian diets. Beyond that, phytates in cereals may decrease the availability of other minerals.

For less strict vegetarians, milk, cheese, and eggs take care of the calcium and B_{12}. If vitamin D-fortified milk is used, it provides that nutrient. If not, there is no dietary alternative because the amount of vitamin D in egg yolk isn't significant enough to make a difference. For growing children and for those like elderly shut-ins who have little exposure to the sun's rays, a supplement at the level of the Recommended Dietary Allowance and no more is the only way to get enough vitamin D, especially during the winter months. Since the vitamin is extremely toxic in large doses, be sure to keep to the recommended level.

For strict vegetarians, extra emphasis on dark green vegetables like broccoli, collards, kale, mustard and turnip greens, legumes, and some nuts and seeds such as sesame seeds helps contribute calcium. As for vitamin B_{12}, the most dependable ways to insure adequate supplies are by regularly using B_{12}-fortified foods or by taking a supplement.

Getting enough iron, always a problem, is more complicated for vegetarians because the best dietary source is animal flesh. Iron in plant foods is absorbed less efficiently. Including foods rich in vitamin C improves iron absorption. But in some cases, blood tests indicate that a supplement is necessary to maintain iron stores.

Clearly, a vegetarian diet can be as healthy as one which includes meat, if planned with an eye to good nutrition. However, vegetarian diets for infants and young children should be used only under the guidance of a pediatrician, perhaps along with a registered dietician. People whose nutrient needs may be elevated, such as pregnant and lactating women, and those who are chronically ill, also might benefit from guidance in menu planning to make sure that their diets are, in every way, nutritionally shipshape.

COFFEE, COKE, AND CAFFEINE

For millions of Americans, the day begins with a fresh cup of steaming-hot coffee. Some drink it blithely, unconcerned about hazards rumored to be linked to excessive intake. Others sip guiltily, nagged by thoughts of potential health risks.

The concern centers not on coffee itself but on its infamous ingredient, caffeine, a drug that acts as a stimulant to the central nervous system and can cause irritability, insomnia, and anxiety, as well as disturbances in heart rate and rhythm. It also appears to affect blood pressure, coronary circulation, and secretion of gastric juices.

Coffee is certainly not the only dietary source of caffeine. The drug also occurs naturally in tea and cocoa, and finds its way into numerous foods prepared with coffee and chocolate, such as baked goods, frozen dairy desserts, gelatins, puddings, pie fillings and candy, and it appears in many soft drinks.

But coffee is still the substance most often associated with caffeine, and the caffeine-disease connection has prompted a hefty body of research. Issues raised include birth defects in children born to mothers who drank coffee in pregnancy; certain types of cancer; cardiovascular disease; behavioral disorders; reproductive problems; fibrocystic disease, or noncancerous breast lumps; diabetes; gout; peptic ulcer; and even cirrhosis of the liver.

However, pinning down relationships between caffeine and various diseases has proved difficult. Individual reactions vary widely, and it is hard to obtain accurate information about caffeine intake. Coffee brewed in different ways contains varying amounts of caffeine, and the same is true for other caffeine-containing foods. Also, much of what we know about caffeine's effects comes from animal studies, and it's unclear whether humans would react the same way.

Some potential risks of caffeine have been studied more deeply than others, for example, possible harm to the unborn fetus. In 1980, the FDA warned pregnant women to avoid or moderate consumption of caffeine, which travels through the placenta to the unborn child. The warning stemmed from a study showing that one of every five offspring of rats force-fed a single dose of caffeine through a stomach tube displayed permanent birth defects, mainly missing or extra toes, and delayed bone development, a condition found to be temporary.

At the time this red flag was raised, the FDA acknowledged that humans might metabolize caffeine differently from animals, thus casting a shadow of uncertainty over the study. A direct link between caffeine consumption and birth defects in humans was not demonstrated, and subsequent studies have lessened concern about the harmful effects of caffeine on the fetus. In a later experiment, the caffeine was put in drinking water and birth defects did not occur, although the animals were born with delayed bone development, which reversed itself, as in the earlier study.

Findings from human studies have proved inconsistent, with some pointing to low birth weight and prematurity among heavy coffee drinkers. One recent study of over 4,000 mothers found that the risk of low birth weight rose with increasing amounts of caffeine. Moreover, among those who consumed the caffeine equivalent of more than 3 cups of coffee a day, birth weight at delivery was about 3 ounces lighter than among those who consumed none. Until all safety questions are resolved, the FDA continues to advise moderation.

As for the caffeine-heart disease link, a flock of studies over the past 20 years have produced inconclusive results. One report collected data from over 1,900 men in the Chicago Western Electric Company Study. After 19 years, more deaths from heart disease had occurred among those who had reported drinking 6 or more cups of coffee daily at their one-year follow-up visit. The deaths could not be explained away by smoking, alcohol, or diet. However, their level of coffee consumption throughout the years of the study had not been tracked. Clearly, the final chapter has yet to be written.

The purported link between caffeine and fibrocystic disease has also gone unconfirmed, as have caffeine's associations with behavior problems in children and cancer of the pancreas. Finally, animal studies have failed to tie reproductive problems to caffeine intake.

What it all boils down to is that caffeine is a central nervous system stimulant, to which some individuals are more sensitive than others. Scientists have not identified amounts at which it might be harmful under certain conditions. Meanwhile, moderation is the wisest path.

Questions and Answers

Q. Is methylene chloride used in some water processes for decaffeinating coffee? Could you explain how coffee is decaffeinated?

A. Based on the results of extensive studies, the FDA in 1985 concluded that any risk associated with using methylene chloride to extract caffeine was so low "as to be potentially nonexistent."

Several processes are used to decaffeinate coffee beans. In the water method, the beans are steamed to add moisture, then soaked for an extended period in a mixture of water and coffee solids. That removes 97% of the caffeine. Finally, the beans are dried to remove excess moisture, and roasted. The water extract used in the soaking process contains noncaffeine solids which affect the quality of the final product. So some manufacturers remove the caffeine and reuse this extract with the next batch of beans. Methylene chloride may be used for this purpose. However, after the caffeine is extracted, the solution is steamed to remove the solvent.

Caffeine may also be removed directly by using methylene chloride, ethyl acetate, a substance found naturally in fruits and vegetables, carbon dioxide, or coffee oil. After direct extraction with methyl chloride or ethyl acetate, the beans are steamed to remove remaining solvent, dried, and roasted. Again, the extract is mixed with water to remove caffeine. Both the solvent and the water extract may be used over. Oil expressed from coffee grounds is yet another solvent. Its effectiveness relies on the fact that caffeine is water-soluble.

Finally, carbon dioxide under high temperature and pressure may be used to extract caffeine. By that method, steam is used to add moisture and draw the caffeine to the surface of the beans before they are exposed to the carbon dioxide.

Q. Is it true that caffeine is sometimes used as a flavoring agent by commercial food manufacturers?

A. Yes. It is used to flavor some gelatin puddings and fillings, soft candies, baked goods, and frozen dairy desserts. When used for this purpose, current regulations state that manufacturers need not declare it on the label. However, the level at which caffeine is used—just 400 parts per million—is considered too small to be significant.

Q. To what extent do brewing methods affect the amount of caffeine in coffee?

A. The latest figures available from the FDA indicate that, on average, a 5-ounce cup of coffee prepared by the drip method contains 115 milligrams of caffeine, while the same amount of coffee made in a percolator contains 80 milligrams. If you choose to use the instant variety, you'll get only 65 milligrams.

However, brewing methods may not exert as strong an effect on the amount of caffeine you're likely to get from an individual cup of coffee as the strength of brew. In fact, differences narrow considerably when we consider the ranges of values. A cup of brewed coffee has been shown to contain anywhere from 60 to 180 milligrams; drip coffee, 40 to 170 milligrams; and instant, 30 to 120 milligrams.

Q. Does tea contain caffeine or theobromine?

A. Tea (like both cocoa and chocolate) contains caffeine as well as both theobromine and theophylline, other related chemicals of the family of compounds called xanthines. Just how much it contains can vary significantly, depending on the variety of tea leaf, where it is grown, and the size of the tea leaf cuts, as well as on the method and length of brewing. That helps explain why figures on caffeine content which appear in print vary so much.

Published figures for a 5-ounce cup brewed either from loose tea or from bag tea for one minute range anywhere from 9 to 33 milligrams caffeine. If brewed for three minutes, the range rises to between 20 and 46 milligrams. But if brewed for five minutes, the low value remains stable while the maximum value rises by only 4 milligrams. To put those figures into perspective, 5 ounces of brewed coffee can contain from 64 to 150 milligrams of caffeine.

Q. Is it better to drink herb teas than regular tea and coffee?
A. Perhaps the most important point is that most herb teas have not really been studied extensively.

Herbs contain a variety of chemical compounds which are extracted when hot water is poured over them. Some are potentially harmful. Thus, drinking herbal tea to avoid the known effects of caffeine may expose individuals to thousands of chemicals about which we know far less.

If you do use herb teas, do so in moderation. Do not depend on them as substitutes for medical care. Home-brewed herbal remedies can range anywhere from ineffective to fatal.

ALCOHOL HAS LITTLE TO RECOMMEND IT

Drinking trends, like eating patterns, change over time. Americans these days are not only turning down hard liquor in favor of "lighter" alcoholic beverages, but they are also choosing drinks with no alcohol at all. Instead of Manhattans and martinis, today's cocktails are more likely to be small glasses of dry wines, sometimes mixed with soda water, and large glasses of nonalcoholic fruit or tomato juices.

No, the nation has not gone dry. While surveys suggest that about a third of American adults seldom or never have an alcoholic drink, another third has up to three drinks a week, and the last third consumes four or more. Statistics show that out of every ten drivers on the road at night, one is drunk.

The disadvantages of alcohol far outweigh any benefits. We can cite only two positive aspects. Some people like the way alcoholic beverages taste, particularly fine wines and good beers. For all drinkers of alcohol there is another evanescent pleasure. As a spirited elderly lady of our acquaintance said on being introduced to a martini, "I hate the way it tastes, but I love the way it makes me feel!" But even that good feeling can be fleeting, as anyone with a hangover knows. And the rest of the alcohol story is bad news.

Ethanol, or pure alcohol, is a central nervous system (CNS) depressant. Low doses cause blood alcohol levels to rise, bringing a temporary feeling of euphoria. However, after more time, CNS function becomes depressed, and the alcohol begins to act as a sedative. Ethanol is highly soluble in water, which means it is easily absorbed from the gastrointestinal tract and distributed throughout the body.

Several factors control how fast ethanol is absorbed and explain the diverse effects alcoholic beverages have on different people. Variations in body fat, muscle mass, and body water, genetic and biologic differences, the type of drink consumed and its concentration of ethanol, and the fullness of the stomach all figure in the equation.

One 2-ounce martini will have a greater influence on a small person than on a large one. Drinking on an empty stomach usually produces rapid intoxication because the ethanol is absorbed quickly, whereas imbibing on a full stomach or eating while you drink means slower absorption and therefore less dramatic effects.

Since alcohol is distributed throughout the body, it can damage more than the central nervous system. Indeed, it is considered directly toxic to many body tissues. A prime target is the liver. While some ethanol is eliminated in sweat, urine, and even breath, the bulk is metabolized in liver cells which convert it to less toxic substances which are then broken down to carbon dioxide and water. The liver, however, cannot speed up alcohol metabolism, so the more alcohol that is consumed, the longer the liver takes to break it down and excrete it. Excessive alcohol consumption over time can produce alcoholic hepatitis and eventually irreversible cirrhosis of the liver.

Continual overindulgence in alcoholic beverages can also result in gastrointestinal disturbances, pancreatic inflammation, heart and blood vessel abnormalities, and nutritional deficiencies. These deficiencies come not only because people who drink excessively tend not to be interested in a good diet, but also because the metabolism of alcohol requires extra amounts of some nutrients, especially some of the B vitamins. Add to that the digestive upsets, malabsorption, diarrhea, vomiting, mineral losses through the kidneys, and you can end up with serious nutritional and medical problems.

Of course, there are people who do not overindulge and will never become problem drinkers. For them the major disadvantage is that alcoholic beverages contain a flood of calories and essentially no other nutritional value. Such drinks are prime examples of "empty calories." Alcohol has 7 calories per gram, more than either protein or carbohydrate (4 calories per gram) and slightly less than fat (9 calories per gram).

These drawbacks apply as much to wine and beer as to hard liquors like scotch and vodka. Beer may be only 4% alcohol, and wine 12%, while 100-proof liquor is 50% alcohol, but the calories add up. One 12-ounce glass of regular beer or ale costs you 140 to 150 calories. Three ounces of table wine contains 75 calories, and a dessert wine, like sweet vermouth, about 120. An ounce of cordials or liqueurs will carry anywhere from 70 to 115 calories. A 1½-ounce jigger of gin, rum, vodka, or whiskey contains between 100 and 125 calories, depending on the proof. If you add to that the calories in the mixers, which can be considerable, the total comes to more empty calories than most people need.

Frequent quaffing can add insidious, unwanted pounds. If you are drinking and dieting, it is hard to stay within the caloric boundaries and still get proper nourishment. So if you like the taste of alcohol, sip slowly and let a little go a very long way.

3 THE NUTRITIONAL AGES OF MAN

The French have a saying: The more it changes, the more it's the same thing. No matter what your age, good nutrition matters, and no matter what your age, the same principles of good nutrition apply. Toddlers, grandparents, and everyone in between would do well to follow the same general guidelines for prudent eating and getting their appropriate measure of exercise. It takes surprisingly little tinkering to adjust our diets to different stages of life.

Yet throughout the life cycle some of our nutritional needs do reflect aspects of change, rising during periods of rapid growth, such as infancy (the greatest period of evolution) and adolescence, holding steady when we have reached adulthood, and undergoing certain transformations with old age. In the elderly, the need for some nutrients may rise, while for others it may fall. But one fact is clear: with the slowdown in metabolism and the decrease in physical activity that often accompanies advancing age, our need for calories declines.

Herein we can appreciate the rhythm and balance of physiological makeup: at stages when we need more nutrients for growth, we also need proportionately more calories than at times of nongrowth or slowdown. Provided we eat a healthful diet, the more calories we consume the more likely we are to receive the array of nutrients needed to build muscle, bone, and tissue. Hence, from our voracious need for growth-promoting nutrients in infancy to our declining caloric requirement in old age, we come full circle nutritionally and, if all goes well, achieve a harmony of supply and demand that serves us in good stead for the complete span of our lives.

Getting a good nutritional start in life begins *in utero.* Pregnant women who already eat a healthy diet need only boost their intake of certain key nutrients to do the best for their babies and themselves. Those whose diets have been less prudent can learn to adjust their eating habits in ways that will benefit them during and after pregnancy as well. But eating for two doesn't mean eating twice as much—nor is it the time to go on a weight-loss diet. As for infants, breast-fed is best fed, nutritionally speaking, but when that is not an option technology has provided highly acceptable alternatives.

Although the introduction of solid foods to babies can be a harrowing process, following a few simple tips may ease the transition. Childhood is the time to instill sound eating practices that will last a lifetime. Adolescence, often the parent's last chance to get a word in edgewise about nutrition, is another potentially challenging stage; the teenager in question may be either a bottomless pit or a chronic dieter. Lastly, the elderly frequently have specific concerns tied to their years and needs. But whatever your age or stage, a healthy, good-tasting diet is a worthwhile—and usually attainable—goal.

EATING FOR TWO DOESN'T MEAN EATING TWICE AS MUCH

A woman's diet during pregnancy has been traditionally the subject of jokes which refer to wild cravings for pickles and ice cream or outlandish combinations like tuna fish with chocolate sauce. This attitude reflects the view that being pregnant is some sort of abnormal condition, during which the moonstruck mother-to-be acts totally out of character and consumes mammoth quantities of often bizarre foods.

While pregnancy certainly does entail profound physiological and emotional changes, it is also a perfectly natural state. And nutritionally speaking, although more of certain key nutrients are needed, a woman's diet during pregnancy does not have to differ radically from her regular eating pattern—provided she is accustomed to eating a well-balanced diet based on a variety of fresh and lightly processed foods. On the other hand, if her prepregnant diet left something to be desired nutritionally, now is the time to build better eating habits that will benefit her unborn child and carry over into her post-delivery life.

The cornerstone of a healthy pregnancy, then, is a sensible diet which restricts empty calories, sugary desserts, heavily salted foods, and fat, especially saturated fats, and emphasizes lean meats, fish, dairy products, whole grains, and plenty of fresh fruits and green and yellow vegetables. A pregnant woman's diet should result in a gradual weight gain of around 2 to 3 pounds per month, monitored by a physician. Eating enough roughage, drinking lots of fluids, preferably fluoridated water, exercising as prescribed, and forgoing cigarettes and alcohol are also important measures. And as we said, there are stepped-up needs for certain nutrients. Check your meal plan to make sure you are getting enough of the following nutrients.

Protein. The demand for protein during pregnancy escalates from 50 to 60 grams a day. Much of this should come from high-quality sources such as meat, fish, eggs, milk, and milk products like yogurt and cheese. To get maximum protein mileage, when high-quality vegetable protein such as dried beans is used, it is best to eat a small amount of animal protein at the same time.

Folic acid. Requirement for this B vitamin also doubles during pregnancy, rising from 400 to 800 micrograms a day. Folic acid is found in many foods, especially whole grains, liver, and green leafy vegetables. However, it is destroyed by heavy processing, removed from highly milled white flours and other grains, and not restored by enrichment of these products. Since Americans tend to eat a lot of heavily processed foods, folic acid deficiency is commmon. Because folic acid is essential for formation of red blood cells in both mother and fetus, many obstetricians recommend folic acid supplements.

Iron. As with folic acid, iron is necessary for proper construction of blood cells. Deficiency is common among young American women who have trouble fulfilling the 15-milligram daily allowance unless they eat liver once or twice a week. As a result, many physicians prescribe iron supplements during pregnancy.

Calcium and Vitamin D. Requirements of calcium go up substantially during pregnancy, from 800 to 1,200 milligrams daily. Calcium, along with vitamin D (of which you need 400 International Units a day) and phosphorus, is essential for bone formation. The best single source of calcium and vitamin D is fortified milk, either whole or skim. A pregnant woman should drink at least three glasses of milk a day or eat the equivalent in cheese (preferably hard cheeses) and yogurt.

Vitamins A and C. Although requirements for these two nutrients (as in the case of vitamin D) do not increase markedly during pregnancy, many women do have to take care to get enough of both. Some of the best sources of vitamin C are citrus fruits, cabbage, melon, and berries. Whole or fortified low-fat milk and dark green and deep yellow vegetables are excellent sources of vitamin A.

Calories. Scientists' conception of ideal weight gain during pregnancy has fluctuated over the years. We now know that for the baby to attain its optimal birth weight, and for the mother to have adequate nutrients, she should gain, on the average, 24 pounds. A good range is 18 to 30 pounds, with very thin women encouraged to gain as much as 30 pounds, and heavier women restricted to the lower limit of 18.

Following the above recommendations will give your baby the finest start and help put you in peak condition too. So if you are pregnant and you already eat well, keep it up. If not, take this chance to put yourself and your child on solid nutritional ground. At the end of the day, ask yourself the following questions: Did I eat two servings or at least 4 ounces of animal protein foods like meat, eggs, fish, or poultry, or high-quality vegetable proteins from legumes and dried beans as partial substitutes? Four servings of milk or milk products? Four of breads or cereals? One serving of vitamin C-rich fruits and vegetables? One serving of dark green vegetables, plus one more serving of other fruits or vegetables? If you can answer yes to all these questions, you'll know you're on the right track.

Questions and Answers

Q. I have been a lacto-ovo vegetarian since I was 16 years old. Now I am 24, married, and expecting my first child. My mother is concerned that I may not be getting enough protein. Can you reassure her?
A. Indeed we can. Assuming you are eating a varied diet which includes adequate amounts of dairy products, fruits and vegetables, and whole-grain or lightly processed breads and cereals, there is little cause for concern. But perhaps a few figures will be more convincing.

The Recommended Dietary Allowance for protein for an average nonpregnant adult woman about 5′ 4″ tall and weighing 128 pounds is 46 grams. To provide for the increased demands of pregnancy, an additional 14 grams should be added, bringing the total to 60 grams a day. What people tend to forget is that foods we generally think of as "carbohydrates" also contribute important amounts of protein. If a variety of these foods, such as cereal grains and dried peas and legumes are eaten together or with dairy or egg protein, the body can use them just as efficiently as it can use animal proteins alone.

Thus, while 3 cups of milk containing 27 grams of protein and 2 ounces of cheese providing 14 grams of protein might supply over half the day's requirement, the rest could easily come from a bowl of oatmeal and a slice of toast at breakfast (7 grams), from the peanut butter and bread in a sandwich at lunch (12 grams), and from the beans and rice in the casserole which also contains cheese (18 grams). Broccoli served with the casserole contribute about 5 grams more. In fact, these vegetable protein sources would provide a total of 42 grams of protein, bringing the day's intake well beyond the target of 60 grams.

Q. During the early weeks of my first pregnancy, I suffered quite a bit from nausea. I kept dry cereal or crackers by my bed and ate a small amount of one of them before getting up. This seemed to help somewhat. I am anticipating having a second child soon and wonder if you could suggest what else I might do if I have the same problem a second time?

A. Several measures seem to help minimize, if not eliminate, the nausea that is a common problem in early pregnancy. First, if you are the traditional three-meal-a-day type, you may be more comfortable if you switch to several smaller but more frequent meals. You may also find it helpful to take liquids apart from solid foods, between ½ to one hour before or after the meals.

It is also a good idea to avoid highly spiced foods, strongly-flavored vegetables such as cabbage, broccoli, onions, and turnip, and deep-fried foods, and to cut down on fat in general, by taking such measures as substituting skim for whole milk.

Happily, the nausea and vomiting that commonly occur early in pregnancy usually begin to subside after about the 12th week. While these symptoms may limit your food intake during the early weeks, it is extremely important to work toward resuming a diet that will meet the nutritional demands of pregnancy as quickly as possible.

Q. Are prenatal fluoride supplements of benefit to a baby's teeth?

A. Available evidence suggests that they are not. Any benefit from prenatal fluoride, either as consumed in the water supply or when taken in a vitamin-mineral supplement accrue only to the deciduous, or so-called "baby" teeth. Moreover, it is believed that the amount of cavity prevention provided by prenatal fluoride supplements is probably not significantly greater than when fluoride supplements are started shortly after the baby is born. There is, however, no evidence that prenatal fluoride supplementation is, in any way, harmful.

Q. I am well aware that alcohol abuse and pregnancy don't mix. But so far, everything I've read seems to give less than satisfactory answers to the question of whether moderate amounts of alcohol are dangerous. Why is that?

A. There are several reasons that make this an increasingly difficult question to answer. First, most studies are based on self-reports of drinking and thus there is a strong possibility of underestimation. Second, most results are expressed as "average" daily intakes, revealing nothing about consumption patterns, or differences between those women who drink a consistent amount regularly and those who binge. Finally, there is no single definition of just what the term "moderate" really means. The studies reported in the literature have defined the term in various and sometimes opposite ways. Some merged heavy and moderate drinkers. Another chose to pair so-called moderate drinkers with those who abstained. Data from such studies obviously cannot be compared.

In other words, what we have is a series of observations which do not permit us to draw any firm conclusions about safe levels of alcohol intake during pregnancy. It is hoped that future research will determine whether there is a level of maternal alcohol intake below which there are no effects on the unborn fetus. Until such information is available and while that issue is still in doubt, prudence indicates abstinence.

Q. Is it true that taking multivitamins during pregnancy reduces the risk of birth defects.

A. The results of the most recent and largest study of that question suggest that one vitamin in particular, folic acid, seems to protect a type of problems, known collectively as neural tube defects. One of these is anencephaly, a condition in which major parts of the brain are missing. It results from the incomplete closing of the upper portion of the spinal cord. The other is spina bifida, the incomplete closing of the bony casing that surrounds the lower portion of the spinal cord. Both defects occur early in pregnancy, after the first month of conception, but often before a woman suspects she is pregnant.

In a survey of nearly 23,000 pregnant women, those who did not take folic acid-containing vitamins during the first six weeks of pregnancy were more than three and a half times as likely to have a child born with a neural tube defect as those who did. Starting folic acid containing multivitamins at seven weeks or more of the pregnancy conferred no benefit, however. The researchers who conducted the study theorize that a genetic predisposition interacts with an essential nutrient, to cause the problem. That nutrient may well be folic acid. As they point out, however, the benefit is conferred by the amount in standard multivitamin preparations. There is no evidence that more is better, and large doses of some vitamins are harmful to the unborn child.

This question will receive continued research attention. However, current evidence provides a good argument for women to take a supplement containing 100% of the U.S. Recommended Dietary Allowances for essential vitamins during their child-bearing years. Certainly, if you are planning to become pregnant, this is something to discuss with your doctor.

Q. I am, by any definition, obese, though not as much so as I was before I began dieting several months ago. I followed a very sensible diet, and feel that I have really improved my eating habits. I am now pregnant. I realize that I need to consume enough of the right nutrients, and that I will gain some weight. But I really do not want to gain back all that I lost. Will I be jeopardizing the health of the baby?

A. No. Recommended weight gain during pregnancy can vary considerably, anywhere from about 18 to 30 pounds. On an individual basis, the specific recommendation must take into account prepregnancy weight. Obviously, women who are overweight when they become pregnant will want to limit the number of pounds they add, while those who are underweight should try to gain more. For women like yourself, the usual goal is to gain only the weight associated with the pregnancy, that is the infant itself, the placenta, increased body fluids, and some increased tissue. That way, shortly after the baby is born, your weight should be the same as it was before you became pregnant.

We would emphasize that restricting calories during pregnancy means maximizing the nutrient density of the calories you do consume. So it becomes increasingly important to plan menus carefully to insure that they include adequate amounts of all the nutrients essential for your baby's growth and development and to protect your own health. Your obstetrician will, of course, monitor your weight gain carefully as part of your prenatal care.

NUTRITION AND PMS

Presumably, from time immemorial, women have been experiencing physical and emotional changes and discomfort during the week or so before the onset of a menstrual period. But it is only recently that "premenstrual syndrome," or PMS, has received widespread publicity. Not surprisingly, with greater focus on the problem has come an increase in the number of claims for remedies, many of them calling for vitamin and/or mineral supplementation, often at "megadose" levels. Do any of these nutritional treatments really work, and are they safe? The evidence for the effectiveness of any of these remedies is, at best, equivocal. Some are potentially harmful.

Most women have probably experienced some form of PMS during their reproductive years, since over 150 different symptoms have been linked to the syndrome. They commonly fall into two categories: psychological problems, including depression, anxiety, irritability, and aggression; and physiological symptoms, among them breast swelling and tenderness, acne, constipation, tiredness, bloating, weight gain, and headaches. To be considered as associated with PMS, the symptoms must appear in the second half of the menstrual cycle, 10 to 14 days before the next period begins, last for several days, and disappear with the onset of menstruation.

For most women, these changes are, by and large, quite tolerable, requiring little more than a few aspirin, a mild laxative, or perhaps some extra time in bed. But for some, the symptoms are severe enough to cause a disruption in everyday life and thus warrant medical attention.

A number of vitamin and mineral supplements have been popularly recommended for the treatment of PMS. Of these, vitamin B_6 is "prescribed" most frequently. Unfortunately, it is potentially more problematic than it is a promising therapy. The vitamin is important for the synthesis of a number of brain chemicals, and low levels of one of these, serotonin, has been associated with depression. So it seems logical to suspect that B_6 supplementation might correct at least some of the psychological problems associated with PMS.

While anecdotal reports of improvements with B_6 abound, scientific evidence for its effectiveness is not so convincing. Only a few well-designed studies have been conducted. In these, neither the investigator nor the subject knows when the pill contains the vitamin or when it is a placebo or "sugar pill." This helps prevent expectations of a particular result from interfering with reporting or recording actual symptoms. Under these conditions it is not unusual for as many as 50% of women on placebos to report improvement. The so-called "placebo effect" makes it even more difficult to draw conclusions about the effectiveness of B_6.

Out of five such scientifically sound experiments, two found no effect and one found improvement only in nausea and dizziness. Of the remaining two which reported a positive effect, one involved just one woman, and the other used levels of the vitamin that have since been found to be potentially harmful.

It is this last aspect of B_6 therapy that has worried health professionals, especially since many women put themselves on supplements without consulting a physician. Although in the past it was assumed that excess amounts of B_6 would be readily excreted in the urine, doctors have in the last five years identified nervous system disorders, including numbness in the hands and feet, burning and tingling sensations in the skin, and impaired muscle coordination in women taking doses as low as 500 milligrams a day—an amount readily available in pharmacies, supermarkets, and health food stores, and well below the 2,000 milligram dose sometimes recommended.

Another vitamin frequently used to treat PMS is vitamin E. Even less research has been done to examine its effectiveness. In one study actually set up to look at whether vitamin E affected benign breast disease, researchers found that it alleviated some PMS symptoms, including bloating, anxiety, and irritability. However, this is hardly adequate evidence on which to base recommendations for therapy.

Vitamin A has also been touted for PMS therapy, even though there is not a shred of evidence that it is of benefit. And it can be toxic at levels just ten times the Recommended Dietary Allowance.

The mineral magnesium has also been use to alleviate PMS symptons, but there is no evidence that it is effective, either. The popular recommendation that calcium intake be simultaneously reduced "to maximize magnesium's effectiveness" is potentially harmful in an era when many women do not get nearly enough calcium in their diets and when osteoporosis is a serious problem in later life.

Finally, among the more exotic nutritional "remedies" is evening primrose oil, which, through a series of leaps of unsubstantiated reasoning is claimed to help alleviate premenstrual pain.

In short, there is no nutrient cure all for PMS, and some that are popularly recommended may even be dangerous. If you do suffer from the condition, it is your gynecologist who should prescribe any treatments, and not the popular press. Any claims that sound too good to be true probably are.

Questions and Answers

Q. Is there any evidence that food cravings are associated with menstrual periods?

A. Several studies have addressed that question over the years. One reported a few years ago found that women consumed about 500 calories a day more for the ten days after ovulation than in the ten days preceding it. Other studies have found increased appetite and cravings for sweets premenstrually, and an association between premenstrual tension or depression and cravings for food and/or sweets. Flaws in the design of the latter group of studies limit the usefulness of some of the conclusions. Finally, a recent study found that women tended to crave chocolate more during their menstrual periods than at other times of the month.

Q. I am in my midforties and have recently become troubled by premenstrual edema. A friend told me that asparagus is an effective diuretic which can relieve this problem. Is that true?

A. This piece of advice falls into what we might call the bottomless reservoir of nutritional mythology. It is true that asparagus itself is low in sodium and therefore will not promote sodium retention. Regretably, however, neither it nor any other of the vegetables which have been proposed over the years, ranging all the way from celery to watermelon, promotes "natural diuresis."

If water retention is causing you discomfort, we suggest you discuss it with your doctor. He or she may recommend one dietary measure which can help control fluid balance and that is, of course, to cut down on salt.

BREAST-FEEDING: A HEAD START ON HEALTH

When it comes to feeding a newborn infant, we don't beat around the bush: breast milk is best. Nature's design has not and probably never can be improved upon by people. Ironically, for many years here in the United States, breast-feeding was officially discouraged in hospitals. Unless a woman clearly specified her will to nurse, she was often automatically given a shot of estrogens to "dry her up," and the baby was fed scientifically-devised formula based on cow's milk and believed to be superior to mother's milk.

We're happy to say that this trend seems now to have reversed itself. It flew in the face of the millions of years during which the human race survived thanks in part to the nurturing powers of breast-feeding. Whereas in 1971 only one-quarter of women nursed their babies in the hospital, by 1985 the figure had risen to 60% and it continues to climb. This return to breast-feeding is heartily endorsed by nutritionists, physicians, and a host of medical organizations including the American Academy of Pediatrics and the American Medical Association.

Our point is not to alarm the small minority for whom breast-feeding is not a possibility. For the babies born to these women, artificial feeding is acceptable and necessary. There is little doubt that babies can be reared satisfactorily on formula feeding. Also, we recognize that variable family situations and schedules may enter into the decision not to breast-feed.

From the purely nutritional standpoint, however, breast milk is ideally suited to young babies. Research has shown that it has characteristics quite distinct from cow's milk. For instance, cow's milk contains about twice as much protein and six times as much mineral matter as human milk. This is not surprising since the growth rate of the calf (until relatively recently the only consumer of cow's milk) is much faster than that of the human infant, so the calf needs those extra nutrients fast. But the protein of breast milk has a more favorable composition and a higher biological value, meaning it is utilized better than cow's milk. So even with a lower protein and mineral content, it permits good growth for an infant.

Manufacturers of infant formulas have largely mastered the challenge of transforming cow's milk into a product that closely mimics human milk. But certain features of human milk cannot be bottled. For instance, the composition of human milk changes during a single feeding, with the milk at the end of the session containing considerably more fat than at the beginning. It's possible that the high fat content later in the feeding helps the baby feel satisfied and stop eating when he or she has had enough.

Breast milk offers more than balanced nutrition. It is beautifully engineered to bridge the gap between birth and the maturation of the baby's immune system at around six to eight months. Human milk contains components of the adult immune system that may protect the baby against bacteria, viruses, fungi, and parasites. Over the years, scientists have identified anti-infective substances in human milk that may fight respiratory and gastrointestinal infections, and such devastating conditions as acute inflammation of the intestines and colon to which premature infants are particularly vulnerable. Breast-fed infants appear to have a lower incidence of middle-ear infections as well.

Colostrum, the first yellowish substance that precedes breast milk, contains substances that attack hostile bacteria from the environment. It also contains many antibodies against viruses, bacteria, and other disease-causing organisms. It is especially effective against pathogens to which the mother is exposed, like the polio virus and streptococcus. Human milk is also rich in infection-fighting white cells. Lactoferrin, a protein in both colostrum and mature milk, inhibits the multiplication of harmful bacteria by tying up the iron they need for growth and making it available to the infant.

In addition, breast-feeding may decrease the frequency of allergic reactions and reduce the severity of childhood asthma. And it's thought that breast milk stimulates the growth and development of the intestinal lining and of its enzymes, improving digestion and absorption of nutrients.

Once they become accustomed to it, many women find breast-feeding quite convenient. However, it does link their own nutritional status together with the baby's. Nursing mothers should be sure to get adequate protein and calories as well as the necessary vitamins and minerals. Because breast milk provides only small amounts of vitamin D and iron, most pediatricians recommend supplements of vitamin D within the first month and iron by six months.

The postpartum period is not a good time to go on a crash diet to shed extra pounds gained during pregnancy. Nursing a baby, however, will help a mother regain her figure more quickly by promoting the contraction of her uterus to its prepregnancy size and encouraging gradual weight loss. It is also important to remember that in addition to all the good things a mother passes to her baby through breast milk, undesirable substances can be transmitted as well. This is especially true for drugs and for fat-soluble pesticides such as PCB's. (Contamination with fat-soluble pesticides should be of concern only to mothers who have experienced industrial exposure or who have eaten large amounts of game fish taken from water containing high levels of these industrial pollutants.) Moreover, since the baby's liver and kidneys are not fully developed, these organs cannot effectively remove or detoxify the substances. A nursing mother should consult her pediatrician before taking any prescription medication and should read warning labels on all over-the-counter preparations.

The decision to breast-feed is best made before the baby is born. This allows the mother to choose a hospital and pediatrician supportive of the practice, as well as to identify community resources such as the La Leche League or the Nursing Mother's Counsel who can provide advice during the first few weeks after the baby is born. These services are especially useful for women who lack family or friends nearby. They can offer extremely helpful tips such as how to insert two fingers to remove the baby from the breast without causing sore nipples.

When it's time to make the decision, above all, feel comfortable with it. Those mothers who give breast-feeding an honest try but have difficulty should feel reassured that even short-term breast-feeding is of benefit. And whichever way you feed your baby, if you keep him or her clean and dry, and treat him gently and kindly, you can relax in the knowledge that you are providing him or her with best kind of start in life.

Questions and Answers

Q. I have heard that breast-feeding women should not eat chocolate. Is that true or is it just an old wives' tale?
A. The idea that nursing mothers should avoid chocolate has been around for a long time. Perhaps some justification for that idea comes from the fact that chocolate contains a caffeine-like substance called theobromine which can be transferred to the milk. However, it is unlikely that a reasonable amount of chocolate would cause a problem.

There has really been very little systematic study of the relationship between foods in a nursing mother's diet and undesirable effects on the infant. And there really are no general rules for foods to be avoided when nursing. Strong flavors such as garlic and onion can be transferred to the milk, but these are not harmful to the infant, and he or she probably won't object. If eating a certain food does seem to upset the baby, obviously you will want to eliminate it.

Q. How efficient is the body in converting the calories I consume into milk calories?
A. Extremely. It is estimated that the mother's body is between 80% and 90% efficient in converting the calories she consumes into food for the infant.

Human milk contains about 70 calories in 100 milliliters, or about 3½ ounces. To produce an average during the first three months of about 850 milliliters, or nearly a quart a day, requires about 750 calories. That does not necessarily mean consuming an additional 750 calories a day during this early period. In fact, the Recommended Dietary Allowance for lactation is set at only 500 additional calories a day. If a woman of normal weight gains somewhere between 24 and 30 pounds or so during a pregnancy, somewhere between four and nine pounds are stored away as fat. It is expected that these fat stores will be drawn upon to contribute 200 to 300 calories a day toward milk production over the first three months of nursing.

If a woman has not gained adequate weight during her pregnancy, if her weight falls too low while nursing, if she is nursing more than three months, or if she is nursing more than one infant, her caloric intake will obviously need to be higher.

Q. I am currently breast-feeding my four-month-old daughter and would like to continue for the next several months until she is ready to drink from a cup. Unfortunately, I gained about 15 pounds too much while I was pregnant and can't seem to lose it. I feel I need to do something to get in shape. I would be satisfied with a very slow weight loss. Can I go on a somewhat restricted diet, say 1,800 calories, and still be able to nurse safely?

A. Yes. In fact, the idea you yourself suggest is an excellent one; namely, that you be content with a very gradual weight loss. To that we would add only that you make sure that you plan your diet carefully.

As you know, the demand for nutrients increases considerably when you are nursing a baby. These increased requirements are reflected in the Recommended Dietary Allowances (RDA's). For example, the RDA's for vitamins A, D, thiamin, and riboflavin and for calcium, phosphorus, and magnesium are increased by about 50% over those for nonpregnant women, while the RDA for protein is increased by 15 grams (the amount in about 2 ounces of meat, fish or poultry) and that for vitamin C and zinc by two-thirds.

A diet which includes 4 cups of vitamin A and D fortified nonfat milk, 10 to 12 ounces of lean meat, fish, poultry, eggs, and low-fat cheese, five servings of fruits and vegetables, including at least one citrus or other good source of vitamin C, one dark green leafy or deep yellow vegetable or fruit rich in carotene, and five servings of whole-grain or enriched breads and cereals will provide adequate amounts of essential nutrients to meet the increased demands of lactation. Such a diet would contain about 1,800 calories. If you remain as active as most mothers do, you should achieve your goal of a gradual but steady weight loss on a diet of this type without compromising your own health or interfering with normal lactation.

Q. I am pregnant and planning to nurse my first child. Lately I have been getting more advice from well-meaning friends that I can handle. Some say that ad-lib nursing, that is, whenever the baby seems hungry, cranky, or restless, for example, is a poor idea—that it can lead to sore nipples and possibly infection. Others tell me that ad-lib feeding is the best way to get started nursing successfully. Can you provide some scientific weight to this debate?

A. As with other matters regarding feeding your baby, we would refer you to your pediatrician for guidance. We can tell you, however, that recent data support the claim that frequent and unlimited feedings in early lactation are associated with more successful nursing and that there is no increase in the incidence of nipple soreness.

Q. I have heard conflicting reports about the relationship between cancer and breast-feeding. Has a link been shown?

A. That relationship has been examined extensively in a number of population studies, but the answer remains unclear. Some showed decreased risk in women who breast-fed their babies, but a larger number did not. Two recent studies suggest that any benefit may accrue mainly or solely to women in their premenopausal years. One which compared over 450 women with breast cancer with nearly 1,400 women who did not have the disease found a negative association between length of nursing and breast cancer risk only in premenopausal women, independent of all other known risk factors. A second study reached similar conclusions and found additionally that among both pre- and postmenopausal women, the risk decreased with increased duration of lactation. But the protective effect was greater among the younger women.

There is much to be learned by more detailed studies of the relationship, but it is premature to advise women to breast-feed specifically to reduce their risk of developing breast cancer.

Q. Is there any evidence that drinking larger amounts of fluids than the 3 quarts which are generally recommended will increase the volume of milk produced?

A. One recent study conducted by the Department of Pediatrics and the Clinical Research Center of the University of Iowa Hospital evaluated the effects of increased fluid intake on volume of milk produced in 21 mothers whose normal healthy infants ranged in age between three and four months. Baseline information suggested that the women were consuming, on average, 3 quarts of liquid, and considerably more in their food.

They were then asked to consume at least 25% more than they normally did (they actually consumed an average of 59% more). The amount of milk produced did not change significantly, nor could the investigators find a relationship between the percent of increase in fluid volume and change in volume of milk produced or between volume of fluid intake and volume of fluid produced.

The test lasted only two days, however, and it is not known whether increased fluid intake for a longer period would result in greater milk production. Of more importance, it does not answer the question of whether mothers of infants who are not thriving on breast milk would respond differently if they increased their fluid intake. This question warrants further investigation.

Q. My first child had colic, which he eventually outgrew. Now that I am pregnant a second time, I would like to know whether there have been any new discoveries about how to manage it more effectively?

A. While it is hardly the final word on the subject, a recent small study is of interest. Subjects included 21 infants less than three months old. All were healthy, growing normally, and had no history of vomiting or diarrhea. All cried more than 2 hours a day despite parental efforts to stop it, and showed typical signs of discomfort, such as drawing their legs up, hardening their abdomen, and then passing gas. The crying occurred during spells of irritability.

Parents were asked to keep diaries of their infants' behavior for 72 hours. Then the infants were divided into two groups for the first 9-day phase of the study. Those in one group were given written instructions about how to respond to infant crying. Specific examples were provided, using information from the behavior diaries. They were advised to assume that crying was an attempt to communicate needs and desires, among them the need for food, sleep, stimulation, and the need to suck and to be held. They were asked not to let the infant cry, but to try to respond by feeding, holding, giving the infant a pacifier, providing stimulation, or putting the infant down to sleep. They were advised, further, to move quickly from one response to the next if crying did not stop. To allay common fears, they were encouraged not to let concerns about obesity prevent feeding on demand, to let concerns about "spoiling" prevent them from holding the infant, nor to let negative feelings about a pacifier prevent them from offering one to the infant. Parents were asked to continue keeping diaries. They were called twice and given feedback on their progress, based on the diaries.

The treatment for the other group focused on change in diet. Those who were on formula were switched to a hydrolyzed casein formula. Mothers of those who were being breast fed were asked to follow a milk-free diet, the assumption in either case, being that the distress was related to a milk allergy. This group, too, was asked to keep behavior diaries; and in addition, breast-feeding mothers were asked to keep a food diary. These parents also received two phone calls and given encouragement.

At the end of 9 days, there was a significant drop in crying in both groups. However, the effect in those whose parents had received the counseling was far more immediate and dramatic, dropping within the first 3 days, and ebbing to just a little over an hour a day. In the second group, crying time diminished more slowly, and at the end of 9 days, the infants were still crying over 2 hours a day.

The second group returned to the pre-study feeding practices and received the same counseling as the first group. No ill effects related to diet were observed. However, their crying time diminished to the level of those who had received counseling first.

Clearly, the pediatrician is the one to decide whether there is a medical reason for an infant's continued distress. However, this small study suggests that when there is no medical reason, the challenge may well be to determine what it is an infant could tell you he wants if he had verbal skills at his disposal.

Q. Does soy formula reduce the risk of colic in bottle-fed babies?

A. Deciding which type of formula is best for your baby is a matter to discuss with your pediatrician. We can tell you that many studies have shown that growth and development proceed normally in babies born at term who are fed soy-protein formulas.

Current evidence does not, however, strongly support the idea that soy formulas are useful in treating colic. First of all, no one is sure exactly what causes colic, although a variety of dietary factors, including overfeeding, allergy and carbohydrate intolerance have been suggested. Moreover, diet changes only occasionally prevent further attacks.

The Committee on Nutrition of the American Academy of Pediatrics, in reviewing the use of soy milk formula, recently stated that any conclusions about the best type of formula to use with colicky babies must be considered tentative, pending the results of further research. Fortunately, in most cases, colic is a problem which seems to solve itself by the time babies are about four months old.

Q. Does breast-feeding protect against middle-ear infections?

A. Perhaps. It has been suggested that milk is more likely to drain into the middle ear and that middle-ear infections, or otitis media, is more likely to occur in bottle-fed babies who are fed in a relatively prone position—and especially in those whose bottle is "propped." Because of inconsistent findings and limitations of study designs, the Task Force on Infant Feeding Practice of the American Academy of Pediatrics believes that further investigation is necessary before a relationship can be firmly established.

Q. I am expecting my first child soon and find that circumstances make it unlikely that I will breast-feed. In looking at formula literature recently, I noticed that some brands advertise different types of protein mixtures. Does one mixture have an advantage over the others?

A. Reaching a decision about which formula to use is something to discuss with your pediatrician. If you have not already done so, you should plan to meet him or her before the baby is born to discuss this and any other specific postnatal questions you might have.

We can, however, tell you about the results of a recent study which addressed that question. One group of infants fed a predominantly whey protein formula and another group given a formula in which the main protein was casein were compared to a group of breast-fed infants. All three groups received essentially all of their calories from formula or milk for 16 weeks, from birth to the end of the study. Parents of formula-fed infants did not know which type of formula they were using.

The fact that all parents were of similar ethnic and socioeconomic backgrounds, and all mothers had received the same prenatal care at a single clinic eliminated major potential explanations for any differences that might be observed. There were no significant differences in weight, length, body fat, or lean body mass at several intervals from the time of birth until the infants were 16 weeks of age.

Q. I have a friend who frequently gives her young son juice, claiming that it provides nutrients he would not otherwise get. My pediatrician has said it is not necessary. He advised that if the baby seems thirsty, I should try a bottle of water. Do you agree?

A. Yes. As for the nutrients juices provide, it is true that they contain some vitamin C, but they are not the only source. Vitamin supplements, which most infants take, commercially prepared infant foods, and infant formulas are all sources of vitamin C.

While we have little doubt your pediatrician will eventually suggest that an occasional bottle or cup of fruit juice is fine, we suspect that he or she had several things in mind when he or she recommended water instead. There are three good reasons to limit the use of fruit juice. Juice sometimes replaces breast milk or formula the baby might otherwise consume. While the two are quite similar calorically, the milk or formula provides both protein and other essential nutrients. Second, bottles of juice are sometimes used quite regularly as "pacifiers." That is, babies are allowed to suck on them for extended periods. This provides the bacteria in the mouth with a continuous supply of sugar to feed on, setting up the perfect environment for tooth decay. Beyond that, some babies with healthy appetites simply do not need the extra calories the juice provides.

Q. What is the latest evidence regarding the relationship between breast feeding and allergic problems in infants?

A. Dr. Michael Kramer of the McGill University Faculty of Medicine recently conducted an excellent, comprehensive analysis of the findings of no less than 37 studies of that problem conducted over the past 50 years. Using a set of 12 criteria to judge the quality of the studies, each was reviewed twice to check for consistency of opinion. Conditions evaluated by these studies included atopic eczema, asthma, allergic rhinitis (upper respiratory symptoms), cow's milk allergy, and other food allergies. The results of his analysis led Dr. Kramer to conclude that the preventive benefit of breast feeding was not significant. He goes on to suggest that the negative results from some of the large, high-quality studies of that question make it quite unlikely that there is a major protective effect.

Dr. Kramer offered several reasons for the failure to find a consistent protective effect of breast-feeding. He suggests that the answer may reside in exploring factors other than breast-feeding itself, among them the mother's diet. For example, several well-documented cases have demonstrated that symptoms in the infant have subsided and then reappeared with the elimination and reintroduction of specific offending foods in the mother's diet. Sensitization to these foods may even occur *in utero.* However, even if such sensitization to so-called foreign protein antigens is important in bringing about allergy problems, attempts to prevent them by altering the infant's diet may be too little and too late. On the other hand, the effectiveness of restricting the mother's diet in the third trimester of pregnancy, in combination with exclusive, prolonged breast-feeding, has not been demonstrated. Even if such a strict regimen offered some protection in children who because of their family history are at particular risk, the difficulty in complying with such a regimen together with the potential nutritional risks involved make it of limited value as a practical preventive measure.

Dr. Kramer concludes that to better understand the relationship between infant feeding and the development of so-called "atopic disorders" will require large, well-designed, well-executed studies, with careful attention to the rigorous details of analysis of the evidence.

Q. What is the offending substance in milk that causes cow's milk allergy in young infants?

A. Cow's milk allergy, which is associated with symptoms such as eczema, colic, and mucous and bloody diarrhea, can be caused by any one of three proteins in cow's milk. These are lactalbumin, lactoglobulin, or casein. However, it is lactalbumin which seems to play the primary role in allergic reactions.

Estimates of just how common a condition cow's milk allergy is vary considerably, ranging from less than 1% to as high as 7.5%, depending on the methods used to make the diagnosis. Fortunately, for those young children who are hypersensitive to cow's milk, adequate milk substitutes are available.

STARTING ON SOLIDS

The convoluted history of infant feeding practices is a testimony to the resilience of our children. During the early nineteenth and twentieth centuries, babies received only milk until the age of ten months. Conventional wisdom recommended such nutrient-dilute items as "beef juice" as appropriate first foods. Records show that tomatoes, beets, and other vegetables were withheld until age two or even later, although our guess is that many an adventurous toddler made a grab for family fare long before it was sanctioned.

In the 1920s more liberal feeding habits began to evolve, and by the 1950s the pendulum had swung to the extreme opposite corner. Some infants endured cereal just days after they were born, and fish when they were barely a month old. Happily, such practices have long been abandoned.

Today's recommendations for introducing solid foods to infants are based on several layers of evidence. We know that a young infant's immature digestive tract cannot handle some foods. Large starch molecules, if given too early, can slip across the intestinal barrier undigested, triggering allergies. Very young babies also lack the motor control to propel food to the backs of their mouths to swallow it. The sucking motions that allow them to take milk from breast or bottle require that they thrust their tongues outward. Faced with a spoonful of food, this same thrusting movement simply propels the puree in the direction of the offerer. Getting an infant to swallow would mean placing the spoon so far back in his or her mouth that he has no choice. Also, at this age, babies are unable to communicate when they have had enough.

Only when an infant can sit with support and control his or her head and neck is he or she ready to step into the world of solid food. Babies will quickly master the art of swallowing thin solids and provide clear cues that they are ready for more or have had enough. All this usually happens between four and six months of age.

When the time comes, it's best to introduce solid foods gradually. Cereals, because they are fortified with iron, are usually the first choice. Except for babies fed iron-fortified formula, the stores they were born with can begin to run low. As the grain believed least likely to cause allergies, rice cereal tends to top the list. Wheat cereal, most often linked to allergic reactions, is held till last. Fruits, generally received with enthusiasm by babies, are added next. Because they are often fortified with vitamin C, serving them with the cereal may improve iron absorption. Next come vegetables, and finally, meats.

Tied to the question of what foods to start when is the issue of homemade versus commercially prepared. Your baby can be equally well nourished either way. Making food at home may be less expensive, and conveniences like microwave ovens and small food grinders can speed the task. However, you must use only top-quality ingredients. If you opt for either canned or frozen vegetables, choose those without added salt. Stick to fresh fruits and scrub them well before using, or use those packed in water, not syrup. Use scrupulously clean implements to prepare and cook foods. Store any foods that will be used later in the refrigerator, but only for a day or two; foods used any longer than that should be frozen in individual portions.

When selecting commercially prepared foods, our advice is to keep it simple. As a general rule, buy jars of individual items instead of mixtures. With fruits, plain is better—without the sugar or modified food starch sometimes added to improve texture or shelf stability. Products that contain no sugar or starch usually say so on the front panel. Commercially prepared sweet desserts are simply unnecessary.

No matter what food you choose, the rules for teaching a baby to eat are the same. Introduce foods one at a time and wait several days between each addition. You'll be able to identify any intolerances that might arise and encourage the child to learn about different tastes. Start with small amounts, perhaps no more than a tablespoon, and gradually increase serving size. Look to the baby for the clear signal that he or she has had enough.

Baby food can be served at room temperature, or slightly warmed. If you use a microwave, follow the food manufacturer's directions, and stir food thoroughly to make sure it is warm throughout but does not have hot spots that could cause serious burns. And always serve portions you think the baby will eat in a dish; never feed an infant from a jar unless you expect him or her to finish it.

The transition from milk to a mature diet is a gradual process. Some foods, most likely the fruits, will be instant hits, while others may meet with unqualified rejection, at least at first. Some may never find favor. Accept the fact that after all, no adult likes every single food, either. Attempting to force unpopular foods will only increase stress and can raise the chances of feeding problems that may last throughout childhood. What it boils down to is that small portions of plain food served with large portions of patience is the menu combination that will yield the big payoff: a well-nourished baby on the road to a lifetime of healthy eating habits.

Questions and Answers

Q. How common are allergic responses to food in very young children?

A. Not very, according to a recent study conducted by Dr. S.A. Bock of the

National Jewish Center for Immunology and Respiratory Medicine in Denver, Colorado. A total of 480 of 501 children over an 11-month period who received their newborn care at a single pediatric clinic completed the study. Children were followed until their third birthday or beyond if adverse reactions to a food continued beyond that age.

At each regular visit parents were asked about the child's current diet and whether any adverse food reactions had been noted. Foods thought to cause problems were eliminated until symptoms disappeared. Then, unless there was a potential danger of a serious reaction, the child was given a small amount of the suspect food, less than that believed by the parent to cause a reaction. The amount was gradually increased either to a point where a reaction occurred or when a usual portion was consumed without ill effect. When these "open challenges" failed to produce objective gastrointestinal or skin symptoms, a blind challenge was administered. That is, the food was administered in dry form, hidden in another food, in increasing amounts until a reaction occurred or until a reasonable amount produced no symptoms.

Open challenges that produced clearly observable symptoms were classified as "probable" sources of reactions, while those that evoked symptoms after a blind challenge were regarded as confirmed. Foods that produced reactions during either test were reintroduced at one- and three-month intervals until symptoms no longer occurred, except in five children whose reactions were severe.

The most commonly reproduced symptoms were associated with fruit or fruit juice, with 56 of 75 children whose parents believed they were sensitive demonstrating a response to an open challenge. Beyond that, of the 133 children whose parents thought they had untoward reactions to food, food sensitivity could be confirmed in 37, or 28%, of them. The food most commonly implicated was milk. Other foods associated with either probable or confirmed reaction were the culprit in only one to four individuals.

Most striking was the finding that the majority of foods could be consumed again within nine months of being identified as the cause of the reaction. However, symptoms associated with fruits and juices, which appeared later, on average at 15 months, tended to last longer.

Q. Is there any reason not to give low-fat milk to infants after they are six months old as long as it's fortified with vitamins A and D?

A. The use of reduced-fat milk during infancy is not recommended. While infants fed as much skim milk as they wanted continue to gain weight, they do so at a slower rate than those fed either whole milk or formula. Moreover, they show a rapid drop in skinfold thickness, an indication that they are using up stored energy. What the implications of this body fat depletion so early in life may be we simply don't know.

Infants given 2%-fat milk—milk with a 2% fat content—ad lib will consume enough milk to take in about the same number of calories as infants fed whole cow's milk or formula. However, it has been suggested that the effect of taking the larger volume of food necessary to get enough calories is not conducive to the establishment of sound eating habits.

Q. Is there any evidence that formula is a better choice than cow's milk for weaning an infant six months or older?

A. The Committee on Nutrition of the American Academy of Pediatrics has outlined a number of unanswered questions regarding the use of whole cow's milk in the second six months of life. They concluded that these unanswered questions must be addressed by well-designed research studies before a firm recommendation can be made concerning the age at which it is safe to introduce whole cow's milk into the infant diet.

Nonetheless, the Committee feels that there is no convincing evidence to suggest that feeding whole cow's milk after six months of age is harmful, if adequate supplementary feedings are given. They suggest that if breast-feeding has been completely discontinued, 6-to 12-month-old infants being fed whole cow's milk should be taking about a third of their calories from a balanced mixture of foods, including cereals, vegetables, fruits, and other foods, in order to insure adequate intakes of iron and vitamin C. They also recommend that the amount of milk allowed be limited to less than about a quart a day. The child's pediatrician should, of course, be the source of more specific advice for an individual child.

Q. Does the type of milk an infant receives affect the color of his or her stools?

A. Yes. Apparently differences in type of protein and in iron content markedly affect stool color. Human milk, rich in whey protein and low in iron leads to yellower stools, while infants getting iron-fortified whey formulas are likely to have greenish stools. And those who are getting formulas rich in casein, the main protein in cow's milk, will be likely to have stools that are yellowish-brown or brown. However, we should point out that while these are the tendencies, there are wide variations.

Should stools change color without any change in diet, it is a good idea to check with your pediatrician. Bright red or tarry stools can signal blood loss, and in that case it is important to consult your pediatrician at once. Happily, that occurs only rarely in infants.

Q. My ten-month-old son recently had his first bout of flu. The doctor prescribed a commercially prepared solution for him to drink for the first 48 hours of his illness. My mother was visiting at the time he got sick and

asked why the apple juice, ginger ale, and liquid Jello diet she used successfully to nurse my sister and me through similar episodes had been replaced. I had been so busy listening to the doctor's instructions for taking care of the baby that most of his technical explanation slipped by. Can you explain?
A. It is certainly true that many an infant has been successfully nursed through acute episodes of vomiting and diarrhea with such things as Jello, apple juice, carbonated beverages, and other clear liquids.

However, infants are particularly prone to dehydration and imbalances of the so-called electrolyte minerals, sodium, potassium, and chloride. And while Jello, apple juice, and carbonated beverages provide adequate amounts of energy, they contain too little of these minerals to replace those lost in vomiting. Moreover, the concentration of carbohydrates in these foods may exceed the infant's ability to absorb them. If that happens, losses of water and electrolytes will actually increase. Plain tea and water, both commonly used to treat diarrhea and vomiting, lack both carbohydrates and electrolytes, while homemade solutions of sugar or salt can vary considerably in their composition.

The commercial solutions which are usually used for 24 to 48 hours may be more expensive than basic items on the kitchen shelf. But when used according to the instructions from your pediatrician, which take into account your child's age, weight, and health problem, they provide the proper balance of energy, water, and minerals.
Q. Is well water potentially dangerous to young infants?
A. Unfortunately, it can be. A couple of years ago, the Journal of the American Medical Association reported a case in which a healthy infant girl, who had been breast-fed at first, began to receive supplementary feedings made with powdered formula mixed with well water. Although she was apparently healthy at the time of her first checkup at one month of age, the mother reported that she had noted transient blueness of the infant's hands and feet and around the mouth from the time she was two weeks old. The mother also noticed that the child sometimes had trouble breathing and occasionally had diarrhea and vomiting. The infant was given progressively larger amounts of formula and her condition worsened. Sadly, the symptoms, unrecognized as methemoglobinemia, went unrecognized. The child's symptoms worsened, and she died.

The problem was traced to well water on the farm where she lived. Concentration of nitrate in that water was 150 mg/liter, 15 times higher than the 10 mg/liter maximum contaminant level set by the Environmental Protection Agency (EPA).

Nitrates, converted to nitrites in the intestine, are absorbed into the bloodstream. There they link up with hemoglobin, the oxygen-carrying pigment in red blood cells, to form methemoglobin, a pigment which cannot carry oxygen to the tissues. Infants under four months of age simply do not have adequate amounts of an enzyme necessary to convert the methemoglobin to hemoglobin. When methemoglobin levels become too high, the infant becomes cyanotic (turns blue because of a lack of oxygen in the blood).

Just how common the problem is we really do not know. However, in rural states, such as South Dakota, Minnesota, Nebraska, and Iowa, a large proportion of the population relies on water from individual wells. Wells which are 100 feet or more deep are more likely to be safe. However, surface waters contaminated with nitrates as well as with chemicals or other microorganisms may infiltrate poorly constructed or improperly located wells. This is especially true of shallow wells, which may be contaminated during flooding, when runoff may contain chemical fertilizers from nearby cultivated fields, and after a heavy rainfall following a drought. Boiling, which may kill harmful bacteria, only serves to concentrate nitrates.

Just how common a problem methemoglobinemia may be is unclear. However, it is certainly entirely preventable. Wells should be tested annually to ensure their safety, and especially before new parents return home with their baby. If there is any question at all about the safety of the water, an alternative source should be used.

BEYOND THE BIB: FEEDING TODDLERS AND YOUNG CHILDREN

Anyone who has done it knows—and those about to do it for the first time will quickly learn—that feeding your preschooler can be both a delight and a challenge.

Before we delve into specifics, it's wise to note this very salient fact: between the ages of two and six, growth in weight slows faster than growth in height. Thus, preschoolers are usually thinner than they were as infants. As growth slows, appetite also falls off.

It's not surprising, then, that many parents find the process of feeding a two-year-old to be a running dispute, if not downright war. A lot of the mealtime havoc stems from the inevitable conflict between the child's ego and the demands of civilized behavior. There's not much to be done about that, except to combine polite gentleness and firmness, and wait it out.

It also helps to keep in mind the basic goal: youngsters should eat wholesome meals that provide essential nutrients as well as sufficient—but not excessive—calories. Along the way, they should be establishing healthy eating habits that will last into adulthood. Fortunately, this is not nearly as difficult as it sounds.

The same foods that make up a healthy diet at any age should be the mainstays of your toddler's bill of fare—only in the child's case, portions will be smaller, and cut in smaller pieces. The daily menu should provide milk or its equivalent in other forms (yogurt, cheese, ice cream); meat, poultry, fish, eggs, dried beans or nuts; whole grains and cereals; and plenty of fruits and vegetables. The latter group should include citrus fruits and leafy green and yellow vegetables.

If these types of foods are the centerpieces of your meals, you are on the right track nutritionally. Relying on heavily processed foods will make it harder, not easier, for your toddler and your family to eat well.

But let's say you do focus on fresh and lightly processed foods, and yet you worry because your toddler does not, shall we say, take full advantage of the benefits of your cuisine.

Our advice is not to be harsh on "finicky" eaters. Children are entitled to some likes and dislikes, within reason, of course. Instead of wrangling with them, take the opportunity to offer them different foods with approximately the same nutrients, and introduce new foods consistently so they gradually acquire new tastes. On the other hand, make no assumptions about which foods young children will turn down. We have watched many a toddler enthusiastically munch on broccoli the first time it was offered. Yet broccoli is often regarded as "too strongly flavored" for young palates.

Remember, too, that young children need to eat more often than adults. Since snacks will eventually make up about one-quarter of their daily caloric intake, teach them how to nibble wisely: on a peanut-butter sandwich, fresh fruit, raw vegetables, nuts, or a slice of whole-grain bread.

Many parents face so-called "food jags"—seemingly endless periods when a child restricts his diet to only a few foods. This behavior is not unique to food, however. Consider the way small children often become fascinated by a single story, wanting to hear it over and over again for a time. And while a couple of weeks of finicky eating will not bring on malnutrition, a great deal of fuss about it may well prolong the problem. Gently set some limits, and wait for the phase to pass.

That brings us to another point: never punish a child for failing to eat what you have served. This is the stuff of which eating problems are made. Forcing preschoolers to clean their plates may induce overeating and instill dislike of mealtimes altogether. Instead, let them serve themselves so they will learn to choose portion sizes that their appetites can handle.

Some so-called feeding problems are not problems at all. Parents of toddlers are often concerned that their child eats like a canary, forgetting about the growth slowdown that cuts energy needs. Also, a child's activity varies from day to day, and so, too, may his or her appetite.

Part and parcel of building healthy habits in your young child is encouraging exercise. Outdoor activity in particular should be promoted. Childhood was designed to be a physically active time, and lack of exercise can mean excess fat. Overweight children may grow into obese adults, and so pay the price twice for a sedentary lifestyle.

The good news is that if you do encourage exercise, limit sweets and other junk foods, and serve a fresh, varied diet, no matter what hurdles arise at your preschooler's mealtimes now, he or she has a solid chance of growing up strong and active, equipped with healthy habits that will last a lifetime.

Questions and Answers

Q. What is the Feingold hyperactivity diet?

A. The Feingold diet, developed by the late Dr. Ben Feingold about 15 years ago, was based on his theory that hyperactivity was part of an allergic reaction. Since substances in foods cause allergic reactions, he postulated that diet therapy could improve behavior in hyperactive children. Later he theorized that certain compounds had a direct toxic effect, although he never proposed how this worked. His "elimination diet" proscribed all artificially colored and flavored foods. Foods naturally containing salicylate, a chemical closely related to the main ingredient in aspirin, were also banned. That list included almonds, apples, apricots, berries, cherries, cucumbers, grapes, oranges, peaches, plums, and tomatoes, and all products made from these foods. Obviously, the diet was highly restrictive, prohibiting most processed and quick-serve foods. Yet despite the time, effort, and sacrifice called for by Dr. Feingold's prescription, his book became a best seller.

Many parents claimed the diet to be helpful. yet controlled studies of its effectiveness—difficult to design and conduct—have failed to demonstrate any consistent effect, applicable to significant numbers of hyperactive children.

Nutritionally, there is nothing inherently dangerous about it, although the taboo against so many fruits might make it more of a challenge to meet the daily requirement for vitamin C. On the other hand, it does not recommend megadoses of vitamins or minerals, and the wide-ranging avoidance of processed foods is in line with many people's desire to switch to more "natural" fare. The Feingold diet should, however, never be seen as a substitute for expert medical attention and evaluation when an attention-deficit disorder is suspected.

Q. My three-year-old daughter has rejected all vegetables except raw carrot sticks. So far I have gone along with it, but is there some nutritional reason that I should be more forceful in suggesting other kinds of vegetables?

A. Keeping a low profile as you are doing is usually the best strategy. A confrontational approach may well prolong the resistance. Besides, the simple fact is that while vegetables contain many essential nutrients, there are none that can't be supplied by other foods in the diet.

Let's look at several examples. Many vegetables other than carrots are rich sources of carotenes the body changes into vitamin A. But carotenes are also present in a number of fruits, particularly yellow peaches, apricots, and cantaloupe. And besides, only strict vegetarians depend exclusively on fruits and vegetables to meet their vitamin A requirements. Nonvegetarians also get vitamin A, itself, from such foods as whole or vitamin A-fortified low-fat or skim milk, hard cheeses, liver, and eggs.

The same is true for iron. While some vegetables contain significant amounts, meat, fish, and poultry are important sources. Dried fruits, as well as whole-grain and enriched breads and cereals also contribute to the day's intake.

Several vegetables including kale, turnip greens, and broccoli provide appreciable amounts of calcium in a form the body can use. (In others it is tied up in a way that it cannot be absorbed.) Most fruits do not provide very much calcium. However, young children can depend primarily on dairy products to meet the major portion of their calcium needs. And they can also get some from canned salmon and small fish, if eaten with the bones, and from tofu, or soybean curd.

Finally, raw or lightly cooked vegetables contain lots of fiber, which is essential for normal bowel function. But fruits, whole grains, and legumes are also good sources of fiber.

So while it is true that the wider variety of foods one eats, the better the chances for a nutritionally adequate diet, eliminating vegetables does not mean that your daughter's diet will necessarily be nutritionally inadequate.

We suggest you continue to offer other vegetables, especially those that tend to be more popular with young children—green pepper rings, tomato wedges, and even raw green beans—along with the carrot sticks she is already eating. Chances are that as she sees you and her playmates who come to visit eating them, she'll soon follow suit.

Q. What is the latest evidence on the relationship between sugar and hyperactivity?

A. There are simply no data to support the idea that sugar plays an important role in hyperactivity.

In an interesting study reported several years ago, Dr. Mortimer Gross of the University of Illinois Medical Center's Department of Psychiatry designed a simple method of exploring the effects of sugar on children with hyperkinetic syndrome. Over a two-year period, each mother who reported that sugar either caused her child's symptoms or made them worse was invited to participate in a blind study which compared the effects of sucrose sweetened lemonade and lemonade prepared with saccharine. The first 50 mothers who agreed were given two separate quarts of lemonade, one with each of the sweeteners. The jars were coded to conceal the identity of the sweetener.

Mothers were instructed to give one-third of the contents of one jar at a time the child could be observed for several hours, and then to rate the behavior on a scale ranging from –5 (much worse) to +5 (much better). This was to be repeated until all the lemonade was consumed. None of the 36 boys and 14 girls, who ranged in age from 5 to 17, showed any consistent response to sugar.

There are certainly good arguments for limiting sugar intake, not only in hyperactive children, but in those without behavior problems. But sugar, the "honey of the reed," generally does not seem to affect behavior adversely.

Q. My pediatrician found that my one-year-old son was slightly anemic and prescribed an iron sulfate preparation. I have been a little reluctant to use it since I have heard that iron supplements are sometimes associated with constipation. Is my concern justified?

A. Constipation does not appear to be a common problem in young children given iron supplements. For example, in a recent study, one group of one-year-old infants without evidence of anemia were given iron sulfate drops and a second group were given a placebo. Constipation, while not uncommon in both groups, was actually reported with a slightly greater frequency in children receiving the "dummy" drops. And in general, there was no significant difference in the frequency of vomiting, diarrhea, or fussiness between the two groups.

While none of the children in that study had low hemoglobin levels—evidence of anemia—at the beginning of the study, iron storage levels were improved at the end of three months in those given the supplement.

Q. Does apple juice cause diarrhea in very young children?

A. Apparently it can. A study of a possible link was triggered by reports of a worsening of diarrhea after drinking apple juice from parents of several young children, ranging in age from just over a year old to about 2½. The amount the children consumed was not enormous, anywhere from 1 to 1½ cups.

The children first underwent tests to determine whether they were able to digest lactose, or milk sugar. A rise in breath hydrogen levels would indicate that the sugar had reached the bowel undigested and was being broken down by bacteria. Clinically, it would indicate that they lacked adequate amounts of the enzyme necessary for digestion of the sugar. Results of these studies were all normal, but when given 7 or 8 ounces of apple juice after a 12-hour fast, the results were different. Breath hydrogen levels began climbing within just 30 minutes. In some children, they continued to rise for as much as two hours. And, not surprisingly, each of the children experienced diarrhea.

It is believed that the explanation for the problem is related to the presence of undigested sorbitol, a sugar alcohol. In later studies, pear and grape juice were associated with symptoms in some children.

If you think apple or any other juice is causing GI problems in your child, you will certainly want to either avoid it or serve only small amounts at one time. In general, however, we would emphasize that parents of children with chronic diarrhea should seek and follow carefully the advice of the doctor.

Q. Are bananas constipating for young children?

A. No. Why bananas should be singled out as a fruit associated with constipation is a mystery. Moreover, while there is nothing nutritionally unique about them (they provide small amounts of B vitamins, vitamin C, and iron, as well as generous amounts of potassium), most children do like them, sliced on cereal or eaten "as is." So it is rather a shame to restrict them unnecessarily.

The absence of fruit and other sources of dietary fiber, particularly vegetables and whole grains, rather than the inclusion of one fruit in particular is a more plausible explanation for constipation. Increasing both the amount of these foods in the diet and fluid intake is a first step in normalizing bowel habits.

Q. Despite the efforts of his parents to convince him otherwise, my eight-year-old grandson refuses to eat meat, fish, or poultry. We are concerned about whether this will create problems in a growing boy.

A. If that's all he's missing, he should do just fine. Milk, cheese, and eggs contain all of the essential amino acids (the building blocks of protein) he needs to meet the demands of growth and to repair body tissues. In fact, a boy your grandson's age will have nearly met his amino acid requirements for the day if his diet contains an egg and a total of 3 cups of milk or yogurt, or 3 ounces of hard cheese.

However, these are not the only potential sources of protein in his diet. Dried beans, nuts and seeds, and vegetables also contain important amounts. To be sure, the quality of the protein in these foods may not be as good as those found in animal foods. However, when eaten at a meal containing dairy products or eggs, the protein in those foods contributes the missing amino acids, improving their quality and making them more useful to the body.

Depending upon his reasons for avoiding animal flesh, the boy may, in the future, decide to eat meat, fish, and poultry. For the moment, the best course of action is first, to respect his preference and second, to insure that in addition to the foods we've already mentioned, his diet contains vegetables and fruits which are good sources of vitamins A and C.

One last hint: since vitamin C improves iron absorption, it is a particularly good idea to serve vitamin C rich fruits and vegetables, such as citrus fruits, broccoli, strawberries, tomatoes, peppers, kale, and dandelions with iron-rich foods. These include such foods as legumes, whole-grain or enriched breads, and cereals and nuts and seeds.

Q. What is the appropriate role of snacks in a toddler's diet?

A. Snacking really has three components: the selection of suitable foods, the issue of timing, and the way in which snacks are served.

More than providing calories, snacks should contribute important nutrients to the diet. The best choices remain such foods as fresh fruit or juice, vegetable sticks, peanut butter on crackers (and preferably crackers lowest in salt), unsalted pretzels, milk, dry cereal, popcorn, cheese cubes, yogurt with fresh fruit, and occasionally such treats as oatmeal-raisin cookies and ice cream. Many of these basic foods can easily be made into a variety of other items, for example, melted cheese on English muffins, grated cheese on popcorn, or "milkshakes" of milk, fruit, and perhaps a bit of vanilla flavoring. Of course, the youngest children should never be left alone with foods on which they might be likely to choke.

Timing is important. Snacks should be placed well apart from meals, so that children are hungry enough to eat when lunch or dinner rolls around. If it appears that dinner appetite is lagging, try serving the afternoon snack somewhat earlier. If your family mealtime is later, two afternoon snacks may be needed, with the second, which is closer to dinner, relatively small.

Finally, snacks should be well-defined "happenings." Children should sit down, eat their snacks, and be done with it. Random nibbling, often while doing other things, does little to encourage sound eating habits. Clearly you have control over the types of foods that come into your home, and therefore over the foods available for snacks. However, as your child gets older, he or she will be visiting homes where the choice of snack food may not always be what you would prefer. There is really little you can do about that, without it becoming more of an issue than it should be.

Q. My son and daughter-in-law give their two children nonfat powdered milk. Both children are quite slim, and I am concerned that their parents are not doing the right thing. What is your opinion?

A. First, many perfectly healthy children are naturally quite slim. As long as their pediatrician feels that their weight is within normal limits for their ages, there is no reason to be concerned.

As for the nutritional value of vitamin A- and D-fortified nonfat dry milk, the only thing it lacks is the fat and the calories from the fat in whole milk. Thus, while a cup of whole milk contains about 150 calories, a cup of reconstituted nonfat dry milk contains a little over half that amount.

In these days of continuously rising food costs, vitamin A- and D-fortified nonfat dry milk continues to be one of the best buys in the supermarket. A family in which two children consume about 3 cups of milk a day and the adults about half that amount would save well over $100 a year on their grocery bill by choosing it over the least expensive whole milk in the market.

TEENAGE DIETS: FILLING THE BOTTOMLESS PIT

Ask the mother of a teenage boy to describe her son's eating habits, and she'll probably sketch out a human bottomless pit, perpetually poised in front of an open refrigerator complaining, "There's nothing to eat in this house."

Given the same question, the mother of a teenage girl may well express the opposite concern: that her daughter, obsessed with thinness, seems to consume almost nothing but diet soda.

Both views might be exaggerated, but it's likely that the son, because of the volume of food he devours, will be meeting his needs for essential nutrients. In contrast, weight-conscious teenage girls who narrowly restrict their intake risk getting too little of the nutrients they need.

For both sexes, healthy eating is critical during adolescence. The last growth spurt, almost as rapid as that of the unborn fetus and newborn infant, occurs in the second decade of life. The sea change of puberty, with its profound physiological and hormonal adjustments, also unfolds during the teen years.

Until they are about ten years old, boys and girls follow parallel growth lines, gaining weight and growing taller at similar rates. Afterwards, different patterns emerge. By the time girls are 12 or 13 their growth rate has already slowed. Boys have another couple of years of slow, steady growth. Their spurt occurs between 12 and 14, and they usually grow taller and heavier than girls. They also develop more lean tissue and heavier skeletons, and their ratio of fat to lean tissue lessens. Women naturally have a greater proportion of fat tissue in their bodies.

During this period of rapid growth, the need escalates for energy, or calories, as well as for other nutrients, especially those involved in building bone and tissue. Both boys and girls require more calories than all but the most active adults. Exact requirements depend on activity level. The recommended allowance for boys between 11 and 14 is about 2,700 calories, rising another 100 calories after that. But, depending on how active they are, boys between the ages of 15 and 19 may need as few as 2,100 or as many as 3,900 calories a day.

For the early growth spurt, girls between 11 and 14 may need about 2,200 calories. Again, depending on activity level, they may need as few as 1,200 or as many as 3,000 calories. Once the growth spurt has slowed, caloric requirements drop a little.

During adolescence, the Recommended Dietary Allowances for all nutrients rise to at least adult levels. For calcium and phosphorus—crucial elements in bone growth—it is higher than it will be ever again, except in pregnant or nursing women. The demand for high-quality protein reaches adult levels for young men and even beyond for young women.

The onset of menstruation steps up a girl's need for iron to 15 milligrams a day for the rest of her reproductive life. Because rapid growth for both sexes raises the demand for more blood to transport nutrients to new tissues, young men need as much iron as young women during adolescence.

What type of diet meets all these demands? One not very different from that at other stages of life. Active young people are likely to satisfy needs for other nutrients as they meet their caloric quota. But those who are less active and therefore require fewer calories must be sure to eat nutrient-dense foods.

To provide the essential nutrients, a daily diet should include at least three servings of fruits and vegetables—either a leafy-green or deep-yellow fruit or vegetable, a citrus fruit or other good source of vitamin C, and one other. It should contain two or three servings of milk or other products rich in calcium; two servings of meat, fish, poultry, eggs, dried beans or peas; and several servings of whole-grain or enriched breads or cereals. Additional calories should come largely from these same foods, particularly those rich in complex carbohydrates and low in fat.

Another word about the differences between the sexes. For women, weight control and dieting often loom large. Young women who think they are overweight should talk with a doctor and come up with a reasonable program, including exercise and planned weight loss of no more than a pound a week. Crash diets are bad at any age; during periods of rapid growth, they can spell long-term disaster.

For young men, the teen years are a time when serum cholesterol starts rising. Yet teenage boys commonly consume mountains of fat-rich cheeseburgers, fries, and milkshakes. On occasion these foods are fine, but for long-term heart health it's best to steer toward heftier portions of foods such as baked potatoes, pasta, rice, and whole-grain breads. And contrary to popular belief, it's exercise that builds muscle tissue, not large amounts of protein from red meat or supplement powders.

Questions and Answers

Q. Pizza seems to be a dietary staple for many teenagers. Yet it is often categorized as "junk food." Is it?

A. No. Too often, foods like pizza which are sometimes sold as "fast foods" or commonly eaten as snacks are regarded as "junk foods." Obviously, neither the speed with which a food is prepared nor the time at which it is consumed has anything to do with its nutritional value.

Pizza is a perfectly fine food. The cheese contributes high-quality protein, as well as some vitamins, calcium, and other minerals. And the crust, made with enriched flour, provides B vitamins and iron in addition to some protein. Alas, by the time the small amount of tomato sauce reaches the consumer, some of the vitamin C has been destroyed. Even so, according to available data, two wedges would still provide about 10% of the day's nutritional requirement. In fact, our only criticism of a basic pizza is that in many cases the cook is just too generous with the oil, which adds unnecessarily to the fat content and consequently to the calories it provides.

True, some of the extra toppings such as salami and sausage do contribute considerable amounts of saturated fat and lots of extra salt. "Extras" such as green peppers or mushrooms and onions are wiser choices.

Q. What, exactly, is anorexia nervosa?

A. Anorexia nervosa literally means "nervous loss of appetite," but that does not really describe the condition. It is, happily, a rare disorder, occurring more frequently in young women than in men. The signs of possible anorexia nervosa include a loss of at least 25% of original body weight, a distorted body image, so that even a thin person sees herself or himself as fat, excessive "business" (either fidgeting or excessive physical activity), and wasting of both fat and lean body tissues, with all the physical changes that accompany that. Oddly enough, anorexics have an obsession with food, describing the major events in life in terms related to food. They also tend to come from families in which the major focus of parental relationships is the adolescent's food intake and health.

Physiologically, patients with anorexia nervosa exhibit endocrine changes, largely related to weight loss. Young women stop menstruating, and boys show a loss of libido.

The patient's history often discloses that they were once fat or chubby, and that an older person whose opinion was important had disparaged their excessive weight. It is at that point that the victim began a strict diet to correct the condition. Many individuals do more than diet, however, engaging in self-induced vomiting, alternating eating binges with extreme fasting. And the use of strong laxatives is common.

Social pressures appear to have something to do with anorexia nervosa, since there is more emphasis on leanness in women than in men and more in adolescents than in adults, and rates are highest among the groups where these pressures are highest. The disease is more common in occupational groups where there is a premium on leanness—ballet dancers and fashion models.

Treatment depends on the severity of the illness. Indeed, in extreme cases artificial feeding is the first step. But, beyond that psychotherapy is the cornerstone of treatment. And that therapy extends to the family. Behavior modification techniques, which reward the patient for eating more and gaining weight are helpful, but without psychotherapy they are rarely of significant value.

Q. What is bulimia?

A. Bulimia is a serious eating disorder which appears to be fairly common especially among adolescent and young adult women. Individuals who suffer from this condition may eat an enormous amount of high-calorie food within a very short period of time (one group of bulimics was found to consume an average of 3,400 calories in about 70 minutes) and then either induce vomiting or take laxatives to quickly get rid of the excess calories and thereby maintain their weight. Some also use diuretics.

While bulimia is not usually life-threatening, the continuous purging can lead to serious health problems. Those who vomit, for example, can erode their teeth, have perpetual sore throats, inflamed esophagi, and swelling of the salivary glands. Excessive use of laxatives can cause disturbances of GI function. And all types of purging can cause mineral losses and disturb the body's acid-base balance. As if all this isn't serious enough, "feeding their habit" puts many a bulimic into difficult economic straits. Unfortunately, many young women who do not meet the diagnostic criteria for the disorder are engaging in bulimic behavior in an attempt to control their weight. That is obviously unwise.

Treatment to control the condition may include a variety of approaches, among them behavior modification, diet counseling, psychotherapy, particularly in groups, and relaxation techniques. Drugs may also be used.

EATING SMART AS WE AGE

"What should a person my age be eating?" No question is asked more frequently than this. The questionner may be anywhere from 60 to 99 years of age, and often requests specific information, usually about nutritional supplements.

The general answer is disarmingly straightforward: do as you have always done, provided you've been following sound nutritional principles all along. If you haven't, now is the time to begin.

Years do bring change—notably, a decreased need for calories. As we age, the amount of lean body mass, which is metabolically more active, declines. Also, older people tend to be less active physically. Calorie control thus becomes crucial to weight control, which aids in prevention and treatment of many diseases common among the elderly. Losing weight can help limit symptoms of maturity-onset diabetes, reduce the need for medication to control high blood pressure, and relieve stress on arthritic joints. But note: eating less makes it even more important to choose foods that pack the biggest nutritional bang for the buck.

Some elderly people ask whether it's too late in the game to bother eating a prudent diet. When it comes to chronic disease, particularly cardiovascular disease and cancer, the benefits are indeed unclear. However, other factors make it more than worthwhile. Take fat. There are several good reasons to cut down, but for older individuals the strongest incentive is that fat is a potent source of calories. Restricting fat to control calories and weight makes perfect sense. Likewise, eating plenty of whole grains and other complex carbohydrates is sensible from various viewpoints. These foods, along with fruits and vegetables, provide numerous essential vitamins and minerals and fiber. A high-fiber diet helps promote normal gastrointestinal motility and prevents constipation, common in older people. As for low-fat dairy products, we don't know the extent to which abundant calcium intake helps thwart bone loss in later years, but it seems wise to consume at least the Recommended Dietary Allowance of 800 milligrams a day.

On to the question of vitamins. Do daily requirements change as we age? Should older people take supplements? In their quest to establish a category of RDA's for older people, researchers from the USDA Human Research Center on Aging at Tufts University examined the evidence to date. They were able to classify vitamins into four groups: those for which requirements might actually decline; those for which need seems to rise; those where requirements apparently stay the same; and those for which there is insufficient information to draw conclusions.

Among those for which need may lessen with age is vitamin A, essential for normal vision, healthy tissues, and resisting infection. It seems that older people who consume less than the RDA actually maintain body stores. Yet more information is needed about the role of both vitamin A itself and the vegetable precursor, beta carotene, before any change in requirements is made.

Requirements for folate, or folacin, the vitamin necessary for making DNA and RNA, may also decline. Age does not reduce absorption, and while many older people apparently consume less than the RDA, no more than 7% of elderly living on their own have low blood levels. Ironically, with the loss of ability to produce stomach acid needed for folate absorption, bacteria growing in the small intestine may produce enough of the vitamin to meet the need.

At the other extreme, older people may have a greater need for vitamin D. Decreased exposure to sunlight, a drop in the production of vitamin D in the skin, and a slowdown in the body's ability to convert the vitamin to its active form all suggest that more may be needed. And while anywhere from 50% to 90% of the elderly may be consuming the RDA for vitamin B_6, research indicates age-related changes in B_6 metabolism. Finally, it may be that some elderly, especially those whose gastrointestinal tracts absorb B_{12} less efficiently, may need more of that vitamin.

However, there seems to be no greater call for vitamin C, thiamin, or riboflavin. As for vitamin E, the suggestion that it may prevent some age-related changes remains highly speculative. There is also no evidence that advancing age necessitates adjusting recommended allowances for niacin, vitamin K, biotin, or pantothenic acid.

In fact, the advice to healthy older Americans closely resembles that for the younger crowd. A well-balanced and varied diet, including plenty of fresh and lightly processed foods, low in fat, light on salt and sugar, and rich in fiber, is the first line of nutritional defense. A single, inexpensive daily supplement providing no more than 100% of the U.S. RDA for essential vitamins and minerals adds a measure of insurance. Supplements targeted especially toward older people are not the best choice—unless they happen to cost less than other products on the shelf.

Good nutrition is hardly a fountain of youth. Don't tell the cosmetics industry, but as Ponce de Leon discovered when he explored the Florida swamps, no such miracle exists. On the other hand, coupled with regular exercise, adequate rest, and enough social contact to meet one's needs, eating well can help you live a long and healthy life.

Questions and Answers

Q. Is there any truth to the claim that nucleic acid supplements retard the aging process?

A. Not a single wrinkle's worth, even though that idea has been around for some time. In fact, a number of years ago nucleic acid-rich sardines were the star ingredient of a longevity diet.

Nucleic acids have been promoted, not only as an anti-aging factor and as a cure for degenerative diseases, like atherosclerosis and senility, but they have also been used in countless beauty products to prevent hair from graying, improve skin quality, and perform other external miracles. Not surprisingly, there is no scientific evidence to support any of these purported benefits.

Nucleic acids like DNA, which carries the genetic code and RNA, which transmits the information on DNA to other substances in the body, are manufactured in the body. The nucleic acids taken in from food or in supplements cannot even be absorbed intact. They must first be broken down by the digestive tract. Moreover, oral supplements of nucleic acids may not simply be a harmless waste of money. Large amounts can raise blood levels of uric acid and are a particular risk to individuals predisposed to gout or kidney disease.

Q. What is a reasonable conditioning program based on vigorous walking for an individual 60 years old?

A. In order to benefit the cardiovascular system, exercise should be vigorous enough to raise the heart and breathing rates to between 60% and 75% of your maximum rate for 15 to 20 minutes at least three times a week. Exercising below 60% does not provide enough conditioning for your heart and lungs and at greater than 75%, it may be too strenuous.

How do you know whether you are at that level? For a 60-year-old the target zone is between 96 and 120 beats per minute, a figure you can check by taking your pulse. Having provided that information, we would add three caveats. First, if you have not been exercising regularly, start out gradually, at around 60% of maximum rate and work gradually toward the higher level. Second, be sure to include periods of warmup and cooldown in your walking program. It is a good idea to stretch or walk slowly for about ten minutes before accelerating your pace, and to slow your walking, perhaps adding some stretching at the end. Finally, if you have not had a checkup recently, you should visit your physician, who may well suggest that you take a stress test before you begin your conditioning program.

"Target zones" for 60–75% of maximal heart rate for other age groups 50 and above are 102–127 beats per minute for 50-year-olds, 99–123 for 55 year olds, 93–116 for those who are 65, and 90–113, if you are 70 years old.

Q. Many older people take vitamin B_{12} shots, believing they are truly necessary for older people. Is there any truth to that?

A. No. There are just two indications for B_{12} supplements. Since it is found only in foods of animal origin, vegetarians who eat no animal products do not have a dependable source. They should take either a supplement containing the Recommended Dietary Allowance of just 3 micrograms a day or use a food, such as soy milk, to which the vitamin has been added.

The other group, for whom B_{12} by injection is indicated, are individuals who have pernicious anemia. Because they lack a substance called "intrinsic factor," they are unable to absorb the vitamin, either from food sources or in a vitamin supplement.

Q. I understand that the number of calories we burn decreases with age as a result of a decline in both muscle tissue and in physical activity. I am 65 years old and have not cut my food intake appreciably. I remain physically active, but it still seems that I should be gaining weight, and I'm not. My doctor says I'm fine, but nonetheless I worry that maybe there's something wrong with me. Is that possible?

A. If, as you say, you have been examined and deemed healthy, there is an alternative explanation. While body functions, including basal metabolic rate (the number of calories the body burns in a resting state) do decline with age, the rate at which this decline occurs varies considerably from one individual to another.

Thus, while on average there is a 15% decrease in basal metabolic rate between 40 and 80 years of age, some individuals in their 80s may have metabolic rates as high as the average 40-year-old. This normal physiologic variation (together with your apparently high level of physical activity) may well explain why you can still enjoy the same number of calories as you did when you were younger without the insidious addition of unwanted extra pounds.

Q. I am a 70-year-old woman who lives alone. I find microwave ovens to be a great convenience. I can prepare favorite dishes I enjoy and freeze them in individual table-ready serving dishes. I have less waste and feel that I am eating better, without spending a lot of time and energy preparing my meals. My daughter, who will not own one, says that what I am doing is not in my best nutritional interest. She says that cooking in microwave ovens destroys enzymes in food. Is that true?

A. Food enzymes are destroyed in microwave ovens, but that is hardly unique to that cooking method. It is heat, and not the type of heat, which destroys enzymes. Besides, the destruction of food enzymes is not intrinsically bad, anyway, and for two important reasons. For one thing, enzymes in food are not the same ones the body uses in its many metabolic processes. Those are produced in the body and are not obtained from food. In addition, while enzymes do have essential functions in foods, they outlive their usefulness. In fact, the process of blanching vegetables before freezing them is designed specifically to destroy enzymes which would otherwise cause undesirable changes during storage. Clearly, mother knows best.

Q. Over the past several years I have had both an ulcer and diverticulitis. Now I have been told that my blood cholesterol is somewhat elevated and that I am anemic. Each problem has brought dietary modifications. I now have several diet lists to follow, and many foods allowed on one list are not allowed on another. The result is that I am left with very few foods in my diet. Can you tell me what I can and cannot eat?

A. Not without knowing more about the details of your medical condition. We suggest that you make an appointment with a registered dietitian. The first thing she (or he) will do is to check with your current physician to determine which modifications are still necessary, which can be liberalized, and whether some can be abandoned.

The problem you describe is quite common. Over the years people are placed on a diet for a medical condition. For a variety of reasons, they continue on an unnecessarily restrictive regimen well beyond the point that it is needed. Ulcers are an excellent example. People may assume that once the problem has occurred, a diet is always necessary, and they never ask about what is reasonable once it has healed. Yet research evidence has led to considerable changes in ideas about effective dietary modifications. The ironic result is that an individual whose condition improved long ago may be following a more restrictive diet than someone recently diagnosed as having the same disease.

There are several ways to find the type of professional help you need. Your doctor may work with dietitians who do patient counseling. The Dietetic Association in your state may maintain a listing of dietitians who do private consultations. The dietary department of your local hospital may also provide these services. If they do not, they will be able to refer you for professional help.

Anyone with several problems requiring dietary modifications should review the need for each periodically. Certainly, no one wants to follow any more restrictions than absolutely necessary.

4 NOT BY DIET ALONE: Weight Reduction and Fitness

One out of every five Americans is overweight, many of them obese. Despite the millions of dollars spent each year in effort to shed extra pounds, the number who actually achieve their ideal weight is small, and the number who remain there even smaller.

Creative minds willing to play fast and loose with science dream up all sorts of reasons to explain why we gain weight, and they offer totally improbable solutions for getting rid of it. Some, like pills designed to numb the tongue and theoretically dull the appetite are harmless, if ineffective; others, like the perennial low-carbohydrate, high-protein diets are potentially harmful; and occasionally there emerges one, like the commercial liquid protein diets popular several years ago, which proves downright deadly.

The truth is that progress in understanding the complex mechanisms that govern weight has been slow. Yet the basic formula rests on scientific principles that have stood the test of time over centuries. In this uncertain world, here's one fact you can count on: if you take in more calories than you burn, you will gain weight. Dieting is not easy even under the best of circumstances; obviously, it would be better to prevent the problem in the first place. That requires a combination of prudent diet and regular exercise to keep the energy intake-and-output pendulum in balance.

Unfortunately, exercise, despite its many physical and mental benefits, is often neglected. Although our bodies were built for action, many of us have sunk into sedentary lifestyles. Yet there are numerous ways to get exercise and tailor it to our own schedules and preferences. We can't all become serious athletes, but those who do often have questions about how diet can affect performance, and recent research has shown that some specific recommendations can be made.

Dieting is not as much fun as exercise, but if approached realistically and attentively, it need not be torture, either. However, crash reducing diets are often recipes for failure. Weight loss may occur initially, but if eating habits are not reshaped, the pounds will be regained, increasing disappointment. You can, however, break through the wall of frustration and achieve your goal. In order to have a chance of succeeding, your diet should be designed specifically for you. It should begin with an assessment of the status quo, and then take into account lifestyle factors and individual likes and dislikes. It should be the last diet you will ever need.

Going beyond balanced diets and exercise, extreme obesity may lead to the possibility of more drastic measures, such as medically supervised liquid diet regimens and surgical procedures. Anyone who is considering these pathways needs to be able to evaluate potential risks and benefits of taking them on.

KEEP MOVING—THE MANY BENEFITS OF EXERCISE

Many of us regard exercise as a somewhat inconvenient way to achieve the trim, muscular look that is so popular in today's America. While there is nothing wrong with wanting to become as attractive as possible, a good exercise program offers more than cosmetic beauty—it may help extend your life.

The well-publicized studies of Dr. Ralph Paffenbarger of the Stanford University School of Medicine and the Harvard School of Public Health, which followed 17,000 male Harvard alumni for approximately 20 years, suggested that an active lifestyle—expending 2,000 calories or more a week in physical activity—added two years of life up to age 80.

Regular exercise appears to reduce risk factors linked to coronary heart disease (CHD), such as high blood pressure and diabetes. In addition, it tends to bring down total levels of blood cholesterol and to raise the levels of HDL's (high-density lipoproteins) in proportion to LDL's (low-density lipoproteins). A high ratio of HDL's in comparison to LDL's is tied to lowered incidence of CHD.

Vigorous exercise keeps the blood vessels around the heart large, more open, and more elastic. It may also open and enlarge other peripheral blood vessels, so that if you do have an artery suddenly blocked by cholesterol deposits or by a blood clot, the blood will have an alternative, lifesaving route to follow.

Decreased risk of death and heart attacks may be the most dramatic payoff, but there are other benefits to exercise, as well. These include weight control and reduced symptoms of anxiety and mild to moderate depression. Also, emerging evidence suggests that exercise has a beneficial impact on other psychological conditions, controls hypertension, and helps prevent osteoporosis.

Despite this wealth of benefits attached to physical activity, and the high visibility of health clubs and joggers notwithstanding, a surprisingly small segment of the population engages in regular exercise. If you are in the sedentary majority, we urge you to consider getting on the move. We say this not in a chastising spirit, but to encourage you to do yourself a favor. Human beings were made for action, and by moving into the active range we are working with, not against, the body's natural internal order.

When we are very inactive, the appetite-satiety mechanism that controls our food intake is no longer trustworthy. We, therefore, may be more likely to overeat, thus compounding any possible weight problem.

The amount of energy that can be used up in most types of activity, which involve only certain parts of the body. It is also directly related to how much a person weighs in the first place. A tennis player, for instance, uses up very few calories moving his or her racket. Most of the calories are burned up as the player moves around the court. Since it takes a lot more effort to move a 200-pound object around a tennis court than it does to move a 150-pound one, a heavier man is going to get rid of more calories in an hour than his slimmer opponent. As a result, he would lose more weight—unless, of course, he ate more. So, the heavier the person, the more results he or she will get from the same activity.

Any physical effort represents some caloric expenditure. Even just dressing and undressing, which most people wouldn't think of as using any energy at all, uses up 40 calories an hour. However, we normally don't spend an hour putting on or taking off our clothes. By comparison, walking for an hour will use up between 100 and 300 more calories than just sitting still; bicycling, up to 500 calories; swimming and skating, up to 600; skiing, up to 900. If you are a well-trained athlete, rowing can get you up to a caloric expenditure of some 1,300 calories as the clock ticks off an hour.

Few people fall into the super-athlete category, but there are a variety of ways to step up physical activity. First, for weight control and just to feel good, we recommend sustained, moderate exercise every day. An hour's brisk walk is ideal. Second, two or three times a week or as often as you can, take part in some form of harder, steady exercise like swimming, jogging, tennis, or bicycling. Third, get three or four periods of hard exercise each week, lasting at least 15 minutes each—something that sets the pulse to racing at about 110 beats a minute, like running, gymnastics, handball, or squash.

The first two sets of exercise will be helpful to people with diabetes or hypertension. Harder exercises—swimming and the like—should be undertaken only after checking with your physician and, for diabetics on insulin, only with the doctor's supervision. People with heart disease need medical approval before engaging in any exercise other than walking, and everyone should get a checkup before beginning the third type of exercise.

For some individuals it is more feasible to increase physical activity by integrating it into the day's set routine. You might try using the stairs instead of the elevator at work, or walking to your job or to stores. Other people prefer to take up sports; if you're in that group, be sure to pick something you enjoy and can realistically do. Remember, too, that it is important to begin slowly and gradually work up to a more vigorous level of activity. And finally, if weight loss is a goal, keep in mind that to lose a pound, you must burn off about 3,500 calories over and above what you consume.

Whatever road you choose, build activity into your life. Chances are you'll live longer and stronger—and you may well enjoy yourself more.

Questions and Answers

Q. My husband and I had a dispute which you can resolve. He says that in walking or bicycling it is the distance travelled and not the intensity of a particular exercise which affects the number of calories burned. I thought the intensity of the exercise figured into the equation, too. Which one of us is right?

A. Your husband. Larger individuals do burn more calories doing the same amount of exercise than smaller people. However, the same individual walking three miles slowly or quickly will burn the same number of calories. The effect of the intensity of exercise on the number of calories burned in the same period of time is considerable, however. For example, a woman weighing 58 kilograms, or 128 pounds, will burn about 175 calories in an hour travelling at the rate of two miles per hour. Quickening her pace to three miles an hour, she will burn about 230 calories. And going faster yet, at the rate of four miles an hour, she will burn about 300 calories. Moreover, while walking at the more leisurely pace does burn calories, the advantage of a more vigorous step is that it contributes to aerobic fitness.

Q. Is there any evidence that those who are more active physically are less likely to be depressed?

A. Apparently so. That was the conclusion reached by Kenneth E. Powell and co-workers at the Centers for Disease Control who recently reviewed what is known about the relationship. As they point out, the difficulty in defining the relationship begins with the fact that the criteria for diagnosing depression are far less precise than for other chronic disease, such as coronary heart disease or cancer. Beyond that, unlike these two conditions, the disease only rarely has a fatal outcome. Less than 1 percent of those who suffer from clinical depression commit suicide. So, in the overwhelming majority of cases, changes in symptoms are what must be measured, and that is far more difficult to do.

Several different types of inquiry have been conducted since the beginning of the decade. Four population surveys, three of them from Canada and one from the United States found that people who were more active were happier. Additionally, one of the Canadian studies, which also obtained information about household chores found a diminished association between activity and positive affect scores, or a happier mood, when both chores and leisure activity were considered together. This suggests that leisure time activity, assumed to be self-chosen may affect mood more positively than obligatory activity.

Other studies have compared the therapeutic effects of exercise to standard therapy in depressed individuals. Those randomly assigned to a jogging program improved as much or more than those assigned to other forms of therapy, including group therapy, counseling, or meditation with a therapist. Conclusions about the effect are limited by the fact that a therapist participated in the group. In two studies of women college students, aerobic exercise and swimming were found to improve depressive symptoms, when compared to women who did not exercise or swim, and in the study where aerobics was used, in comparison to those who attended a meditation program.

Finally, a follow-up study of the first National Health and Nutrition Examination Survey (NHANES I) reported that women classified as not active at the time of the original survey were twice as likely to be depressed eight years later than those who were active. A similar, though not significant, pattern was observed for men. The reason for the weaker effect is not clear. As the authors of this review conclude, while available evidence suggests that physical activity reduces depressive symptoms and improves mood, a clearer definition of the relationship depends on improvements in study design, including better definitions of depression and measurements of physical activity.

ATHLETES AND THEIR DIETS

Some years ago a football coach who had heard that royal jelly, a substance produced by bees, could improve a team's performance, asked us if this was true. When we told him the only proven function of royal jelly was to feminize bees, and that its effect on humans was unknown, the coach quickly lost interest.

Weekend sports enthusiasts and competitive athletes alike hungrily consume such substances in hopes of bolstering their prowess. Each year millions of dollars go toward amino-acid mixtures, "energy replacers," and vitamin and mineral supplements for which there is no proven or even likely benefit.

In the past two decades, research on maximizing human physical capacity has intensified. Much effort centers on gauging the merits of the "training" diet. Recently the American Dietetic Association issued a position paper on nutrition, physical fitness, and athletic performance for adults. The bottom line stated in the paper is that while we now know more about the physiology of exercise, sensible dietary recommendations for competitive athletes have changed little over time.

One fact is clear: athletes whose weight is normal need more calories than sedentary individuals of the same size. While it is generally recommended that we all eat more complex carbohydrates and less fat, this is particularly true for the competitive athlete. Complex carbohydrates help promote storage of glycogen—muscle starch—which is important in endurance contests. Increasing glycogen stores enhances performance by providing greater energy reserves to draw on during competition. That allows the athlete to maintain a high intensity of exercise. But advice regarding "carbohydrate loading," or packing the muscles with glycogen, has been modified.

As originally prescribed, athletes first depleted their muscle stores and then ate enormous amounts of carbohydrate for several days before an event. But there were side effects: repeated loading was associated with depression, lethargy, and loss of muscle tissue. Because chest pain, abnormal electrocardiograms, and other problems were also reported, the procedure was modified.

Nowadays, athletes are advised to consume hefty portions of carbohydrate throughout the training period, and to use carbohydrate loading judiciously. Beginning a week before a competition, they are counseled to taper their activity, with complete rest the day before the event, and to slowly increase carbohydrate consumption from about 350 grams a day to as much as 550 grams, or 2,200 calories of carbohydrate, for the three days prior to the event. To put that figure into perspective, a pound of spaghetti contains 340 grams of carbohydrate. Athletes whose caloric requirements are very high may need to consume more.

Carbohydrate loading has specific uses. It is beneficial only in endurance events lasting more than 90 minutes or in multiple competitions. It should be used only three or four times a year, and it should not be practiced by young children or teenagers, or without medical consultation by athletes who have diabetes or hypertriglyceridemia.

Unlike carbohydrate loading, packing the diet with protein has no known benefit, despite the plethora of products suggesting otherwise. Research indicates that current Recommended Dietary Allowances for endurance athletes may be slightly higher than for nonathletes. But athletes who eat enough calories to meet their energy needs are consuming well above that amount anyway. The idea that very high protein diets are necessary for muscle building is totally unfounded and possibly harmful.

Similarly, athletes don't need special vitamin and mineral supplements except in very specific, highly individualized situations. For example, young women athletes who do not menstruate regularly may be at risk of losing calcium from bone, and might be prescribed supplements to offset losses. Anemia is another common problem facing women athletes. But again, it is recommended that supplements be prescribed only after an evaluation of an individual's iron stores and should not be viewed as self-help measures by weekend athletes. Meganutrient capsules and powders are unnecessary for either competitive athletes or for those who simply enjoy regular physical activity.

Adequate fluids are also essential to athletic performance. Because vigorous exercise may blunt the thirst mechanism, regular fluid consumption should be scheduled. Athletes are advised to take 2 cups of fluid about two hours before exertion, and another 2 cups, 15 to 20 minutes before endurance exercise. If it is especially warm, small amounts of fluid should be consumed every 10 to 15 minutes. For most people who are undertaking normal exercise at moderate temperatures, the fluid of choice is plain, cool water. Heavy exercise or extreme heat may call for a low-dose supplemental electrolyte replacement during endurance competition.

To summarize, athletes need more food and fluid than sedentary people. They need a well-balanced diet, but do not have unusually high requirements for protein, vitamins, and minerals. Those involved in endurance exercise should consume generous amounts of carbohydrates. In the last analysis, training, not commercial performance enhancers, is the key to athletic success.

Questions and Answers

Q. I understand that fluid replacement is important for distance runners, but does the temperature of the fluids make a difference?

A. Yes. Cold liquid reduces the stomach temperature and this may increase the gastric motion and rapid flow through to the intestine where it is absorbed. For example, in one study, half of a solution taken at 5°C (41°F) left the stomach within 15 minutes, while only 27% of a solution of the same drink taken at 35°C (95°F) left the stomach in that amount of time.

Volume also seems to have an important effect on fluid absorption. Increases in fluid intake of up to about 20 ounces cause a progressively greater emptying rate and consequently promote more rapid restoration of fluids to the body.

Q. Is cold beer a good post-exercise fluid replacer?

A. It may be thoroughly enjoyable to relax over a cold beer and rehash the details of a vigorous game of tennis or racquetball, but it is not the best choice as a fluid replacer. Beer, like other alcoholic beverages, and most of the mixers that go with them, contains dissolved particles which slow the rate at which the liquid leaves the stomach. For that reason, it is best to take a large drink of water to replace body fluids before settling back to enjoy a post-game beer.

Q. My teenage son, who is on the high school swim team, has been trying to convince me that bee pollen, sold in the health food stores, might help improve his performance. What is your opinion?

A. Bee pollen is just one of a number of so-called "ergogenic" aids sold with the promise that it will improve athletic performance. The fact is that there is no reason to believe that it will help your son finish his next race even an arm's length ahead of his competitors. Nor is there evidence to support claims for improving the performance of runners or any other athletes.

Despite the fact that bee pollen has been touted as "the only perfect food," and a source of youth and health, it provides no extraordinary nutritional benefits. Moreover, several observations might raise some skepticism about it. First, and least serious, there is no real assurance that all that is labeled as "bee pollen" is truly pollen gathered by bees. Of potentially greater concern, however, is the fact that bee pollen contains nucleic acids and should not be used by individuals predisposed to gout or kidney disease. And finally, since pollen can be allergenic, questions have been raised about the possibility of serious reactions in allergic individuals.

Q. I have read different opinions about whether it's a good idea to take salt tablets when exercising vigorously in hot weather. Can you please explain when salt supplements are indicated?

A. Your primary nutritional priority should be water and not salt. In fact, athletes who engage in endurance competitions plan to drink large amounts of fluid prior to and during events, even though they do not feel thirsty. They may take as much as 3 cups of fluid in the two hours before an event and a pint of plain water right before the competition. If exercise is prolonged, it is also a good idea to take small amounts of fluid during the competition. It won't totally replace all of the lost fluids, but it will reduce the risk of getting overheated.

Salt lost during heavy exercise can then be replaced by using the salt shaker with a somewhat heavier hand at the next meal. Salt tablets are not recommended, however. They can cause nausea, vomiting, and gastric distress. Excess salt can also increase the workload of the kidneys and, if taken without adequate amounts of fluid, will make the dehydration worse.

TEN REASONS WHY DIETS FAIL

Many people engage in an annual Olympic event: their personal weight loss diet. Sadly, few medals are won, because most attempts end in failure. The basic reason is the same: an imbalance in the equation between caloric intake and expenditure. But underlying the failures is a minefield of common mistakes. If you are about to try to bring your weight under control, here are ten pitfalls you should try to avoid:

1. Errors in judging portion sizes. For example, such small mistakes as an overestimate of ¼ cup of raisin bran at breakfast, a 3″-diameter apple rather than one measuring 2½″ across at lunch, and an extra ounce of meat and an extra teaspoon of butter or margarine on a potato add up to about 185 calories. You must eliminate 3,500 calories to lose a pound, so errors of that ilk would produce an additional pound every 19 days. The antidote: arm yourself with a set of measuring tools, preferably including a small scale, at least until you are sure your estimates are on target.
2. Errors in adding excess calories while preparing food. Usually, this means extra fat. To keep fat in check, use low-fat or skim milk dairy products and lean meat whenever possible. Use a minimum of fat in cooking, and drain and trim all visible fat from prepared food before you put it on the table. You know your own weak spots; if chicken skin is an irresistible temptation, why not discard it before cooking or before you even sit down?
3. Choosing a diet plan that is out of step with your lifestyle and preferences. If you choose a diet plan with preset menus, pick one you can live with. Are the lunch suggestions feasible given your work schedule and environment? Would you be happier with a plan that includes three small meals and two snacks a day rather than one with three regular meals? If you find it hard to go to bed without a snack, you may have more chance of succeeding with a diet plan that allows for one.
4. Choosing a diet plan that is imbalanced with respect to carbohydrate, protein, or fat, or one that sounds too good to be true. It may be possible to lose seven pounds in seven days on such a diet, but that weight loss is

almost all water. Once the diet is abandoned, the weight will return, and with it a feeling of failure. These diets tend to be unpalatable, and they are nutritionally unsound.

5. Picking a diet that is calorically too restrictive. It's hard to plan nutritionally adequate diets containing fewer than 1,200 calories. Besides, most people find it difficult to restrict their intake so narrowly. The possible exception, the Very Low Calorie Diets, are not for amateurs. They should be used under medical supervision and in the context of a larger program that includes the eventual adoption of a more liberalized, nutritionally balanced diet.
6. Failing to build in a regular program of physical activity. Exercise is crucial to weight loss and maintenance, and while its role is often downplayed, consider that adding a daily brisk walk for 45 minutes will amount to the loss of an additional pound every 17 days.
7. Failing to plan for special events. Life does not go on hold for the duration of a diet. For many busy people the normal course of business may include lunch and dinner meetings, a drink after work, and social obligations. If your life fits this type of mold, victory in weight loss will depend on planning. Inventory the day before it begins, so as to pace your caloric intake. Plan your luncheon meeting at a restaurant with low-cal options—and choose something light when you get there. Order calorically more dilute drinks at cocktail hour and opt for carrot sticks over peanuts, or have tomato juice at the bar if you want wine with dinner.
8. Stepping on the scale too frequently. Nothing is more frustrating than waiting for the needle to drop. When it doesn't or worse, when it rises, many people react by abandoning their diets. Weigh yourself no more than once a day, in the morning after you have gone to the bathroom. Remember that fluid retention, especially premenstrually, may up the reading. If you see no change after several days, and you believe you've been following your diet, you might have to cut back on calories and increase your exercise level.
9. Failing to allow for personal vulnerability. It's often hard to follow a diet to the letter every day. An occasional overindulgence need not mean disaster, but responding with a series of overindulgences will. Learning to accept the fact that there are times when things do not go exactly as planned will help get you back on track more easily.
10. Failing to build in rewards for your efforts. Dieting is never easy, and it should be rewarded. Find other ways to be good to yourself. Take time to go to a movie, buy a small gift for yourself, or make a long-distance phone call to someone you miss. Above all, choose something just for the pleasure of it.

Questions and Answers

Q. I have noticed that there is considerable variation from one calorie chart to another for what appears to be the same food. Why is this?
A. There are several possible explanations. One explanation is that the difference in the portion of food being described may or may not be significant. For example, supposing the individual who constructed one calorie chart chose an apple 2½" in diameter as "an apple" while those who constructed a second chart chose an apple measuring 2¾" across. The former would provide 52 calories and the latter 68 calories. A difference of only 16 calories is not considered significant. And without a scale few of us would be able to discern which was the slightly larger piece of fruit anyway. On the other hand, one chart might list a hamburger as providing 245 calories while a second lists it as providing 325 calories. A difference of 80 calories is significant, and, in this case, is explained by a difference of an ounce of ground meat. Clearly, if you are deciding to buy a calorie chart, it is important to choose one in which portions are carefully specified and to make sure that when you use it, you are making your estimates of calories per serving based on the portion specified.

Ingredients, and consequently, caloric value of commercially available mixed dishes can vary considerably from one manufacturer to another. So, whenever possible, it is better to depend on nutrition labeling information rather than on calorie charts for brand-specific information.

WHY NOT A QUICK FIX?

When your scale shows an extra ten pounds, it's a very normal reaction to wish them off immediately, if not sooner. Like fairy godparents with magic wands, a steady stream of "experts" oblige with fail-safe advice about how to realize that goal effortlessly, even happily, and if not overnight, surely within days, or, at most, weeks. Their credentials as authorities on weight control are nothing if not varied. There are movie stars and television personalities, both those who remain eternally thin and those whose weight change is more erratic than New England weather. There are also a few physicians who forget what they learned about basic physiology in some of the nation's finest medical schools as they design diets that promise far more than they can deliver. And finally, there are the self-styled diet preachers, whose expertise is limited to the fact that they number among the formerly fat.

So-called "new" diets are really just a few basic themes endlessly reshaped and repackaged and trotted out as "revolutionary," rather like dresses from the '20s reworked for the '90s. If we were to award a prize for the one recycled most often, it would probably go to the low-carbohydrate, high-protein diet created more than a century ago by British surgeon William Harvey for his patient, William Banting. Banting, so overweight he had to back down the stairs, immortalized his success story in a publication called "A Treatise on Corpulence Addressed to the General Public." That was in 1863. In more recent times the low-carbohydrate, or ketogenic, diet has periodically been a best-seller as the Pennington or DuPont Diet, although the DuPont Company has always protested the use of its name. Similarly Air Force officers disowned any connection to it when it appeared as *The Air Force Diet.* It was also the basis of *Calories Don't Count.* With martinis it became *The Drinking Man's Diet;* later, with water, it was the "Stillman Diet.' In the '70s there was *Dr. Atkin's Diet Revolution.* And that is only the beginning of the list.

The basic claim is that on a low-carbohydrate diet the excretion of ketones, products of incomplete combustion of fats, leads to greater weight loss. It is true that at first, weight loss is rapid, not, however, because of greater fat loss, but because of a temporary loss of body water. It is also apparently true that many people who have been used to eating lots of carbohydrates lose their appetites when they suddenly cut way down. As a result, they lose weight simply because they restrict calories. Once they get used to the diet, however, their weight levels off or even goes back up, despite biochemical mumbo jumbo to the contrary. As for the claim that calories are "wasted" by incomplete fat combustion, the number of calories lost turns out to be extremely small, representing about two-thirds of an ounce a day. This certainly is not enough to account for much of anything. Finally, the fact that these trendy diets are often high in fat, and especially in saturated fat, makes them particularly unwise for anyone concerned about reducing their risk of cardiovascular disease. We cannot predict the exact nature of a recycled version of the low-carbohydrate diet for the '90s. However, we can be sure that whatever form it takes, it will be no more effective than any that have gone before it in producing long-term weight loss.

At the other extreme are diets excessively high in carbohydrates. One of the most commercially successful of those was *The Beverly Hills Diet.* Not only was it nutritionally imbalanced, but it was based on scientific nonsense and nutritionally imbalanced. Food enzymes were promoted as the key to weight loss. Claims for food enzymes as adjuncts to weight loss did not originate with the Beverly Hills diet. They appeared long before, even as part of low-carbohydrate diets, and remain with us to this day, in the form of grapefruit pills and a printed diet to go with them. (The most recent form of that diet that we have seen would lead to weight loss—because it provided about 500 calories a day!) The truth is that enzymes in food in no way affect the digestive process. That must be accomplished by enzymes secreted by the body. Moreover, contrary to the main thesis of the book, undigested food, claimed to turn to fat, cannot be absorbed, and therefore provides no calories. As for the diet itself, it was basically a low-calorie fruit diet, lacking in a number of essential nutrients. On diets that are low in protein, the body must break down protein tissue in muscle and body organs to get enough of the amino acids it needs. Moreover, some individuals who followed the diet reported severe diarrhea, muscle weakness, and dizziness. Long-term successes among those who hitched their star to the Beverly Hills diet, if any, remain anonymous.

Not all diets focus on energy nutrients. Others emphasize one or a very few foods. There are yogurt diets, salad diets, liquid diets, high-fiber diets, fish diets, and of course, fasts of varying duration. To be sure, it is possible to lose weight on any one of them—as long as you consume fewer calories than you burn. If you choose one that is especially restrictive, you may lose weight even faster than on a more traditional diet. Then, why not choose one of these diets? For one thing, many fad diets, like those we have described, can be downright dangerous. Clearly, it makes little sense to jeopardize your health for the sake of shedding a few pounds. In the absence of some systematic retraining of the eating and exercise habits that led to weight gain in the first place, those pounds, shed with at least some pain, will return at least as quickly and perhaps even faster. Moreover, recent evidence suggests that repeated cycles of weight gain and loss, which one of us (JM) long ago called "the rhythm method of girth control," make new attempts at weight control even more difficult. The parade of fad diets and weight-loss gimmicks is not likely to stop. But the next time you find yourself tempted by one of them, ask yourself one simple question. "Does it sound too good to be true?" If the answer is "yes," it probably is.

Questions and Answers

Q. A chewing gum, claimed to act as an appetite suppressant, contains benzocaine, which I thought was an anaesthetic. How is it supposed to help dieters?

A. Benzocaine *is* an anaesthetic. The idea behind putting it into diet aids is that it will act directly on the taste buds to numb them, dull the sense of taste, and therefore supposedly cause the dieter to want to eat less. Manufacturers have put benzocaine into chocolates and sucking candies, too.

In our opinion, addressing the problem of trying to lose weight by eliminating the pleasure of tasting the food you eat attacks the problem from entirely the wrong direction. To us, it seems far more important to concentrate on developing techniques to help you learn to enjoy and feel satisfied by your diet. Success in achieving that goal will not only help you stay on your diet, but it will also help you to maintain your weight loss.

Q. Are any safe and effective drug treatments being used to treat obesity these days?

A. At present, there are neither prescription nor over-the-counter drugs which can be regarded as safe and effective in producing long-term weight loss. In the short term, drugs that interfere with appetite can increase the rate at which weight is lost. However, over a longer period, patients may experience serious problems, including both side effects and addiction. Drugs such as thyroid hormone were commonly used in an earlier era in the hopes of increasing energy consumption, but they, too, led to serious side effects.

Bulking agents, such as methylcellulose and guar gum have often been promoted to aid the weight-loss process. The theory is that they will fill the stomach with indigestible material and thereby decrease food intake. Results indicate that the use of these products does not lead to weight loss and that those who try them may suffer from intestinal gas.

Q. I received an advertisement for a plastic body wrap which was supposed to take off inches instantly. Are these of any value, or are they just one more fraud being foisted on the vulnerable overweight population?

A. Body wraps of every description have been around about as far back as anyone can remember. Some are "site specific"—that is, they are meant to be worn around a particular part of the body. Others are whole suits designed to cover the entire body. Some are designed to be inflated, while others are to be used with heat. And some direct the user to apply a lotion or cream to the body before using the wrap. The one thing they all have in common is that none of them work.

Contrary to the claims which are made for these products, they don't "melt fat," no matter how much heat you use with them. Any reduction in a body measurement or any dramatic weight loss immediately after using a body wrap is not due to true weight loss, but to the effects of perspiration. That effect will disappear just as soon as the individual rehydrates his or her body with liquids or foods.

Q. Why doesn't spot reducing work?

A. Spot reducing can't work because hormone-sensitive lipase, the enzyme necessary to release the fat from storage, is present in all fat cells.

In response to the demand created by burning more calories than are available from your diet, this enzyme is released in fat cells all over the body. It cannot be directed to a specific region. While thighs, for example, may get thinner, and toning exercises can help to firm the muscles, there is no way to program the removal of fat from your thighs or any other specific part of the body.

Q. I have seen advertisements for diet aids in which the active ingredient is glucomannan. What is it and does it work?
A. Glucomannan is an indigestible polysaccharide, or starchlike compound, made up of two simple sugars, glucose and mannose. In watery solutions it forms a gel. Thus, it has been claimed that in part it is effective because it creates a feeling of fullness. The dieter who feels full faster would theoretically feel satisfied sooner and eat less. However, evaluations of bulking agents have found no clear evidence that these products were of benefit in weight-loss regimens.

The pitch for glucomannan, however, has gone beyond its gelling properties. It is also claimed that it causes food to travel through the digestive system faster, with the result that fewer calories are absorbed. In addition it is supposed to inhibit the digestion of fat.

Glucomannan powder has been sold in Japan for a number of years and, like countless other diet aids, it has brought profits to producers and distributors if not more streamlined bodies to consumers. In fact, there is no evidence that it is an effective weight-loss aid or that it acts in the way that is claimed.

A HANDY GUIDE TO WEIGHT REDUCTION

For the truly fashion conscious, the ultimate in clothing is not bought off the rack but tailor-made to fit to perfection. Similarly, when it comes to losing weight, the diet with the best chance of success is one that is custom-designed to take into account your personal taste preferences and lifestyle. In other words, a diet is not superimposed willy-nilly on your life and habits, but grows out of what you are already doing. A program that requires you to eat cottage cheese and grapefruit will fail if you abhor those foods.

Of course, many would-be dieters do need to make serious changes in their eating patterns. If, for instance, you are used to grabbing a doughnut and coffee for breakfast, a double burger, fries, and a shake for lunch, and dining on roast beef, gravy, and ice cream at night, it's true that you'll have to do more than simply eat smaller portions in order to put yourself on the right weight-loss track. But for many people, even though their customary diet and inadequate exercise has led to the accumulation of extra, unwanted pounds, a closer look at eating habits may reveal much that is worth salvaging, and that is where diet planning should begin.

No matter where your taste preferences lie, in the end, any weight loss boils down to a matter of calories. Only by calculating calories are you likely to lose weight and maintain proper nutrition. And it's reassuring to note that you need not be Albert Einstein in order to master calorie counting. You can begin with a very simple equation: namely, that 3,500 calories per week cut out of your food allowance will mean a loss of one pound of body fat provided that you do not, at the same time, cut down on your normal activity.

At the beginning of your diet, you lose excess body fluid as well as fat, so you will actually lose more than a pound for each 3,500-calorie reduction in food. As time goes on, you will be losing only fat, and you will be using fewer calories to propel your smaller body through its daily routine. As a result you will have to increase your activity moderately in order to continue to lose each pound.

To calculate a lower-calorie diet, begin with the number you will need each day to maintain proper nutrition. Usually, a woman should not drop her calorie intake below 1,200 a day, and a man should not let his fall below 1,600. Teenagers are in a period of rapid growth and thus need more nutrients. Teenage girls should get 1,400 to 1,600 calories a day, and teenage boys, 1,800 to 2,000. If you are relatively active physically, you may want to make your diet more generous than the minimums given above.

Once you have established how many calories you need per day, the next step is to calculate how many you are presently consuming. We suggest you start by getting a calorie counter, available at any bookstore, and then keeping a careful record of all the food you eat each day for a week. Also, start weighing yourself every day. If your weight is stationary, you are balancing calorie intake and expenditure.

Now you are ready to begin cutting back on calories. Suppose you have determined you now consume 2,100 calories per day, and you want to cut back to 1,600. Rather than indiscriminately eliminating foods, look over your food record for nutrient and calorie content.

Circle those foods that are empty calories, such as candy and soft drinks, or food which are high in calories but low in nutritional value, such as strawberry shortcake. Eliminate the empty calories—the sugar, cake, and whipped cream—and keep the strawberries, which are a good source of vitamin C and other nutrients but are relatively low in calories.

Next, analyze your menus for fat content. We need some fat in the diet, but ounce for ounce, fat contains almost twice as many calories as do proteins or carbohydrates. By cutting down on cooking and table fats, and high-fat foods, you can save calories without sacrificing nutritional value.

Then, check your revised menus for the basic foods that will provide the 40-odd essential nutrients you need to maintain health. Your daily plan should include:

- At least three servings of vegetables—at least one serving of leafy green or deep yellow vegetables.

- At least one serving of citrus fruits, tomatoes, cabbage, or other good source of vitamin C.
- At least one additional serving of potatoes or other vegetables.
- Two servings (or about 6 oz.) of lean meat, poultry, or fish, with dried peas and beans as alternates.
- Two servings of whole-grain breads and cereals, and other foods made with whole grains.

Bear in mind that serving sizes can vary considerably. A kitchen scale will help you keep portions in line. Be as meticulous about figuring portion size as about figuring calories. Portions bigger than those listed in the calorie counter will provide more calories than you counted on. And where you can, replace a food of high caloric value with one with fewer calories and the same nutritional value. Make sure to strike out sauces and gravies, notorious sources of calories.

Now, add up your total calories again. How many have you cut out? If you are near your goal of 500 fewer calories per day, try following the new menus for a couple of weeks. Since you are eliminating a total of 3,500 calories per week, you should lose a pound a week.

If you find you are not losing enough weight, go over your food list again, cutting more calories and building up nutrients, until you hit the weight-loss program you want. For your health's sake, however, don't go under the calorie minimum. Instead, step up physical activity.

A good "budgetary" rule for the would-be dieter is this: daily income, 2,000 calories; daily expenditure, 1,800. The result: misery. But if your daily expenditure is 2,000 calories and daily expenditure 2,100, the result is happiness.

Questions and Answers

Q. Is there any evidence that eliminating snacks is associated with more successful dieting attempts?

A. No. It is important to keep in mind that measures which make the dieting process easier vary from one individual to another. For example, some people prefer to eat just three times a day. For one thing, caloric intake is lower than what they have been accustomed to. Having to "save" some calories for snacks reduces the amount they can eat still further, to a level where the amount of food they can eat at mealtimes (with the exception, of course, of such things as raw vegetables and fat-free broths, which are very low in calories) is unacceptably low. Beyond that, some dieters feel that they are better able to stay within their limits if they restrict the number of times they eat and are not involved with food at other times of the day. At the other extreme are dieters who prefer to divide their calories into six or even eight small servings, feeling that they are better able to stay within defined limits if there are only short intervals between eating occasions. Still others find that one snack a day is critical to maintaining their regimen. For example, it may be that a small snack before beginning to prepare dinner prevents constant nibbling before the meal is ready.

We should add that when calories are limited, it is especially important to include nutrient dense foods in a diet, that is, foods which provide a lot more than just calories. Otherwise, the diet may well be lacking in essential nutrients. So while a reducing diet allows little room for snacks of such things as candy and potato chips and other fried snack foods, as long as you stay within your caloric limits there is no reason to give up eating between regular meals.

Q. Is it true that celery is a poor food to eat while dieting because it causes fluid retention?

A. That idea has been around as long as we can remember. While we cannot say for certain, it may be linked to the fact that celery is one of several vegetables which are relatively high in sodium. Others in this group include artichokes, beets, carrots, white turnips, spinach, and most other dark-green leafy vegetables. This is of little practical importance, except where sodium intake must be sharply limited. In those cases, which are now rare, the amount of all of these vegetables is restricted. But for dieters who like it, celery is perfectly acceptable.

Q. Several years ago a lot of attention was directed to the so-called "fat-cell" theory of obesity, which linked fat-cell number and size to the likelihood of successful weight control. I've heard nothing about it lately. Has it been discarded?

A. No. It is more than 15 years since researchers Jules Hirsch and Jerome Knittle reported that individuals with adult-onset obesity had much larger fat cells (hypertropy) than normal-weight individuals, and that individuals who became obese as children had an increased number of fat cells (hyperplasia). In fact, while obese children tend to have both cell hypertropy and hyperplasia, cell size may be normal, while cell number can be increased as much as fivefold.

It was once believed that nutritional and genetic influences early in life could lead to hyperplasia, but that the number of fat cells stabilized in adolescence. If this were true, weight gain and loss in adults could occur only by change in cell size, not cell number. It is now known that cell number can increase in adults—perhaps as existing cells reach an upper limit of size as a result of caloric imbalance over a long period. Conversely, cell number may decline when individuals lose weight and keep it off for a long time.

According to the fat-cell theory, weight loss will be extremely difficult for obese individuals with an excess of fat cells because of biologic pressure to keep those cells supplied with energy. To attain so-called "ideal weight," the individual must reduce cells to subnormal size by depleting them of fat. This may create symptoms similar to that experienced by normal-weight individuals experimentally placed in a state of starvation—persistent hunger, preoccupation with food, and a number of psychological symptoms. It has been suggested that cell size presents a biological limit beyond which weight loss is exceedingly difficult, and that fat-cell number determines body weight at which this limit is reached.

Confirmation of this theory must wait for the results of further studies. One of the most important aspects of the story is that fat-cell size, more than cell number and more than weight gain per se, appears to be important in obesity-associated risk for medical problems. Thus, an individual with too many fat cells may lessen risk by reducing fat-cell size to normal even though he or she remains overweight by society's standards.

Q. What is the relationship between having a so-called "sweet tooth" and becoming obese?

A. Surprisingly enough, there does not appear to be one. While there are several good reasons to use as little sugar as possible, it is linked to the development of obesity only to the extent that it contributes to caloric excess. And contrary to what you might expect, the few studies that have been done indicate that obese individuals do not have an innate fondness for sweeter foods. Not only do they prefer less-sweet foods than their leaner counterparts, but that preference continues even after they have lost weight. Like obese adults, obese children also prefer less-sweet foods. However, when these children lose weight, their preference for sweetness is the same as that of normal children.

Q. I have a reducing diet which gives a recipe for making a low-calorie salad dressing with mineral oil. Doesn't mineral oil contain calories? And is it really safe to use mineral oil in salad dressing?

A. Mineral oil is a by-product of the oil refining process, one of a group of chemicals called hydrocarbons. While hydrocarbons can be used as a source of food to grow some single-cell organisms such as yeast, the human body lacks enzymes to break it down. Therefore, it does not provide any calories. Despite that fact, however, it is not a suitable substitute for regular vegetable oil.

Beyond the fact that mineral oil is not terribly palatable, it is not totally innocuous. It acts as a solvent for fat-soluble vitamins, carrying them through the body without allowing them to be absorbed. And since it has an affinity for carotene, the plant substance which the body converts to vitamin A, using mineral oil dressing on your salad will prevent you from absorbing much of the carotene which salad greens and other vegetables pro vide. Mineral oil also acts as a laxative.

There are many low-calorie salad dressings you can make using yogurt or tomato juice as a base and altering the seasonings for the particular salad you are serving. If you want an oil-and-vinegar or oil-and lemon-juice dressing, you will be far better off to adapt your taste buds to a more tart mixture.

Q. A television commercial for a "high-protein" cereal says that women who are dieting need plenty of protein so they will lose fat and not muscle. Does dieting increase protein requirements?

A. No. The only situation in which protein becomes an issue is in individuals following protein-sparing fasts. Of those diets, generous amounts of protein prevent the breakdown of lean tissue, especially body organs.

It is extremely unlikely that anyone following regular low-calorie diets of 1,200 or even 1,000 calories will fail to consume adequate protein to build and repair body tissue. Protein not used for these purposes is simply burned for energy or stored as fat, as are excess calories from other energy sources.

Cereal with skim milk and a glass of vitamin C-rich fruit juice make an excellent, nutrient-dense breakfast for dieters and nondieters alike. But the decision about what cereal to choose need not be based on its protein content, even when restricting caloric intake.

Q. If one is following a very strict reducing diet, are vitamin supplements necessary to provide extra energy?

A. Taking a supplement providing no more than 100% of the Recommended Dietary Allowance for each of the nutrients it provides does help insure that you are getting adequate amounts of essential nutrients. Beyond that, the concept that vitamins provide energy is simply untrue. Energy, or calories, comes from carbohydrates, proteins, fats, and alcohol. In order for the body to burn those so-called energy nutrients, adequate amounts of vitamins and minerals must be present. In their absence, deficiency symptoms may appear.

Fatigue is a symptom commonly associated with nutrient deficiencies. So it is natural that among the purveyors of nutrient supplements there are those who suggest, as directly as they can while remaining within the limits of the law, that vitamin and mineral supplements provide pep and energy. But the truth is that these preparations eliminate fatigue only if the source of that fatigue is a nutrient deficiency.

Q. Can you please explain the "set-point" theory of obesity?

A. The set-point theory says that weight is set at a relatively constant level. Individuals are obese because their set point is abnormally elevated, and conventional efforts to lower and then maintain body weight will fail because regulatory mechanisms which determine the set point will compensate.

Support for the theory comes mainly from studies with animals, especially rats. If allowed to eat all they want of a regular diet, they maintain a fairly constant weight. When made experimentally obese or thin, they simply maintain their new weight.

Several other lines of evidence are used to support the argument that humans have a weight set point. First, it has been observed that individuals maintain their weight within a fairly narrow range over long periods, despite often marked variation in both caloric intake and energy expenditure. Second, one group of investigators has found that when normal weight volunteers were put on reducing diets, their weight returned to normal once they were allowed to eat as they wished, while a second group found a similar effect in normal volunteers made experimentally obese. Finally, estimates put the number of dieters who regain the weight they lost as high as 95%.

Dr. Thomas Wadden of the University of Pennsylvania School of Medicine summed up the value of the set-point theory by observing that it helps explain several common problems which plague the successful management of obesity: the high drop-out rate; the negative emotional responses to treatment; the limited success; and the regaining of weight lost in treatment. But, as he has pointed out, there are other explanations for each of these problems. And practically speaking, there is no way to determine human set points.

The bottom line is that obesity therapy must continue to focus on those factors we can manipulate—and chief among them are diet and exercise.

THE VERY LOW CALORIE DIET IN THE TREATMENT OF OBESITY

We are all impressed when a friend or celebrity—such as Oprah Winfrey—sheds mounds of pounds in a short period and emerges, like a butterfly out of a cocoon, with a brand-new body. As long as we live amid an abundance of fattening foods, such feats will be met with admiration, envy, and a desire to get on whatever dietary bandwagon is credited with producing the weight loss. Unfortunately, not all regimens are medically or nutritionally sound, and some can be downright dangerous if followed for long periods without medical supervision. Very low calorie diets are a case in point.

Over 20 years ago, a modified fasting technique was first used to treat people who were considerably overweight. Since then, researchers studying the method have learned more about where it fits into the inadequate armamentarium of weapons used to battle obesity.

Very low calorie diets, or VLCD, were designed to eliminate the serious, undesirable physiological effects of eating nothing at all. Total fasting does lead to rapid and significant weight loss. But more than body fat is shed, and much of what is lost can be lean tissue from vital organs. Furthermore, once the individual resumes a normal diet, restoration of lean tissue is usually accompanied by the accumulation of extra body fat and weight gain.

In contrast, the VLCD usually contains anywhere from 200 to 800 calories, primarily from protein of top quality. In fact, protein intake is often set quite high—at almost twice the Recommended Dietary Allowance for nonpregnant, nonlactating adults. Supplements of vitamin and minerals, including the "electrolytes" essential for fluid balance, are generally prescribed. These calories may come from a chemically defined powder or formula, or from the so-called Protein-Sparing Modified Fast. That includes animal protein foods, limited amounts of low-carbohydrate vegetables, and lots of fluids, along with appropriate nutritional supplements.

The approach offers several advantages. First, rapid weight loss encourages individuals to stick to the diet. And, ironically, well motivated patients seem better able to follow the well-defined VLCD than conventional diets. Loss of hunger, which occurs for somewhat mysterious reasons, seems to make the task easier. On the down side, the regimen is not without possible side effects. Some people experience symptoms of low blood pressure for the first week to ten days. Other problems include constipation, dry skin, mild fatigue, hair loss, intolerance to cold, and emotional symptoms.

In the short run, results seem encouraging. On average, men lose 3 to 5½ pounds a week and women, 2 to 4½ pounds, primarily fat tissue. Average losses of between 15½ to 22 pounds at 4 weeks, 44 pounds at 12 weeks and anywhere from 68 to 90 pounds at 24 weeks have also been reported. The process does not pose the dangers associated with the infamous liquid protein diets which claimed several victims in their heydey about a decade ago. (You may remember liquid proteins as the stars of the popular "Last Chance Diet.") The VLCD regimen is safe for 12-week periods if used by appropriate candidates and under proper supervision. There are no data which evaluate their safety and effectiveness for longer periods, but concern has been raised about potential harm if used for more than three consecutive months.

The VLCD seems best suited to individuals who are at least 30% above ideal weight, but less than 100% over that level, a group for whom success with conventional methods is generally unlikely. Among those more than twice their ideal weight, the VLCD simply does not seem to lead to permanent weight loss, although it is useful in trying to help them shed some weight to reduce the risks associated with surgical treatment for the condition.

Even among those who do fall into the correct weight category, there are many contradictions to using the VLCD. It should not be followed by people with certain circulatory problems or those who have recently suffered a heart attack, by individuals with juvenile-onset diabetes, by pregnant women, when certain drugs are being used, and when particular emotional problems are present. Also, it should not be attempted by elderly individuals.

As described by Dr. George Blackburn of Harvard Medical School, the regimen actually begins with an extensive evaluation and a low-calorie balanced diet providing between 800 and 1,200 calories. This program promotes gradual loss of body water and thereby prevents the rapid fluid loss associated with abrupt institution of the VLCD. Next, the individual is put on the very low calorie regimen and followed weekly by medical personnel knowledgeable about the metabolism of fasting. Key indicators of body functioning are monitored on a regular basis, many of them weekly. In the third phase, a normal weight maintenance diet is gradually reinstituted.

Since weight maintenance is the goal, a comprehensive program to prevent an individual from regaining pounds once he or she is back on a regular diet should be provided and should include nutrition education, mental reconditioning, behavior modification, relaxation techniques, and exercise.

Even with all these inputs, there is no guarantee of success and long-term weight maintenance. In one study, subjects regained an average of 14 of 46 pounds after two years, and in another, they regained 35 of 50 pounds after five years. The conclusion is that a VLCD regimen should be used only under the guidance of an experienced medical team, in a setting that provides a comprehensive program to prevent regaining lost weight. It is not for amateurs and should never be adopted as a self-help panacea.

WHEN IS SURGERY THE ANSWER TO OBESITY?

That overweight and obesity are caused by a disharmony between caloric intake and expenditure is beyond debate. It follows, then, that correcting the imbalance should set the problem straight. But as anyone who has ever tried to diet knows, this is more easily said than done. In the annals of nutrition, the frequent failure of methods to help people shed excess weight and keep it off is quite large.

For many who make repeated attempts to lose weight, using either safe or dangerous means, the end of each effort is marked by regaining all the weight lost and then some. The tragic sequel can be so-called morbid obesity, defined as at least 100 pounds over desirable weight, or, in people less than five feet tall, 100% or more over ideal weight.

These unfortunate individuals are often beset by a swarm of problems. Many are unable to work or find jobs because of their size. They are more likely to have diabetes, hypertension, and heart disease, as well as foot and other orthopedic problems. The simplest accident can be extremely dangerous for them, especially if an operation is needed, just because they are such poor risks for surgery. Last, but certainly not least, their food bills, providing for as many as 7,000 calories a day, are enormous. It is for these individuals, whose lives are hemmed in by excess weight, that surgery, despite its risks, offers a ray of hope.

Since the early 1960s, surgery has been used as treatment for obesity. Although surgical methods have improved in the years intervening, they remain far from foolproof. As we noted, surgical procedures carry extra risk for the obese, during both the operation and recovery. Long-term problems may ensue as well, and there is no guarantee that weight gain will not recur. Surgery, then, is not for everyone with an obesity problem. Treatments are usually reserved for those with, or at the greatest risk of developing, serious medical conditions known to be helped by weight loss, and who are unable to maintain weight by other means. Most candidates actually refer themselves for surgery, citing limitations in simply carrying out their normal day-to-day activities.

Nowadays, of the various types of procedures used, all employ one or both of two underlying principles. They either restrict the amount of solid food that can be ingested, or, by bypassing a portion of the digestive tract, they prevent calories from being absorbed; or they do both. Some kinds of surgery are performed entirely in the stomach, others in different portions of the small intestine, and some involve both small intestine and stomach. In addition, a vagotomy, or severing of nerves in the stomach, has been used in conjunction with stomach surgery.

How effective is surgical treatment? Evidence on tap suggests that weight loss is usually about one-third of weight before surgery, or 55% to 60% of the excess, regardless of the type of operation. However, procedures designed to produce malabsorption are generally more effective, with a larger percentage of patients achieving and maintaining weight loss.

Beyond the immediate goal of weight loss, the surgery has been shown to improve serious medical problems, sometimes dramatically. Indeed, the effectiveness of the body's insulin increases and symptoms disappear in most diabetics even before they have lost substantial weight. Several studies have also demonstrated that blood pressure returns to normal after surgery for weight loss. Surgery, like any weight-loss method, has been shown to reduce blood levels of triglycerides, or blood fats, and LDL cholesterol. It also helps lessen respiratory problems related to excess weight.

Harder to assess is the extent to which surgery enhances an individual's quality of life. However, limited studies suggest that those who have the procedure experience improvement in their general well-being.

Sadly, not all the news is so positive. Complications can result. Individuals who undergo gastric surgery, which restricts the size of the stomach, must follow a special diet and eat according to carefully prescribed instructions. Failure to do so can lead to vomiting and/or failure to lose weight. Ironically, the most common problem with gastric restriction is weight gain, related to the so-called "soft calorie syndrome": eating foods that slide through easily.

Surgical procedures that lead to malabsorption are linked to other problems. One hazard is that, without careful monitoring, deficiencies of essential nutrients can occur. Still, in a recent review of the procedures, Dr. John Kral, Professor of Surgery, State University of New York Health Sciences Center at Brooklyn, an expert in this area, observed that the safety of the surgery and the recognition and successful treatment of side effects in cooperating patients has improved greatly over the past ten years.

Once again, surgery, with its many shortcomings and limitations, is the path for only a small percentage of obese people. There remains much to be learned about selecting appropriate candidates and matching them to the right kind of operation.

5 SPECIAL PROBLEMS DEMAND SPECIAL DIETS

Historically, diet therapy has all too often rested on what has been called the "we all know" syndrome: prescriptions based on logic rather than on scientific observations of cause-and-effect relationships. The classic example is the bland milk and cream ulcer diet. Not only did it lack healing power, but it promoted obesity and boosted serum cholesterol levels. Experience has shown that the most dramatically effective diet therapies are those used to treat rare disorders. For example, a diet low in the amino acid phenylalanine right from birth can save an infant with the inborn error of metabolism called phenylketonuria from mental retardation.

On the other hand, diets used to treat such common disorders as hypertension, gout, diabetes, and diverticular disease are much more loosely defined. Two principles should guide all diet therapy: first, the diet should be only as restrictive as necessary; and second, it should be instituted only after a clear-cut diagnosis is made.

Like marriage, good nutrition ought to endure in both sickness and health. Some illnesses, like cancer or AIDS, can pose nutritional challenges brought on both by the disease and its treatment. Yet, although it can provide no miracle cure, a steady supply of nutrients and calories is crucial to maintaining the patient's strength and spirits.

THE NEW LOOK IN DIABETIC DIETS

With the discovery of insulin in 1921, a diagnosis of diabetes no longer meant certain death. Unfortunately, 65 years later, there is no cure, although hope exists both for that and for a vaccine to prevent the disease in children. Meanwhile, researchers and practitioners are working tirelessly to improve the effectiveness of treatment.

According to the American Diabetes Association, nearly half of the more than 11 million Americans who have diabetes do not know it. Too often the diagnosis of the more common type, "non-insulin dependent diabetes," is made only after an individual develops one of the serious complications of the untreated disease. This is tragic, since better methods of treatment have allowed diagnosed diabetics who "live by the rules" to lead longer, healthier lives.

Our understanding of the role of diet in diabetes continues to grow. The revised report of The Committee on Food and Nutrition of the American Diabetes Association, "Nutritional Recommendations and Principles for Individuals with Diabetes Mellitus: 1986," provides an updated road map for nutritional management. Not surprisingly, the guidelines closely parallel those of the American Heart Association and the National Cancer Institute, with the first emphasis on achieving and maintaining ideal weight. The committee also gives more specific recommendations for promoting measures to help normalize blood sugar and blood fat, and to minimize wear and tear on the kidneys.

First, it is recommended that carbohydrates supply between 55% and 60% of total calories consumed. Fiber, important for the general population, is even more critical for those with diabetes because they live at greater risk of cardiovascular disease. Whenever possible, unrefined, fiber-rich carbohydrates should be substituted for refined grains. Foods such as legumes, lentils, roots, tubers, fruits, and vegetables contain water-soluble fibers of particular benefit in normalizing both blood glucose and blood fat levels. Eating fruits and vegetables raw and without pureeing them maximizes the fiber effect. The report suggests that some individuals may be able to have modest amounts of sugar, depending on weight status and whether the diabetes is under control.

Second, unlike those for the general population, these guidelines make recommendations about protein intake. Americans, says the report, tend to consume too much protein. Moreover, diabetics have a heightened risk of kidney disease. The end products of protein metabolism must pass through the kidneys. So to protect those organs, protein intake should be kept to the

Recommended Dietary Allowance of 0.8 grams per kilogram of body weight for adults. (To translate that to your own RDA for protein, simply divide your weight in pounds by 2.2, the number of pounds in a kilogram, and multiply by 0.8).

Third, the risk of cardiovascular disease associated with diabetes makes it especially wise to limit fat intake to less than 30% of total calories, and cholesterol to under 300 milligrams a day, with saturated fat held to less than one-third of that. Recommendations for salt (1,000 milligrams per 1,000 calories, and no more than 3,000 milligrams per day) and for alcohol (moderation) parallel those for the general population.

To assist people with diabetes in following their diets, a joint committee of the American Diabetes Association and the American Dietetic Association has issued a revision of the basic system used in dietary management since 1950. The exchange lists, which categorize nutritionally equivalent foods into calorically similar portions, have been updated and expanded in a new booklist which highlights both foods rich in fiber and those high in sodium. Included is a multistage system to help individuals gradually learn how to manage their diets.

These are just the broad brushstrokes of a detailed set of recommendations, and diet represents only part of the equation of successful diabetes management. Many individuals require insulin or oral hypoglycemic (blood sugar-lowering) drugs to control their condition. Physical activity should be a regular feature of the daily schedule, and aerobic exercise is strongly recommended.

The point, however, is not to offer a road map for self-treatment of diabetes, even if the condition is mild. Individuals with diabetes deserve personalized instruction and periodic reevaluation. What is crucial is to underscore that diagnosis is the first step. The sudden onset of symptoms of insulin-dependent diabetes, which usually occurs in young children or adolescents, include frequent urination and excessive thirst, extreme hunger, rapid weight loss, fatigue, irritability, nausea, and vomiting. They are too severe to be ignored. Symptoms in the majority of adults, who are usually over 40 and overweight, may include some of these, but the condition may be marked by more vague signs such as blurred vision and other sight changes, tingling or numbness in the legs, feet, or fingers, frequent skin infections or itchy skin, slow healing of cuts and bruises, and drowsiness.

If you are experiencing any such symptoms, visit the doctor. If they are related to diabetes, the only obstacle between you and continued good health may be the failure to follow recommendations known to minimize the risk of serious complications of diabetes.

Questions and Answers

Q. About a year ago my husband found out that he had diabetes. He was overweight and out of shape. Since that time he has lost weight, reformed his dietary habits, and begun to exercise regularly. On his last visit to the doctor, he was told that he could have an occasional alcoholic drink. That surprised me, because I had thought diabetics really should not take alcohol. Also, the doctor told him to cut back on his fat intake to allow for the calories from alcohol. Since alcohol comes from fruits and grains, this didn't make sense to me. Could you please reassure me that alcohol is all right for a diabetic and that it is appropriate to cut back on fat intake when taking a drink?

A. While large amounts of alcohol can cause serious problems, particularly for insulin-dependent diabetics, there is no evidence to indicate that small amounts are harmful. However, the calories in alcohol and the mixers that sometimes go with them do have to be taken into account in planning the day's diet.

On the surface, it would seem that since alcohol is derived from carbohydrate sources, it should replace carbohydrate foods in the diet. The fact is, though, that the body metabolizes alcohol in the same way it handles fat. Moreover, since it has been recognized for some time that diabetics are at an increased risk of developing atherosclerotic heart disease, dietary recommendations for diabetics suggest that a larger percentage of calories should come from complex carbohydrates and a smaller percentage from fat, especially saturated fat. Therefore, it makes good sense to cut back on fat in order to keep the caloric content of the diet constant while consuming some alcohol. Your husband's doctor may also have advised him to substitute carbohydrate-containing mixers for other carbohydrates he normally eats.

In people who take insulin, a hypoglycemic reaction (low blood sugar) may be mistaken for intoxication and go undetected if there is alcohol on the breath. It is, therefore, especially important for them to wear a Medic-Alert marker indicating that they have diabetes.

Q. Is it true that diabetics should avoid red beets?

A. No. The most likely source of that widely accepted myth may be the fact that certain varieties of beets (called sugar beets) are grown specifically as a source of sucrose, or table sugar.

The beets that come to our tables as a vegetable also contain sugar, but they're hardly unique in that regard. So, too, do a number of other vegetables as well as all fruits. That's fine. Diabetics, like nondiabetics, need sugars and starches for energy. Moreover, fruits and vegetables provide essential vitamins and minerals as well.

Most individuals who develop diabetes in their adult years are overweight. Those who lose weight and keep it off can often bring the condition under control without medication. But as we get older, our caloric requirements drops. Since we are burning fewer calories, stricter dietary control is necessary in order to lose weight. It is primarily for that reason that the number and size of servings of all foods is usually clearly specified. That includes fruits and many vegetables, not only beets, but a lot of others as well.

Q. My doctor has told me that my blood sugar is too high, but that if I lose weight it would probably return to normal. I'm supposed to see him again in a month to decide whether or not I need medication. I am so afraid that I will eat the wrong thing. Can you give me some guidance about what I should eat?

A. In the first place, losing weight can, as your doctor says, have a dramatic effect on bringing an elevated blood sugar back within a normal range.

Second, there is nothing mysterious about the type of diet you need. No one food will "do you in." In general, you need a well-balanced, low-calorie diet. Because fats are the most concentrated source of calories and because diabetes is associated with an increased risk of heart disease, it makes sense to keep the diet low in fat, especially saturated fat. Since sugar contributes nothing but calories, it has little place in the diet when one is trying to lose weight. So your diet should include skim milk and other low-fat dairy products, lean meat, fish, or poultry, with dried beans as alternates, fresh fruits and vegetables, including some which are good sources of vitamins A and C, and whole-grain or enriched breads and cereals. Eggs, which are high in cholesterol, should probably be limited to no more than three a week.

This general advice must be adapted to your individual situation. Since diet is such an important part of maintaining your health, we suggest that you consider getting professional help in learning to manage it. Perhaps your doctor can suggest a dietitian who can help you tailor a diet that best fits your needs. If not, the dietitian or nutritionist at your local hospital or health department can direct you to competent professional help.

Q. I am a diabetic and follow my diet quite closely. I use sugar only on rare occasions. I was surprised to read that potatoes cause the same rise in blood sugar as does table sugar. Does that mean I would be better off without potatoes?

A. No. Over the past several years, diabetes associations of many Western countries, including the U.S., Great Britain, Canada, Finland, and Australia, have recommended eating more unrefined carbohydrates, especially those rich in fiber, along with a reduction in fat. Beyond that, the question of which carbohydrate foods are best for diabetics remains cloudy.

In short-term studies, it has been found that dried legumes, like kidney beans, red lentils, black-eyed peas, and chick peas—all of which are also rich in good-quality protein—caused a smaller rise in blood sugar than did whole-wheat bread. Long-term studies have shown substantial improvement in diabetic control when these gel-forming fibers are used generously in the diet. Apparently they slow the rate of digestion.

It has also been shown that blood sugar responses to rice, pasta, and All-Bran were higher than for legumes, but less than for bread. Surprisingly, the response to both white and whole-wheat bread was the same.

Potatoes caused a higher blood glucose level than bread, and one similar to that of the simple sugar, glucose. Still other studies have shown that sucrose, given with a meal, raised blood sugar only as much as potatoes and wheat did.

While fiber seems to slow digestion and blunt the rise in blood sugar, it is not the only factor. Wheat in pasta leads to lower responses than wheat in bread and whole rice causes less of a rise than rice flour. Particle size and integrity of structure may, therefore, also be important.

All in all, the main advantage of a diet high in starchy carbohydrate seems to be an overall decrease in the average blood glucose concentration, possibly by making insulin more effective. Indeed, some studies have demonstrated that an increase in low-fiber carbohydrate has benefit. Both bread and potatoes have formed a substantial part of several experimental diets which have, over a period of weeks and months, resulted in improved diabetic control. In one study where insulin-dependent diabetics were given bread enriched with either wheat bran or guar, glucose levels improved to an appreciable and similar extent. So there seems to be no good reason to eliminate whole-wheat bread, potatoes, or other cereals on a sensible diabetic diet. Sugar, on the other hand, is not essential, and overweight diabetics who must continue to restrict energy intake will do well to avoid it.

CONSTIPATION AND OTHER PROBLEMS OF THE BOWEL

In polite company, it may still be considered an indelicate subject. But judging from the swelling size of the laxative industry, constipation seems to be an all-too-common national ailment. Americans spend nearly $400 million on the more than 120 laxative preparations available over the counter. How do these products work, when should they be used, and most important, how do you prevent the problem in the first place?

Laxatives can be grouped into four major categories: softeners and lubricants, osmotic agents, stimulants, and bulking agents. A single product may contain a combination of these ingredients. When the need for a laxative is indicated, it is important to read the label carefully to see exactly what is inside.

Softeners act by facilitating the mixing of intestinal water and the fatty substances in the stool, softening the fecal matter and easing its passage through the intestine. Docosate sodium is the substance most commonly used in these preparations. Lubricants, such as mineral oil, coat the stools, making them easier to pass.

Osmotic agents, which contain magnesium or sodium, alter the fluid and electrolyte balance in the colon. As a result, water is retained in the bowel, and the increased pressure stimulates intestinal movement. Magnesium may also act by stimulating the release into the gut of a hormone called cholecystokinin, which itself promotes fluid accumulation.

Stimulants such as senna, danthron, bisacodyl, phenolphthalein, and castor oil are believed to work by both initiating muscle contractions in the colon and by causing increased intestinal water retention.

Finally, bulking agents derived from polysaccharides or cellulose take on water and swell in the colon, increasing stool bulk and thus encouraging intestinal muscle activity.

Unfortunately, the misconception seems to be afloat that these products are completely safe, perhaps because they are advertised widely and are available without a prescription. Yet they do have side effects. Stimulants, which cause abdominal cramping, are believed to be the most abused of all laxatives. An alarming number of weight-conscious women use these products to try to purge themselves of calories after a meal.

Not only is this an ineffective antidote to overeating, but, more importantly, excessive use of stimulants can lead to fluid and electrolyte imbalances and cause serious, permanent damage to the colon. Mineral oil, when used over an extended period, may impair the absorption of the fat-soluble vitamins A, D, E, and K. And while bulking agents are probably the safest alternatives, they must be taken with adequate fluid to prevent complications.

Individuals using other medications, and particularly the elderly who may be taking several different drugs, should check with their doctor or pharmacist before taking any laxative to make sure there is no risk of undesirable interactions. Some laxatives can decrease the absorption of orally administered medications. On the other hand, some drugs and over-the-counter preparations such as anticonvulsants, calcium-containing antacids, and iron supplements can lead to constipation in some individuals.

Pregnant women, many of whom suffer from constipation, should also be sure to ask the advice of their physician before choosing a laxative. Those containing stimulants are to be avoided. This is true also for nursing mothers, since these drugs will pass into the milk.

As an alternative to laxatives, which carry varying degrees of risk, three nonpharmacological, truly "all-natural" measures can both treat and help prevent constipation. In fact, they are usually the first to be "prescribed" by a physician.

First, increase the consumption of fiber, a food component often in short supply in the American diet. Dietary fiber acts by a mechanism similar to that of the bulking agents, increasing stool volume and thereby stimulating intestinal movement. High-fiber foods include bran, whole grains, fruits, vegetables, and nuts.

Second, get daily exercise. Just walking may be enough. Exercise increases the activity of the intestinal muscles, facilitating the movement of the stool through the colon. Also, get in the habit of allowing a regular time to respond to the urge to have a bowel movement. Often this is a period after a meal.

Finally, we must emphasize that while constipation may be a common condition and one for which treatments are readily available, it can mask far more serious medical problems. Self-treatment of constipation for more than a few days without seeking medical advice is risky business.

Questions and Answers

Q. I developed a pain in my lower right side. The doctor ordered X-rays and then diagnosed diverticulosis. He explained what the condition was and suggested that I increase my fiber intake. Unfortunately, I really was not feeling well and didn't pay close attention to what he was saying. Can you please tell me something about this condition?

A. Diverticula are pouches, or hernias, which push through the intestinal wall. Many individuals develop diverticula as they get older, but fortunately suffer no discomfort. In others, symptoms can include constipation, diarrhea, abdominal pain, and gas. At present, high-fiber diets are generally used to treat this condition. The reason is that the fiber absorbs moisture and produces a larger, softer stool which moves more quickly and easily through the intestine.

Q. Is there any evidence that dietary habits are associated with the development of ulcerative colitis?

A. Since food travels through the gastrointestinal tract, it is logical to wonder whether diet has a role in the development of ulcerative colitis. Recently Drs. Beverly Calkins and Albert Mendeloff of the Johns Hopkins Schools of Hygiene and Public Health and Medicine reviewed the available evidence for an association between diet and both ulcerative colitis and Crohn's disease, another type of inflammatory bowel disease, and found no clear-cut relationship.

Dietary studies to answer that question are difficult to do. For one thing, relevant dietary practices might have occurred years before the disease is diagnosed. Beyond that, dietary practices may change from the point at which the disease develops until it is diagnosed, making it difficult to establish links. So there have been few studies of pre-illness diet.

Diet has been suggested as an explanation for the lower rates of colitis for Jews living in Israel than for Jews in this country. And even in Israel the disease is more common among Ashkenazi Jews than among non-Ashkenazis. And dietary factors have been shown to parallel these differences. American Jews tend to eat more fat and meat and less carbohydrate and fiber than Israeli Jews. And Ashkenazi Jews in Israel consume more meat, milk, and eggs than non-Ashkenazis. But this is hardly evidence to claim a cause and effect relationship.

Early studies suggested that milk consumption was associated with ulcerative colitis, but these studies have not been supported by later research. Finally, questions have been raised about whether the type of infant feeding might play a role. Studies of that question have provided inconsistent findings. It is true that during the era in which the prevalence of breast-feeding was on a steady decline the incidence of inflammatory bowel disease was on the rise. Now breast-feeding has become more prevalent, and the incidence of inflammatory bowel disease has stabilized and may be declining. But the number of individuals with these disorders is simply too small to draw any conclusions. Given the large number of infants fed formula over the past four or five decades and the relatively small proportion who develop inflammatory bowel disease, any effect of formula would be very difficult to identify.

Q. Please explain what irritable bowel syndrome is and what dietary measures are recommended for individuals who have it?

A. Symptoms of irritable bowel syndrome, a common condition, result from abnormal motility of the colon and can include indigestion, cramping, abdominal pain, and diarrhea, which may alternate with constipation.

While restrictive, low-fiber diets were commonly used in the past, today it is recognized that such therapy simply was not consistently effective. Instead, individualized dietary modifications are designed to help provide symptomatic relief.

For example, increased amounts of fiber are often recommended for either constipation or unformed stools. Avoiding coffee, carbonated beverages, and cold drinks, in general, may be of benefit if diarrhea is a problem. Cutting down on fat may also help to relieve symptoms in some individuals. Legumes, cabbage, and other vegetables which are likely to result in gas production are among foods often associated with symptoms. And in controlled studies, tea and coffee, citrus fruits, and dairy products were among the foods associated with symptoms in some, but not all individuals. Some people who have irritable bowel syndrome also have lactose intolerance. Obviously, those individuals who associate discomfort with the consumption of dairy products are well advised to limit them to amounts they can tolerate easily.

Q. What, besides dried beans, causes intestinal gas?

A. While certain foods are known as "gas-formers," intestinal gas actually comes from a variety of sources. It can come from swallowing air "as such" or in air-containing foods. Gases are also produced by interactions between secretions in the intestine or by tissue metabolism. Finally, gases result from the fermentation of undigested food by bacteria in the intestine.

Gases are eliminated in three ways. For example, atmospheric gas may be eliminated by burping it back up through the esophagus. It can also diffuse into the blood, eventually to be exhaled through the lungs. Finally, it can be expelled through the rectum.

To some extent the composition and location of the gas will determine how it is expelled, but other factors may also be involved. In the intestine, how much is diffused into the blood and how much is expelled as flatus will depend on such things as intestinal blood flow, intestinal motility, and on where in the intestine the gas is produced.

ULCERS AND OTHER DIET-RELATED DISEASES

Ask most people to describe someone with a peptic ulcer and they will come up with the picture of a hard-driving executive, under constant stress, who pacifies the pain in his digestive tract with antacids, a constant flow of milk, and a diet of creamed baby foods and soft white bread. In reality, that is a somewhat oversimplified picture. Certainly people under stress do get ulcers. But others, under the same stress, do not. In fact, the role of stress in the production of ulcers remains unclear, although recent research suggests the possibility that people with ulcers handle pressure differently from those without them.

Ulcers as a recognized disease have been with us for centuries. A 2,000-year-old inscription on a pillar of the Temple of Asklepios, the ancient Greek god of healing, describes the case of a man with a stomach ulcer. Yet we still do not know what causes ulcers to develop, or exactly who will get one. They are most common in middle-aged people and, until the 1930s, men were ulcer victims by a wide margin—six to one. Today, in the U.S., the male-to-female ratio is about two to one. It's estimated that some four million Americans suffer from ulcers at any given time, and another six million have had one in the past.

While we don't fully understand why ulcers occur, we do know how they evolve. They develop in membranes lining the walls of the gastrointestinal (GI) tract in what is called the mucosa. Normally the stomach and small intestine protect themselves against ulcers with a covering of mucus through which a neutralizing solution of bicarbonate can pass. Cells exposed to stomach acid have other defenses, too, and when damaged, they are usually replaced. But for reasons that remain unclear, sometimes the defenses are inadequate. In those cases, an ulcer forms when two substances in stomach juices cut through the inner lining of the stomach or intestine and begin boring into the walls themselves. One is the protein-splitting enzyme, pepsin; the other substance, which activates the pepsin, is hydrochloric acid.

Hypersecretion does not fully explain the problem. Many people with ulcers secrete as much as four times the normal amount of gastric acid. Others may secrete a normal amount, but the mucosa in their GI tracts is less resistant to gastric juices. Exactly what causes this lowered resistance has not been identified, but several things seem to be involved, among them low blood flow in the mucosa and a defect in the body's ability to inhibit gastric secretion. Recent studies suggest that a specific bacteria, *Campylobacter pylori,* may be involved in the development of the disease. And aspirin and other nonsteroidal anti-inflammatory drugs used extensively to treat arthritis can lead to ulcers in susceptible individuals.

Beginning in 1911 and for decades thereafter diet remained a cornerstone of the treatment for peptic ulcer. The goal of the "Sippy diet," named after its author, Dr. Bertram W. Sippy of Chicago, was to minimize acid secretion, neutralize what was produced, and protect the damaged area from the abrasive action of coarse food. Ironically, the sickest patients were put to bed and given nothing to eat for several days, leaving the injured area directly vulnerable to the destructive action of the pepsin-hydrochloric acid combination. They then were started on a regimen of milk and cream. That proved a poor idea. Studies have shown that protein and calcium, both abundant in milk, are powerful stimulants of acid production. As a result, the Sippy diet may indeed provide relief—temporarily—but ultimately it causes the stomach to churn out more acid, leading to more ulcer pain. Moreover, because it is high in fat, and especially saturated fat, it is considered unwise for anyone at risk of heart disease.

Similarly, the use of frequent small feedings of bland, soft food has been set aside. With a few exceptions, texture and flavor are probably not relevant. Food does temporarily relieve the gnaw of ulcer pain, and on those grounds, the regimen of eating small, frequent meals could be defended. On the other hand, because practically all foods stimulate acid production to some degree, that recommendation, too, has gradually faded from favor. In fact, modern treatment of peptic ulcer disease focuses on drugs, including both cimetidine and antacids, and, where necessary, various surgical procedures. Dietary modifications, based on more systematic observation of what is and is not effective, are actually quite modest, varying mainly with the severity of the symptoms. First, coffee, cocoa, and tea consumption, including decaffeinated varieties should be limited, and avoided altogether when an ulcer is "acting up." Similarly, alcohol, a direct irritant to the gastric mucosa, should be avoided altogether in the face of symptoms. But at other times, beverages containing less than 12% alcohol may be tolerated. Ground pepper has also been identified as a source of symptoms, though the reasons remain unclear.

The last three recommendations can be summed up under the category of ordinary common sense. Avoid eating before going to bed to prevent oversecretion of acid during the night. Avoid highly acid juices if they cause symptoms. And, finally, avoid any other food that causes discomfort. Attempts to identify exactly which foods they might be have served to demonstrate the ancient adage that one man's meat is another man's poison.

Questions and Answers

Q. What is gluten enteropathy?

A. Gluten enteropathy is an intolerance to gliadin, one of the two fractions of gluten, a protein found in wheat, rye, barley, and possibly oats. The cause of the condition remains unclear, although current evidence supports the idea that immune factors are involved.

In infancy it usually occurs when cereals are added to the diet. It may also appear for the first time in adulthood, mainly between the ages of 20 and 30.

Patients with the condition experience fatty, foul-smelling diarrhea and are unable to absorb essential nutrients efficiently. Fortunately, if followed carefully, dietary treatment can produce dramatic results. Foods containing wheat, rye, barley, and oats must be completely eliminated. Corn meal, as well as flours made from rice, arrowroot, potato, soy, and wheat starch should be used to produce baked goods.

Initially, it may also be necessary to restrict both lactose and fat, but these can be added back once the condition is under control. It can take several months for the intestine to recover from damage sustained before treatment is started.

Q. Why is it that protein is restricted in some people with kidney disease?

A. The principal reason lies in the unique way the body gets rid of the end products of protein metabolism.

Carbohydrates are broken down to carbon dioxide and water. The carbon dioxide is exhaled through the lungs and the small amount of water that is produced during metabolism can generally be exhaled, passed out through the sweat glands, or eliminated in the feces. The body handles fats in much the same way.

In contrast, the major end products of protein metabolism, including urea, uric acid, sulfate, creatinine, and organic acids normally pass through the kidneys and are excreted in the urine. While the breakdown of tissue protein contributes some of these waste products, the main source is dietary protein.

When kidney damage is extensive, these metabolic end products cannot be eliminated efficiently. Instead, they accumulate in the tissues and blood. At that point protein intake must be restricted. Just how severe the restriction will need to be depends on the extent of the kidney damage.

Q. What foods should an individual with gout avoid?

A. Happily the list is short. For several years, diet has taken a solid back seat in the management of gout, both because effective drug treatment is now available, and because our increased understanding of the disease itself makes severe dietary restriction illogical.

Gout results from a disorder in the way the body handles purines. Blood levels of uric acid, a product of purine breakdown, rise too high. Acute attacks of arthritis-like symptoms result when the uric acid crystallizes into salts which are deposited in body tissues, especially around the joints.

Because it was thought that uric acid came only from purines in foods and from the breakdown of tissue proteins, it seemed logical to restrict foods rich in purines. We now know that the body makes uric acid out of such plentiful raw materials as carbon dioxide, ammonia, and glycine, an amino acid. So severe dietary restriction cannot be expected to produce dramatic results.

Dietary treatment for gout focuses first on achieving and maintaining ideal weight. But both fasting and crash dieting are contraindicated, since they can precipitate gouty attacks. Second, drinking large amounts of water, as much as 2 quarts a day, is extremely important. It helps eliminate uric acid, reducing the risk of forming kidney stones and protecting against kidney damage. Beyond that, it is suggested that the diet contain only moderate amounts of protein and relatively little fat. Finally, some authorities recommend that foods highest in purines, including liver and other organ meats, sardines, anchovies, fish roe, meat extracts, and legumes be omitted.

Q. I realize that there are many good reasons to avoid consuming large amounts of alcohol, but why is it particularly important for people with gout? Also, can a person with gout drink coffee and tea?

A. Excessive alcohol consumption can increase the level of urates, crystals of uric acid, in the blood. In addition, individuals with gout often have hyperlipidemias, or high blood fat levels, and these are associated with an increased risk of coronary heart disease. Excessive alcohol intake can exacerbate the problem.

Coffee and tea (and we would add cocoa) do not present a special problem for those with gout. While it had at one time been thought that caffeine and its chemical relatives, the so-called methyl xanthines, were metabolized to urates, it is now known that they form somewhat different compounds which are not deposited in body tissues.

Q. Comfrey-pepsin capsules are sold at a health food store as digestive aids. But are they safe?

A. A letter to the New England Journal of Medicine provides qualitative evidence that you would be well advised to avoid them. Analysis of two brands of comfrey-pepsin capsules, one allegedly made from the leaves and the other from the roots of the comfrey plant, indicated the presence of significant amounts of so-called "pyrrolizidine alkaloids." These compounds are toxic to the liver and some have been shown to be carcinogens (cancer-causing). The letter points out that serious illness had been reported a year earlier in a woman who consumed two comfrey-pepsin capsules at each meal for four months. Clearly the potential risk associated with their use suggests that they are better left on the health food store shelf.

Q. Recently I passed a kidney stone which was analyzed and found to contain calcium oxalate. The doctor told me first to drink enormous amounts of fluid, as much as 3 or 4 quarts a day, and to sharply limit my intake of milk and milk products. Why didn't he also restrict the dietary sources of oxalate?

A. We should begin by reinforcing your doctor's first recommendation. Diluting the urine by drinking large amounts of water reduces the concentration of the offending substances which form the stones, and that makes them less likely to develop.

Beyond that, while diet is theoretically of some value in retarding stone formation, its usefulness as a preventive measure has not been fully established. We can only speculate on the reason for your dietary recommendations and would encourage you to check back with your doctor for a complete explanation. However, calcium, not oxalate, is usually restricted in patients who form calcium oxalate stones and who also have high levels of calcium in their urine. It is only in those patients who do not excrete excess amounts of calcium that restriction of oxalate as well as calcium might be of value.

Q. Papaya enzyme is sold as a digestive aid. Does it work?

A. No Enzymes are proteins. Like other proteins, they are made up of chains of amino acids, which are "wrapped" or packaged into more compact configurations.

All enzymes, both those in foods and those produced in the body, work most effectively within a rather specific range of acidity or alkalinity. When that environment changes markedly, their powers are curtailed. The first step in the digestive process alters their structure, rendering them unable to function as enzymes. Denaturation, as it is called, spreads out the amino acid chains and loosens them, allowing enzymes made in the body to begin dismantling the proteins into their component amino acids, which the body will then absorb.

Enzymes in food are denatured either by the acid in the stomach or by the alkaline environment of the small intestine. Digestive enzymes created by the body meet a fate similar to those consumed in raw foods. Once they have completed their work and moved along to a less favorable environment, they too, are digested. The amino acids from which they were constructed are then absorbed and used by the body to build new proteins.

MAN AND MILK

From the dawn of human evolution up until the recent past, an infant's survival hinged on the ability to get its vital nutrients from breast milk. In light of that, the revelation less than 20 years ago that millions of older children and adults lacked the ability to digest lactose (milk sugar) seemed extraordinary.

The difference, it appeared, was related to culture and geography. Throughout history, many groups have never kept dairy animals and never drank milk after infancy. These have included the aborigines of Australia, the natives of New Guinea, and Native-Americans. Other groups, among them Orientals and natives of West and Central Africa, kept dairy animals but seldom used milk as adults.

The ability of these groups to digest milk sugar may have begun to diminish some 10,000 years ago. On the other hand, among Northern Europeans and some Mediterranean peoples, the capacity to make sufficient lactase, the crucial sugar-splitting enzyme, evolved as a genetic adaptation after early childhood in populations which raised dairy herds and depended on dairy products as important foods in the post-weaning period.

When the problem was first recognized, people wondered whether alternatives to milk should be offered in school-lunch programs serving groups where lactose intolerance was likely to be common. Another question raised was whether milk was an appropriate food to send to developing countries where lactose intolerance might also be widespread. A food as nutritious as milk could not be set aside lightly.

Over the years, a stream of research has helped put the problem into perspective. These studies have drawn an important distinction between lactose intolerance and milk intolerance and have identified other biological, cultural, and physiological factors which also explain differences in milk-drinking habits.

Lactose intolerance is diagnosed by giving an individual a large dose of milk sugar dissolved in water and then making a series of observations. Measuring the rise in blood sugar shows the degree to which the milk sugar has been digested. Smaller increases mean that less has been digested.

Lactose intolerance also produces gastrointestinal symptoms, including gas, bloating, and diarrhea. Levels of oxygen in exhaled air will be also higher, a sign that bacteria are fermenting the undigested sugar in the large intestine. By those measures, only the populations of Northern and Central Europe and some Middle Eastern groups, as well as individuals of European descent in North America, Australia, New Zealand, and elsewhere are likely to "pass" a lactose tolerance test.

But here's a key question: Given that the test for lactose intolerance uses doses of lactose that are much larger than the amount you would usually take in at one sitting, is it really relevant? How does it truly relate to our ability to consume milk and milk products without ill effect?

Recently, Dr. Nevin Scrimshaw of MIT reviewed the enormous body of evidence that had been amassed over nearly two decades. He concluded that milk consumption is influenced more by availability, social attitudes, nutrition education, feeding programs, and cultural factors than by the ability to digest lactose.

It is now clear that the majority of lactose maldigesters can consume the amount of lactose in a glass of milk without ill effect, especially if the milk is taken with meals. In double-blind investigations of symptoms associated with lesser amounts of milk, lactose has not been identified as the culprit in most cases. It is also well recognized that lactose is better tolerated in milk and milk products and when consumed with meals than when the same amount is given with water. And happily, the inability to digest lactose has no adverse effect on the absorption of the essential nutrients in the milk.

Observations from child-feeding programs the world over indicate that while it may take weeks or months in places where it is an unfamiliar food, a glass of milk eventually becomes well accepted even where lactose maldigestion is widespread. Continued intake of lactose in milk does not stimulate the production of the sugar-splitting enzyme; nevertheless, discomfort associated with milk consumption seems to lessen over time. Why this happens is still a mystery. One possibility is that individuals simply become more accustomed to the symptoms and experience less discomfort.

The ability to digest large amounts of milk sugar drops sharply in early childhood for many people across the globe. Many of those who associate milk with unpleasant symptoms may prefer to depend on cheese and yogurt as dairy foods. But the weight of the evidence suggests that few of them need write off "nature's most perfect food" entirely.

HYPOGLYCEMIA

In the hall of fame of medical myths, surely hypoglycemia holds an honored place. If we had a penny for every time the term has been bandied about inaccurately we could have retired long ago to bask in Tahiti.

Part of the problem lies in the signposts pointing toward hypoglycemia: fatigue, weakness, recurrent headaches, and extreme hunger that leads to binges of overeating. These symptoms are somewhat vague and certainly common, and people are always looking for labels to explain what they experience.

All too often, we've heard of individuals diagnosing themselves as having hypoglycemia—or low blood sugar—with barely a rudimentary understanding of what that means. In reality, the condition is both rare and difficult to diagnose.

Idiopathic hypoglycemia is the presence of very low blood sugar without any demonstrable organic disease. Sometimes hypoglycemia indicates a serious medical condition: congenital enzyme deficiencies; involvement of the liver, the adrenal glands, or pituitary gland; or problems of the central nervous system or the pancreas. Cancer of the pancreas, which leads to the overproduction of insulin, is the single most dangerous cause of hypoglycemia. In infants, acute hypoglycemia may signal that the baby is unable to gain access to energy reserves of glycogen (animal starch) stored in the liver. Very occasionally, hypoglycemia results from an overactive pancreas rather than from disease.

What happens during a hypoglycemia attack? Following a meal high in simple sugars, the pancreas reacts by flooding the body with insulin. Sending a surge of glucose into the body cells, the insulin causes blood-sugar levels to drop dramatically. The effect resembles that which occurs when diabetics get too much insulin, and the symptoms are also similar: weakness, trembling, and extreme hunger. In severe cases, there may be hysterical symptoms, convulsions, and ultimately, coma.

Now, let's say you feel tired and weak much of the time, you have frequent headaches, and that you deal with unexplained pangs of hunger by binging on sugary foods. The last thing you should do is to assume that you have hypoglycemia. Diagnosis of the condition is no do-it-yourself proposition. In fact, it requires a special five-hour test. The patient drinks a concentrated glucose solution, after which the rise and fall of blood sugar is carefully monitored at regular intervals. Normally, it takes about three hours for blood glucose to drop back to fasting levels. If diabetes is present, it will take longer. By contrast, where hypoglycemia exists, it could take as little as half an hour. The surge of insulin removes blood sugar very rapidly. Low blood sugar coupled with the simultaneous onset of symptoms is the sign of hypoglycemia.

Supposing you were found to have the condition, the next step would be treatment. The goal there would be to supply the body with glucose—which we need for fuel—without overstimulating the pancreas and sending us on an insulin-induced roller-coaster ride as our blood sugar levels alternately soar and plummet.

The classic diet once suggested for treatment was low in carbohydrate, with little or no readily absorbable sugar, and heavy reliance on protein and fat. Candy, jellies and jams, and sugary drinks and desserts were all ruled out. Meat, fish, poultry, or cheese appeared at every meal, and vegetable oil was used in salad dressing. In severe cases the daily intake was spread out over eight small meals. To be prepared for a sudden attack, the patient was advised to carry crackers and cheese at all times.

The recommended regimen has been updated today to include more complex carbohydrates such as whole grains which are rich in fiber and which the body uses slowly enough to avoid provoking undesirable symptoms. This diet allows for less emphasis on fat and less likelihood of producing elevated serum cholesterol.

Even though it can be treated, nobody would willingly choose to suffer from hypoglycemia. The question then becomes, Why are so many people so quick to assume that they have it? That is a matter for conjecture. If you are experiencing the symptoms—weakness and fatigue, headaches, hunger pangs, and binging on sugary foods—you may indeed have a problem. Chances are, however, that it is something other than hypoglycemia. Only a thorough examination, and your physician, can tell for sure.

YOUR BLOOD PRESSURE AND YOUR DIET

One out of every four Americans—between 50 and 60 million people—has hypertension, or high blood pressure. Among those 74 and older, the figure soars to as many as half. Those who do not have regular medical checkups, including a blood pressure measurement, can live with undetected hypertension for years. While there may be no symptoms to provoke a trip to the doctor, undiagnosed and untreated hypertension raises the risk of both heart disease and stroke. That is especially sad since enormous strides have been made over the past two decades in treating the condition.

But any discussion of the treatment of hypertension, once diagnosed, and of the role of diet in that treatment, is really putting the cart before the horse. The primary focus should, after all, be on prevention. That begins with weight control. While there are lean hypertensives, the condition is believed to be twice as common among obese adults (those who are 20% or more above their ideal weight), than among those who are not. Indeed, evidence from large studies indicates that in populations where weight does not rise with age, neither does blood pressure.

A second step toward prevention focuses on the role of salt, and more specifically, of sodium. Here the picture is somewhat more complicated. The National Academy of Sciences' Committee on Diet and Health, in its recently released and much publicized *Executive Summary of Diet and Health: Implications for Reducing Chronic Disease Risk,* advances a convincing case for reducing salt intake. As they point out, blood pressure levels are strongly and positively linked to habitual salt intake. In populations where salt intake is 6 grams or more a day, blood pressure rises with age and hypertension is frequent; where usual consumption is less than 4.5 grams, the age-related rise is slight or absent, and there is little hypertension. The problem is that while studies indicate that some people are more sensitive than others, and that sensitivity is determined by genetics, we simply have no way of detecting the salt sensitive among us. The Committee's recommendation to Americans is to limit salt to 6 grams a day by using less in cooking, eliminating the salt shaker from the table, and using salty foods sparingly. In making that recommendation, they pointed out that although a greater reduction would probably be preferable for those who are salt sensitive, they chose the higher level as a first goal that could be more readily achieved.

Risk of high blood pressure also rises with increased alcohol consumption. Reducing risk is just one more reason to limit alcohol intake to very moderate amounts.

Evidence for links between other dietary factors and hypertension is less clear. However, data from both population studies and animal experiments provide evidence of an inverse relationship between stroke-related deaths and potassium intake. Indeed, a diet low in sodium and high in potassium, found in abundant amounts in fruits and vegetables, is associated with the lowest frequency of strokes.

An inverse relationship between calcium intake and blood pressure has also been reported, and perhaps given more publicity that it deserves, at least on the basis of evidence now available. Observations come both from population studies and from studies of individuals who consumed calcium supplements. But findings are inconsistent and do not suggest a role for anything more than the Recommended Dietary Allowance of 800 milligrams a day.

So much for what we know about preventing hypertension. For those who already have it, the dietary message is not radically different. Happily, the past two decades have witnessed the arrival of a small army of drugs that doctors can use to help patients keep their blood pressure under control. Yet a role for diet remains. The first step, for those who are overweight, is to reduce. That single measure can lead to a dramatic drop in blood pressure. And even among those who do not succeed in achieving their ideal weight, smaller losses bring significant improvement.

A second step, to which some, though not all, hypertensives respond, is a reduction in salt intake. And while we often refer to it as "salt," sodium is really the target. In some individuals, a combination of moderate sodium restriction, similar to that recommended for prevention, and antihypertensive therapy may permit blood pressure control with fewer medications and fewer side effects. Your goal should be around 2,400 milligrams of sodium per day. Some sources of excess are obvious, but others are less apparent. So, at least at the outset, a regular check of nutrition labels may help identify some of the hidden sodium in your diet. And to make absolutely sure of how you are doing, an audit of your diet and an analysis of its sodium content for two or three days is a very worthwhile exercise.

Finally, use alcohol in very moderate amounts. It is premature to suggest modification of nutrients such as potassium, calcium, and even fiber and fat on the basis of their potential effects on blood pressure. Nonetheless, there is no lack of reasons to eat plenty of fiber-rich fruits and vegetables and low-fat dairy products, to cut back on fat, and to place greater emphasis on unsaturated fats. Preventing and controlling hypertension through diet are just part of the overall message for sensible eating.

Questions and Answers

Q. For several years I have been taking the type of diuretics which require that I make sure I get adequate amounts of potassium in my diet. I was originally advised to take a large glass of orange juice and eat a banana once a day. My enthusiasm for bananas has waned. Where else might I look for potassium?

A. Orange juice and bananas are both excellent sources of potassium, and both are low in sodium. But they are hardly unique in that regard.

Let's begin with some basic figures. Both a cup of orange juice and a medium banana contain over 400 milligrams of potassium, but so does a cup of grapefruit juice, a cup of cantaloupe, honeydew, or canned apricots, and a medium baked or boiled potato. Vegetables providing between 200 and 400 milligrams include half-cup servings (and remember that is considerably less than many people ordinarily eat) of broccoli, brussels sprouts, collards, winter squash, or yellow turnips. A medium tomato and ¼ cup of wheat germ also fall in this range. So, too, do a small orange, a medium peach or pear, and a cup of pineapple chunks. A number of other fruits and vegetables provide lesser amounts, but they all contribute to increasing your potassium intake.

Finally, red kidney beans, an often neglected source, contain over 600 milligrams of potassium per cup. The "rub" is that the canned varieties usually have salt added. So if you are watching your salt intake, cook the dried variety. A good bowl of chili made with a small amount of lean ground meat, onions, and either fresh tomatoes or tomatoes canned without salt, and seasoned with lots of chili pepper, is a wonderful antidote to the perennial complaint against the blandness of the salt-free diet—and it's rich in potassium and a number of nutrients as well.

Q. I have tried to use sodium labeling information to reduce the sodium content of my diet. But I don't know where I'm at with respect to my current intake. I could be a lot more effective in cutting down if I knew how much sodium I was getting in my diet. How do I find out?

A. Determining usual sodium intake takes a little time, but it is worth the effort. First, keep a careful record of everything you eat for at least three days. Write down both the type and the amount of each food. Save labels from processed foods which have information about sodium content. Next, you will need to calculate the amount of salt you're getting if you use it in cooking. Just measure the salt you add, and divide by the number of servings in the recipe to estimate your salt intake from that source. (There will be a slight overestimate from that which gets discarded in cooking water, but it will not affect your results significantly.) Finally, to estimate salt added at the table, put a measured amount into a shaker which you use exclusively over your record-keeping period. At the end of that time, measure what's left, and you will know how much you used.

Now you're ready to calculate your intake. Using sodium labeling information whenever possible, record the sodium content for each food for which product-specific information is available. Remember to make adjustments where the amount you ate and the specific portion listed on the label vary. At this point there will be a number of gaps in your information.

For each teaspoon of salt you added in cooking or at the table, add 2,130 milligrams of sodium. Add your figures, divide by the number of days for which you kept records, and you will have your usual sodium intake. This exercise will not only tell you your usual intake, it will help you learn more about the sodium content of the basic foods in your diet, and provide you with a framework for cutting back to achieve your targeted intake.

Many large supermarket chains now publish booklets which provide information about the sodium content of large numbers of the foods they carry. These are available free, or at very low cost, and they may be all you need to fill those gaps. If you still need further information, you can purchase one of the many guides to sodium content available in paperback at your local bookstore.

Q. Is too much licorice harmful to people with high blood pressure?

A. If you eat quite a bit of licorice and take diuretics which get rid of potassium as well as sodium, it is a good idea to select licorice candy in which anise oil is used for flavoring. Excesses of most things are potentially hazardous, at least to some individuals, and so it is with licorice. Licorice contains a compound called glycyrrhizin which can act like corticosteroids, causing the body to retain sodium, get rid of potassium, and elevate blood pressure. In case reports in the medical literature citing problems, licorice consumption was as much as 2 or 3 ounces of candy a day over a period of several years, or two packages of licorice gum daily for several months. Since nearly all licorice imported into this country is used to produce tobacco, individuals who chew tobacco and swallow their saliva could also be affected adversely.

Q. Our supermarket now sells a variety of salt-free seasonings in which the main ingredient is potassium chloride. Before I buy them, I would like to know what potassium chloride is and whether it is safe?

A. Potassium chloride is chemically quite similar to table salt, the difference being that potassium takes the place of sodium in the molecule. Most people can use salt substitutes, if they like the taste, as an alternative to regular table salt, but some individuals cannot tolerate increased potassium. Therefore, it makes good sense to check with your doctor before you buy them. Beyond that, potassium chloride doesn't taste much like regular salt. It has a flavor all its own, one that people must develop a taste for. Alternatively, many individuals prefer to use herbs and spices more extensively. Garlic, mustard, ginger, cinnamon, nutmeg, oregano, basil, thyme, chives, dill, pepper, and many others are naturally low in sodium and can be used in any amounts. Because salt is a flavor enhancer, in many cases when you eliminate it, you will probably want to use larger amounts of other seasonings than the recipe calls for to achieve the desired effect. Seasoned salts, such as garlic salt and onion salt, contain regular table salt. So if you are trying to reduce your salt intake, avoid them.

NUTRITION AND STRESS

Stress was not invented in the eighties, but perhaps no decade held out more "solutions" to the millions of Americans who feel they suffer from increased pressure at home or work. Given the rising interest in nutrition, it is no surprise that the pharmaceutical and health-food industries have responded with "stress formula" vitamin preparations designed, they say, to help the body cope with the heavy physiological demands of today's fast-paced world.

Usually included in this stress formula are vitamin C, the full complement of B vitamins (thiamin, riboflavin, niacin, B_6, B_{12}, biotin, folic acid, and panthothenic acid), and one or more of a number of food factors such as choline, carnitine, and inositol. All are involved in the formation of neurotransmitters, the chemical messengers that help carry out directives from the brain, and/or in the metabolism or utilization of protein, fat, or carbohydrate—the fundamental processes that keep us going.

Such functions are cited in the advertising literature accompanying the preparations to explain why these nutrients are used in the "stress-specific" formulations. The advertising suggests that the need for these nutrients increases as life becomes more hectic.

But are such supplements worthwhile? Can they help us "convert food energy" and improve our stamina and intellectual capacity under stress? Let's examine the evidence.

The broader definition of stress goes well beyond psychological tension and anxiety and encompasses any event that disrupts normal body functioning. It includes serious injury or illness, such as a severe burn or pneumonia, major operations such as open-heart surgery, pregnancy, and hard physical labor. These physiological forms of stress are the ones that have been most extensively studied with respect to nutritional requirements. In many cases, increased nutrient intake, either in the form of food or supplements, is necessary to enable the body to adapt to the greater strain.

It is not clear whether the same treatment helps with psychological forms of stress. Much of the research in this area, primarily using experimental animals, has focused on the effects of nutritional deficiencies on the response to stress, not on whether supplemental vitamins improve the ability to function in a stressful environment.

For the average American adult, dietary intake of the water-soluble vitamins most commonly found in "stress" preparations is usually adequate. Clinical deficiencies are seen rarely. Yet promoters of supplements often prominently display lists of deficiency symptoms associated with the vitamins. Among them are fatigue and mood changes, such as depression, apathy, and irritability. The implication is that anyone who experiences these common feelings is not meeting his or her nutritional needs and thus needs supplements.

The few clinical studies (most of which were done in the 1940s and 1950s) turned up little evidence in support of benefits of supplemental vitamins on performance under stress. Additional B-complex vitamins had no impact on mental well-being, resistance to fatigue, or recovery from exertion. Nicotinic acid (niacin) was able to prevent an increase in urinary excretion of fat metabolites normally seen during emotional stress, but there was no effect on the excretion of so-called "fight-flight" hormones, epinephrine and norepinephrine, or the associated increase in heart rate or blood pressure.

Although the tissue levels of vitamin C are known to decrease during periods of psychological stress, a double-blind study of medical-school students uncovered no differences in mental and physical well-being between those given the vitamin and those taking a placebo.

It thus appears that taking supplemental vitamins to help you function better in stressful situations is unlikely to do much good. Can it hurt? Most of the preparations that we found on the shelves contained levels of the vitamins at or slightly above the Recommended Dietary Allowances (RDA). A few formulations provided megadoses, amounts ten times or more above the RDA. In one case, the daily regimen suggested on the label contained 125 times the RDA for B_6 for an adult woman, and a thousand times the RDA for thiamin.

In general, because these vitamins are water-soluble, any excesses are excreted in the urine. But prolonged use of high doses may have toxic effects. Neurological impairment following long-term intake of gram amounts of B_6 has recently been reported in the medical literature. Supplemental niacin can cause severe flushing and gastrointestinal problems, and liver damage can occur at excessive levels of intake.

Emotional stress may lead to loss of appetite, and a subsequent decline in the nutritional adequacy of the diet. People who respond to stress by eating less may wish to take a daily supplement. In that case, a multivitamin supplement that covers a range of nutrients at reasonable levels, and not a special stress formula, is the one to choose.

THOSE ELUSIVE FOOD ALLERGIES

If there's one thing the science of nutrition doesn't lack, it's controversy. One of the most controversial subjects is food allergies—how often they occur, the symptoms and diagnostic methods, and the accepted treatment. There is even controversy over whether the word "allergy" is appropriate in describing the problem.

Adverse reaction to food can occur for several reasons. It may result from an enzyme deficiency, as in the case of lactose intolerance. It may also be due to a physiological or a chemical reaction. Tyramine, a substance found in many foods and a potent dilator of blood vessels, can cause such a reaction. Finally, adverse reaction may result from an immunologic source. Only this last type can technically be called a food allergy. "Food intolerance" is probably a more apt term to use when discussing the overall problem.

Reactions to food can range from mild symptoms, such as a bit of nausea, to something as severe as anaphylactic shock, a life-threatening response. They can come within the first few minutes of eating, or they may take a few hours to develop. Reactions can also occur close to where the offending food is (the mouth or gastrointestinal tract) or at a more remote location (skin eruptions or a stepped-up heart rate).

The only truly scientific and unbiased way to determine if a food allergy exists requires a double-blind, placebo-controlled oral test in which patients swallow capsules containing either extracts of the suspected food or a sugar solution. All this is coded, and neither physician nor patient knows what he or she is getting.

Unfortunately, this test is difficult to perform, both because the patient must fast for several days before each test and because only a few food challenges can be made in one day. Since few studies have been done using this technique, most reports are based on what people think is happening to them and are, therefore, open to question. No wonder there is disagreement, not only about the range of symptoms that can be traced directly to a particular food, but also about the frequency with which it happens.

Most physicians agree that food intolerances are more of a problem in children than in anyone else. The most common is intolerance to cow's milk, estimated to occur in 7% to 12% of all children. Other common food allergies include eggs, nuts, and soy. That is why nursing mothers with a family history of allergies are advised to avoid excessive intake of those foods. Fortunately, most children outgrow their food intolerances. For that reason, parents should be encouraged to have their children tested from time to time. However, the longer a food allergy persists, the less likely it is to disappear.

When it comes to reactions in adults, some doctors suspect that many self-diagnosed food "allergies" are psychological. A recent study found that only 4 out of 23 patients thought to be hypersensitive to foods actually had intolerances when given a controlled food-challenge test.

One symptom associated with food intolerance in both children and adults that has received renewed attention in the medical literature is migraine headache. Some experts estimate that as many as one-fourth of all migraines are diet induced. This has led to a laundry list of foods claimed to be associated with these often-debilitating headaches. They include citrus fruits, grapes, pineapple, coconut, tea, coffee, cola, wine, chocolate, milk and cheese, pork, beef, corn, cane sugar, legumes, and yeast. In fact, one study of children uncovered 55 different foods that provoked headache symptoms.

Just what causes dietary migraines is still unclear. One theory is that a host of foods contain substances called amines, which can trigger the release of neurotransmitters and dilate blood vessels. Migraine sufferers may have problems metabolizing amines.

Treatment of dietary migraines and other food intolerances continues to be controversial. Some doctors claim to be able to desensitize patients by injecting small amounts of food extracts. But most physicians believe elimination from the diet of the offending food or foods is the only effective treatment. Unfortunately, for some this can mean a fairly restricted diet.

Questions and Answers

Q. Some wine labels say that they contain sulfites. Could you please tell me why they are now being added to wine if it is known that they cause allergic reactions in some people?

A. There is nothing new about using sulfites in wine making. In fact, as far back as 1933 the Food and Drug Administration set an allowable limit for sulfites of 350 parts per million. What is new is the regulation requiring that consumers be informed of their presence.

Sulfur dioxide, the compound most often used, is employed in several steps in the process. It is sprayed on newly picked grapes and added to newly pressed grape juice to prevent spoilage during transport to the winery. It is used to clean the wine barrels and kill undesirable bacteria, and it is added to the finished wine to improve its flavor and help in the aging process.

The new regulation, aimed at alerting individuals who are sulfite sensitive, applies only to recent vintages. All older wines contain sulfites, even though the label may not say so. While even small amounts of sulfite can be extremely dangerous to those who are sulfite sensitive, a problem more common among asthmatics, not all unpleasant reactions to wine are the result of sulfite sensitivity.

Q. Could you please provide me with an update on regulations regarding the use of sulfites in food?

A. The practice of adding sulfites to raw produce, except potatoes, was prohibited in 1986 to protect sulfite-sensitive individuals at risk of life threatening responses to the additive. It could continue to be used in a number of processed foods. However, as of January 1987, manufacturers had to declare it on the label of packaged items that contained at least 10 parts per million, the smallest amount that could be detected at the time the ruling was made. So ingredients lists for a wide range of products, including dried fruits, juices, canned and dehydrated vegetables, gelatin, dry soup mixes, baked goods, teas, processed seafoods, condiments and relishes, and jams and jellies, all may contain sulfur dioxide, sodium sulfite, sodium bisulfite, sodium metabisulfite, potassium bisulfite, or potassium metabisulfite. A regulation which became effective in January 1988 requires that the labels on beer and wines be labeled "contains sulfites." However, since this regulation is quite recent, beer cans that have been around a couple of years might not have that information, even if sulfites were used in preparing it.

It is estimated that there are no more than 100,000 sulfite-sensitive individuals in this country. Nonetheless, those who are should keep in mind the several situations where sulfites are not clearly identified. Dried fruit, purchased in bulk, and fresh shrimp may contain sulfites. So, too, may foods made with precut and processed potato products. Unless potato dishes are known to have been made from raw, fresh potatoes, the safest course for the sulfite sensitive is to avoid them.

Q. My husband's doctor prescribed a type of drug he called an MAO inhibitor. At the same time he gave him a list of foods to avoid. What is the link between the food and the drug?

A. MAO inhibitors are used most commonly to treat depression and some anxiety disorders, although they have other uses, too. Their effectiveness is thought to lie in blocking the action of enzymes which would otherwise inactivate neurotransmitters in the brain. Unfortunately, tyramine and other so-called "pressor amines" found in varying amounts in certain foods are no longer inactivated either. These compounds can have powerful effects on blood pressure. Toxic levels can cause very serious hypertensive symptoms including severe headache and irregular heartbeat. In the extreme, fatal brain hemorrhage can occur.

Recommendations for foods to avoid are inconsistent for several reasons. One problem is inadequate documentation of reactions. In addition, tyramine content of an individual food can vary considerably depending on processing, incidental contamination, fermentation, ripening, or degradation. For example, in two samples of Gruyère cheese, one taken at the rind had 700 micrograms more tyramine per gram than the other taken just over an inch into the interior.

In an article published a couple of years ago, Beverly J. McCabe, Ph.D., R.D., of the University of Arkansas, provided a rational approach to avoiding tyramine reactions, based on both reviews of case reports and data from food composition tables. Of the case reports published in the literature, 80% involved cheese. So cheese (except cottage and cream cheese) head the list of foods to be avoided. Also on that list are smoked and pickled fish, cured meats, meat extracts, liver, Chianti and vermouth wines, beer and ale, sauerkraut, broad beans, yeast extracts and Brewer's yeast, and banana peels (Banana peels are an unlikely food, although a single case report involved consumption of a whole stewed green banana, including the peel. It is in the peel where tyramine and another amine called dopamine are concentrated.)

Foods to be used with caution, that is, in servings no bigger than a half-cup, or 4 ounces, include avocado, raspberries, soy sauce, chocolate, red and white wines, port wine, distilled spirits, peanuts, yogurt, and cream from unpasteurized milk.

Any foods can potentially develop moderate to high tyramine content if handled poorly or kept for prolonged periods. Since reports of single cases often involve spoilage, it is a good idea to emphasize the use of fresh foods. Resynthesis of monoamine oxidase occurs slowly, and individuals are vulnerable to reactions as long as three weeks after the drug is stopped. Consequently, the diet should be continued for four weeks beyond the time the drug is discontinued.

Q. A friend who relies heavily on health foods claims that certain foods such as flour-based cakes and cookies have a greater tendency to form mucus in the body. The excess mucus provides a fertile environment for some diseases, and therefore, a mucusless diet can have a marvelously therapeutic effect. Is there any truth to that theory?

A. The idea that certain foods produce "mucus," and that mucus is a breeding ground for disease is no more true today than it was when it was first put forth more than 60 years ago.

The originator of the Mucusless Diet Healing System was a man named Arnold Ehret. He believed he cured himself of diabetes on a diet based largely on fruit. To synthesize his theory, he drew on a most diverse collection of resources, among them the writings of Socrates, the Book of Genesis, unidentified Egyptian philosophers, and the late nineteenth-century food faddist, Horace Fletcher.

As a first step in the regimen, Ehret prescribed a three-day fast. Dizziness or headaches, certainly not unlikely symptoms after three days without food, indicated clogging with mucus and toxemias. According to Ehret, that suggested it was time for the mucusless diet. If that failed to alleviate the symptoms, Ehret prescribed a purgative concoction containing buckthorn bark, ground psyllium seed husks, and ground dark fennel seeds.

There is no more reason to believe that the mucusless diet has any basis in fact than there was in the 1920s when it first appeared.

DIETARY RECOMMENDATIONS FOR CANCER AND AIDS PATIENTS

 Making false promises to cancer patients is cruel. Diet provides no miraculous escape from cancer. Yet by bolstering the body's stamina, an adequate supply of nutrients and calories helps fight the good fight against the disease. A well-nourished patient responds better to chemotherapy, recovers more quickly from surgery, and, in general, is better able to withstand the side effects of treatment. Good nutrition also helps the patient maintain his or her strength and ability to resist infection.

Not only is diet an important aspect of therapy for cancer patients, it differs from other forms of treatment because it is under the control of the individual. Unfortunately, complications both of the disease and of the treatment often make it difficult to maintain good eating habits. Over the years, dietitians who work with cancer patients have found that several simple measures can help alleviate the more common problems associated with eating.

It should be noted that many of the problems which affect the eating habits of cancer patients are the same as those associated with AIDS patients (and AIDS treatment). Therefore, the following dietary recommendations can be applied to the diets of people suffering from AIDS as well. Here are some suggestions for coping with the most common problems related to diet.

Individuals frequently suffer from nausea and vomiting as a result of radiation treatments and chemotherapy. If your doctor prescribes antinausea medicine, take it ½ to 1 hour before eating. If you feel nauseous, don't overeat; small, frequent meals are the best way to ensure an adequate intake. Rest after meals but do not lie down for at least two hours after eating. Clear, cool beverages such as ginger ale and cold broths are recommended. Popsicles, gelatin desserts, low-fat foods, and dry or salted foods (pretzels, crackers, dry cereal) are all good choices. Avoid spicy, overly sweet, high-fat, and fried or greasy foods.

Radiation and drug therapies can also cause diarrhea or constipation. In the event of diarrhea, it is important to drink plenty of liquids to prevent dehydration. It is best to drink between, rather than with, meals. Diluted orange juice, fruit nectars and bananas will help replenish lost potassium. Limit intake of milk and dairy products, and avoid caffeine and greasy and high-fat foods. Reduce your fiber intake by eating white rice, white bread, and cooked fruits and vegetables, rather than high-fiber foods. If the diarrhea persists or has blood in it, contact your doctor.

If you are constipated, try adding more fiber to your diet by eating raw fruits and vegetables, whole grains, nuts, beans, and bran. These can be grated or chopped in a blender if you have difficulty chewing or swallowing. Increase fluid intake, especially of fruit juices. Physical activity (walking or other light exercise) sometimes helps.

Mouth sores and pain are another complication which can interfere with eating. These are most often due to surgery, radiation, or chemotherapy. Patients who have recently undergone surgery in the head or neck area will also experience difficulty swallowing.

For mouth pain, limit spices and salt, and avoid acidic foods such as oranges and grapefruits. Dry foods like toast or crackers can make the soreness worse; they should be dipped in tea or coffee before eating. Nonabrasive, moist foods such as puddings, eggs, noodles, cottage cheese, canned fruits, and ice cream are best. Extremes in temperature may be irritating, so it's better to eat food at moderate temperatures. Smoking can also irritate your mouth and throat.

If you have difficulty swallowing, choose soft, single-textured foods such as mashed potatoes, oatmeal, eggs, and yogurt. Add sauces or gravies to meats and vegetables to make them softer. Drink liquids with a straw. Tilting your head back or moving it forward may make it easier to swallow. If your mouth is dry, try sucking on candy or ice cubes.

Some people experience taste changes as a result of treatments they are receiving. Generally, bitter foods taste stronger, sweet foods less so, and meat no longer tastes good. If you are not suffering from mouth pain, try experimenting with spices and herbs to enhance flavors. Meats can be marinated in sweet fruit juices or Italian dressing. Adding bacon bits, ham strips, onions, and garlic will improve the palatability of some foods.

Anorexia is another factor which can jeopardize nutrient intake. The disease, treatments, emotional stress, anxiety, fear, and fatigue all seem to contribute to a lack of appetite and subsequent weight loss. One way to cope with this is to try to create a relaxing and inviting atmosphere at mealtime. If possible, eat with a friend, and choose your favorite foods. Smaller meals eaten more often during the day, frequent snacks, and an instant breakfast shake or milk shake between meals are a few ways to increase caloric intake. If tolerated, fat-rich foods such as butter, mayonnaise, sour cream, and cream cheese can add considerable calories. Most importantly, eat well when you are feeling good to make up for the times when you aren't.

Despite the claims of charlatans, there is no food regimen that will cure cancer or AIDS. But maintaining a nutritionally balanced and calorically adequate diet is crucial to maximizing the value of treatments for these diseases. If you still are not able to maintain an adequate diet after trying these suggestions, consult with your physician or dietitian. He or she may recommend other forms of nutritional support.

Questions and Answers

Q. What is the difference between enteral and parenteral feeding for cancer patients and when are they used?

A. The cancer patient must contend with a variety of complications which result either from the cancer itself or from the medications and treatments being received. Diarrhea, nausea, vomiting, mouth sores, and taste changes are only some of the symptoms which make getting enough nutrients a struggle.

If the patient is having difficulty meeting his or her nutrient needs with a regular diet, other forms of nutritional support may be necessary. Enteral nutrition is a form of support in which nutrients are received directly into the digestive tract. Various nutritionally balanced formulas (for example, Sustacal and Resource Plus) can be used to supplement the regular diet. In some cases, these may even be used as the sole source of nutrition. When oral intake of food is not possible, but the digestive tract is still functioning, enteral tube feeding is a viable alternative.

In nasogastric feeding, nutrients are delivered through a tube placed in the nose. Patients can be taught to place their own nasogastric tube so that feeding may be done in the home. Tube feeding is most often used if the patient is unable to swallow, if there is upper GI tract obstruction, malabsorption, or severe diarrhea or vomiting. If necessary, the tube may also be placed so that the nutrients enter directly into the stomach or small intestine. Special enteral formulas, which require little or no enzymatic activity for absorption, are available for people with malabsorption problems.

Parenteral nutrition is a form of nutrition support in which nutrients are given intravenously. Because of its invasive nature, there is a higher risk of infection. It must be administered by a professional. This type of nutrition therapy is appropriate for patients who are unable to eat and whose gastrointestinal tract is not functioning, eliminating the use of enteral nutrition.

Q. Is there any special diet that can cure AIDS?

A. Unfortunately not. Good nutrition does have an important role in the management of AIDS, but it is not the panacea that some people would like it to be. A well-nourished patient will respond better to treatment and is better able to fight infection, but there is no diet that will cure the disease.

AIDS patients are particularly vulnerable to malnutrition. While nutrient needs may increase, the actual supply of nutrients to the body may decline. Decreased appetite, pain in the mouth and esophagus, diarrhea, nausea, vomiting, and malabsorption are some of the many problems which make it difficult for people suffering from AIDS to get enough nutrients.

To make matters worse, many people have turned to alternative diets (macrobiotic, *Fit for Life,* etc.), herbal remedies, and megavitamin therapies in an attempt to combat the disease. There is no scientific evidence which indicates that any of these so-called remedies are effective in controlling AIDS. At best, they are just a waste of money, but in some cases they may even be detrimental. Fad diets frequently do not provide adequate amounts of nutrients and several vitamins can be toxic if taken in large quantities (ten times the RDA).

Because malnutrition can further weaken the immune system and worsen the effects of opportunistic infections, a well-balanced diet is crucial for the well-being of the patient. There is no clear-cut approach, but eating a variety of fresh fruits and vegetables, whole grains, milk products, and meats is the best way to ensure that you are getting enough nutrients.

For information on how to best meet your nutritional needs and ways to relieve the symptoms that may interfere with eating, write to:

The Task Force at Wang Associates, Inc.
19 West 21st Street
New York, NY 10010

Questions and Answers

Q. What is the current thinking about the value of vitamin C in treating cancer patients?

A. It may be helpful to begin with a historical perspective. In the early 1970s, Dr. E. Cameron of Scotland, joined by Dr. Linus Pauling, reported that large doses of vitamin C had a remarkably positive effect on the survival of cancer victims. In their study, they did not use a treatment group and a nontreatment group. Instead, as a comparison, they used case records available at the hospital. There were questions about whether this research method provided an accurate picture.

Several years later, a group of investigators at the Mayo Clinic, using a controlled double-blind study design, found that ascorbic acid had no advantage over a placebo either in improving symptoms or in lengthening survival time in a group of patients with advanced cancer of a variety of types.

Pauling criticized the study on the grounds that most of the patients had received chemotherapy before they were given the vitamin C. That, he claimed, might inhibit the ability of the vitamin to stimulate natural body defenses.

To put that question to rest, researchers at the Mayo Clinic conducted another double-blind study. This time they chose only patients with colorectal cancer which had spread, and none of their cases had a history of having chemotherapy.

The researchers specifically chose this type of cancer for two reasons. It was the most frequent cancer reported in the study by Cameron and Pauling, and one for which they claimed a striking improvement in survival. In addition, the researchers felt ethically secure since no available chemotherapy had been shown to give symptomatic relief or to prolong life. This disease of the large bowel is, in fact, extremely resistant to both drugs and radiation.

Again their results showed convincingly that large oral doses of vitamin C had no effect on survival or on control of symptoms. How can one explain the positive results of the earlier trials? It is quite likely that the two groups—those who received the ascorbic acid and those who were chosen out of the files as comparable cases—differed in important ways which biased the outcome.

Q. Is there any evidence that macrobiotic diets are effective in treating cancer?

A. No. Although macrobiotic literature contains reports of miraculous cures by the diet, there simply have been no reports in medical journals describing the course of cancer patients following these diets, nor have there been any controlled studies in suitable animal cancer models.

In the macrobiotic theory of disease, "a cancer is seen as an attempt on the part of the organism to create a balance. If the cancer is removed, this overall balance will be disrupted and collapse." Accordingly, to maintain harmony this "natural" phenomenon should not be disrupted either by removing or destroying it. Thus, macrobiotics advocate diet as the main therapy for cancer.

This is downright disastrous. While proper nutritional management is an essential adjunct in treating cancer patients, it is never the main therapy. In a review of macrobiotics in cancer treatment and prevention several years ago, the Clinical Nutrition Research Center of the Section of Gastroenterology and Nutrition Services at the University of Chicago pointed out that diet is not an alternative to conventional therapy. Beyond that, the report states that there are certain elements, inherent in the macrobiotic diet, that make it particularly undesirable for the malnourished cancer patient who needs sufficient calories, protein of high biological value and adequate amounts of vitamins and minerals.

For example, the macrobiotic diet recommends that 50% of each meal consist of whole grains—foods relatively low in calories. Even healthy young adults who go on these diets often lose weight. And because cancer patients with weight loss have a poorer prognosis, concern about the caloric adequacy of these diets is clearly justified. Moreover, cereals contain complex carbohydrates and may be high in fiber, making them less easily digested and absorbed. A diet high in fiber can also impair mineral absorption. And, in patients with bowel obstruction, a heavy influx of fiber might cause additional problems. As for protein, although adequate combinations of amino acids can be obtained with a wide variety of grains and vegetables, cancer patients characteristically have lower food intakes, making this goal harder to achieve. So, especially for those who are losing weight, protein intake may be insufficient. Finally, people who have difficulty swallowing or inflamed mucus membranes may prefer soft or liquid diets. Yet this would conflict with the fluid restriction, a traditional, if ill-advised part of the macrobiotic regimen.

Nutritional support may prevent further weight loss or even promote weight gain in a severely malnourished patient. But it's clear that dietary interventions should be conducted only under medical supervision and within the context of the total treatment plan.

Q. Is there any truth to the notion that certain vegetables like broccoli have the ability to protect against cancer?

A. Evidence suggests that there is. The cruciferous vegetables, such as broccoli, cauliflower, cabbage, and kale, contain naturally occurring compounds called indoles, found to inhibit the formation of cancer-causing chemicals or to reduce cancer susceptibility in experimentation. While the implications of these findings for people are not completely clear, there is every reason to include these vegetables in your diet in generous amounts. They are good sources of a number of vitamins and minerals, and they are rich in fiber. Also, if not smothered with butter or margarine or hidden in a rich sauce, they are delightfully low in calories.

Q. What is the relationship between alcohol consumption and cancer?

A. Alcohol has been linked to an increased risk of certain types of cancer for over 60 years. It has generally been associated with cancers of the upper respiratory and GI tracts. Moreover, a synergistic effect between alcohol and smoking has been demonstrated. But while the connection between alcohol and cancer was first identified some time ago, the mechanism by which alcohol consumption leads to cancer remains unclear.

Pure alcohol does not cause cancer in laboratory animals, which implies that it is not a carcinogen. However, humans do not consume pure alcohol. They drink beverages which are complex fermentation products. And some alcoholic beverages have been shown to contain substances which do cause cancer in laboratory animals. So alcoholic beverages may act as a source of carcinogenic contaminants. Alternatively, it has been suggested that alcohol may act as a promoter or solvent to facilitate the transport of carcinogens across cell membranes. And there are still other theories about how it might work.

One factor that seems to play a role in the development of cancer is nutritional status. Malnutrition can be a particular problem in alcoholics who consume as much as 25% to 50% of their calories from alcohol.

The real point is that while we don't know exactly how alcohol relates to the development of cancer, there are certainly sufficient data available to suggest that moderation is the wisest course.

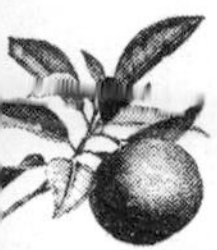

QUESTIONS FROM THE KITCHEN

Breads, Cereals, and Grains

Q. Does salt have a function in making yeast bread, other than in contributing to flavor?

A. Yes. Salt has an effect on both carbohydrate and protein-splitting enzymes and thereby has a significant effect on the texture of the finished loaf. In order to grow and produce carbon dioxide, yeasts need a steady supply of fuel. Initially, that comes from the small amount of sucrose used in making bread, which yeasts are able to break down to glucose and fructose. Once that is used up, they must depend on the flour for their food. Enzymes in the flour are able to split the starch into the disaccharide, maltose, which the yeast can then break down further. A little salt in yeast dough promotes the action of the starch-splitting enzymes in the flour and thus helps maintain a steady supply of maltose to the yeast. Salt also acts to inhibit the action of protein-splitting enzymes in flour which would otherwise weaken the protein and gluten, and affect the texture adversely.

Q. Should regular (that is, not instant) rice be washed before it is cooked? Some package instructions say to wash it while others say not to.

A. The difference in directions relates to the way in which the rice was enriched with thiamin, niacin, and iron. Some rice kernels are coated with a mixture of these nutrients, and that coating is not rinse resistant. In so-called converted rice, however, most of the nutrients originally present in the whole grain are forced into the kernel. But this rice may also be enriched with additional B vitamins and iron, so it is important to cook it according to package directions, following instructions for washing and rinsing.

For maximum nutrient retention it is best to avoid rinsing before cooking and to use only as much water as the rice will absorb. Anyway, rice sold in this country is quite clean, and there is really no reason to wash it before cooking.

Q. I have read that in processing dry cereals, the protein is "denatured" and is less available to the body. What is denaturation, and is that true?

A. Amino acids, the basic units of protein, are linked together by so-called "peptide bonds" to form polypeptide chains. These chains are then linked in a variety of ways. Denaturation is simply a change in the shape or spatial arrangement of these chains without a break in the bonds.

Among the items which can cause this rearrangement of protein molecules are acid, salt, and heat. In the case of dry cereal, the dry heat used to toast or puff the grains leads to the formation of extra linkages between the amino acids in adjacent chains. That may decrease the digestibility of the protein in the cereals to some extent. However, in this country, where our diets generally contain generous amounts of protein, this is of little practical importance.

Q. Is there any nutritional difference between spinach pasta and regular pasta?

A. None of any practical significance. In fact, what is commonly available in supermarkets is really not pasta (that is flour, water, and vegetable), but spinach egg noodles.

The government has an official recipe, or Standard of Identity, for noodles made with vegetables. It specifies that when vegetables are used—and they may be fresh, canned, dried, paste, or puree—they must contribute at least 3% of the finished weight of the product. That is quite a small amount, just under 2 grams, or less than half a teaspoon in 2 ounces of dried noodles. In most cases, this means that the nutritional contribution of added vegetables, even if a somewhat more generous amount is used, is really too small to be of practical importance. Providing difference in cost is not a factor, the reasonable basis for choosing these noodles appropriately focuses on aesthetics, including both taste and color.

Q. What are the differences between white bread flour, all-purpose flour, and cake flour?

A. While all three come from the starchy endosperm of the wheat kernel, how much is used varies with the type of flour being produced. "Patent" is the term used to describe the amount of endosperm used to make the flour. "Long-patent" flour contains a higher percentage of endosperm, including the more crush-resistant portions. It is higher in protein. So while all white flours are calorically equal, long-patent bread flour contains a little more protein than either of the other two. "Short-patent" cake flour contains the least amount of endosperm and is lowest in protein, while all-purpose flour lies in the middle.

The nutritional importance of differences in protein content in the flours in this country may be insignificant, but it is quite important to providing the desired effect in baked products. Higher amounts of protein in bread flour develop into a gluten with the necessary strong, elastic qualities. The gluten that develops in all-purpose flour is less strong and elastic. And the highly starchy cake flour develops a weak gluten appropriate for the delicate texture of cakes.

A second difference relates to particle size. Bread flour has the largest particles and is coarse and gritty compared to cake flour, which is fine and powdery, with all-purpose flour falling somewhere in the middle.

Finally, there is a difference in the type of wheat used. Bread flour is produced mainly from hard wheat, while cake flour is made from soft wheat. All-purpose flour is usually a blend of flours, combined to provide the desired protein content.

Cheese

Q. Recently a house guest brought me some very special cheddar-type cheese. Unfortunately it was more than I could use within a reasonable period of time. I put half of it in the freezer, but since then a friend has told me that cheddar should not be frozen. Is that true?

A. No. Cheddar and other types of cheeses can be frozen quite successfully. Exactly how long they can be kept before they begin to deteriorate, however, will depend on the variety involved. In one study, while cream cheese showed no deterioration at the end of six months, cheddar kept more than six weeks began to lose color and undergo undesirable texture changes. But even if the cheese does become crumbly and difficult to serve "as is," it is still perfectly fine to use in cooking.

The quality of frozen cheese has not been evaluated extensively, but according to one source, cheeses which seem to freeze most successfully include Camembert, Port du Salut, mozzarella, and Liederkranz-type cheeses, as well as Parmesan.

Eggs

Q. What causes a blood spot in an egg?

A. Eggs are formed from the inside out. That is, the yolk is formed first in the chicken's ovary, and then drops into the mouth of the oviduct, the tube through which it must travel in order for the hen to lay it. As it does, it is covered with layers of egg white from tissues that secrete albumin. Next comes the formation of a membrane; and finally, at the bottom of the oviduct, the shell is deposited.

Blood spots are the result of ruptures in the wall of the ovary or the oviduct which occur before these layers are added. Eggs with blood spots may not be aesthetically pleasant, but according to information from the American Egg Board, they are safe to eat.

Q. I have noticed that when I hard-boil eggs, the outside of the yolk turns a greenish-gray color. What causes this and is it harmful?

A. The green color is the result of a series of two chemical reactions which lead to the formation of a compound called ferrous (or iron) sulfide. Sulfur occurs in roughly equal amounts in the white and the yolk, but the sulfur in the white is more sensitive to heat. It is readily combined with hydrogen to form hydrogen sulfide during the cooking process. The hydrogen sulfide then reacts with the iron in the egg yolk to form ferrous sulfide.

While you may find a greenish-gray yolk esthetically unattractive, it is not harmful. But there are several measures to prevent it from happening. First, rather than cooking eggs in rapidly boiling water, simmer them at a somewhat lower temperature. Second, avoid overcooking them. And finally, cool them promptly. This latter step will also help them to peel more easily.

Q. Can egg whites and yolks be frozen?

A. Yes. Egg whites can be frozen "as is" and will whip to the same volume as if they were fresh. If you are freezing more than one at a time, 2 tablespoons are the equivalent to the white of one large egg. Egg whites should be thawed in the refrigerator. Remember, however, that regardless of whether you are using fresh egg whites or egg whites that have been frozen, you can be assured of better volume if you warm the eggs to room temperature. That is perhaps best done by putting them in container set in a pan of warm water for just a few minutes.

To freeze egg yolks, you must add either a small amount of sugar or salt as a stabilizer to prevent them from becoming gummy and viscous when they are thawed. Which one you choose will depend on how you are likely to use them once they are thawed. Use 1 tablespoon of sugar or corn syrup, or ½ teaspoon of salt per cup of egg yolk. A tablespoon of yolk is about the amount in a single large egg. Obviously, if you are freezing just one or two yolks at a time, you would use just a pinch of either one.

 Q. Why is cream of tartar sometimes used in whipping egg whites?

A. Cream of tartar makes the foam more stable. Ironically, however, both cream of tartar and salt, often added to egg whites for flavor, delay the formation of foam in the first place. For that reason, directions in many recipes specify that you whip the egg whites to a foamy stage before adding either of these ingredients.

Cream of tartar is derived from tartaric acid, which occurs naturally in fruits, particularly in such things as currants and grapes. In fact, in making wine, the tartrates normally present in grape juice must be removed before it is bottled. If not, tartrate crystals gradually form as it sits on the shelf.

Q. Why do overbeaten egg whites become stiff and dry and look almost curdled?

A. The effect is caused by changes in the structure of surface proteins in the film surrounding the air cells, which render them insoluble and inelastic. The protein in overbeaten eggs actually behaves as though it had been cooked.

Adding sugar, as you would do in making a meringue, creates a more stable and shinier foam. This shininess is due in part to preventing the protein from coagulating. The addition of sugar makes it possible to beat egg whites for quite a while longer without producing undesirable changes. And while foam beaten alone must be used at once or it will break down, when sugar is included, the foam (or meringue) can stand for some time without deteriorating.

Q. I have noticed that egg yolks vary considerably in color. Do those which are deep yellow have more cholesterol than paler ones?

A. No, color is not an indicator of either differences in cholesterol level or of nutrient content. Two factors contribute to the color density of egg yolks. One, heredity, is of relatively minor importance. The other, type of feed, exerts a more powerful influence.

Many egg producers control the amount of greens they provide to their hens in order to produce egg yolks with a medium color intensity. Hens can convert pigments in the greens to vitamin A, and the deep yellow color of yolks is a sign of the presence of that nutrient. However, hens may be given vitamin A-supplemented rations, and thus the yolks of the eggs they lay, even though pale in color, may contain just as much of the vitamin as those which are considerably more yellow.

While heredity plays a minor role in determining the color of the egg yolk, breed is the sole factor that determines shell color. But like egg yolk color, shell color has no effect on nutritional value of the eggs, or for that matter, on grade, flavor, or cooking performance. Paying a premium for one shell color or another is a waste of money.

Milk

Q. Does freezing milk affect its nutritional value?
A. No, although you should be sure to rotate the stored containers so that you will use the milk on a first-in–first-out basis. Also, milk should be kept in the freezer only about a month.

Nutritional considerations are only part of the story, however. Freezing does cause quality changes in milk. It weakens or ruptures the protein film that helps emulsify the fat globules. As a result, fat globules tend to stick together in clumps. Similarly, the dispersion of protein and calcium phosphate in milk is disturbed by freezing, causing them to settle out when the milk is thawed. Therefore, for most people, evaporated and nonfat dry milk are more satisfactory backups than frozen milk. Obviously, milk that has been frozen should be shaken well before it is used.

Q. In comparing labels of fresh skim and nonfat dry milk, the fresh milk has more calories. Why is that?
A. The caloric difference is probably explained by the fact that in all likelihood, the producer of the skim milk you checked adds nonfat milk solids to give a bit more body. In fact, many people who use nonfat dry milk at home do exactly the same thing by reconstituting it to a stronger constituency than directions on the package state. Nutritionally, the net effect is a small increase in carbohydrate, protein, and therefore, in calories.

Q. What causes a skin to form on the top of milk when it is heated?
A. When milk is heated in an uncovered pan, water gradually evaporates from the surface allowing casein, the main protein in cow's milk, to concentrate. The skin is a mixture of the casein, along with some fat and calcium compounds.

You may have noticed that once a skin forms, milk tends to boil over. That is because steam forms under the skin layer. It is possible to prevent skin formation by whipping the milk occasionally as it heats. Not only will you save yourself a stove-cleaning job, but you will conserve the nutrients that would be discarded with the skin.

Fruits and Vegetables

Q. Is there a way to handle the tomatoes available in the supermarket during the long months when the marvelous locally grown fruit is not available, so that they will taste a little fresher?
A. Yes. It is, unfortunately, impractical to let tomatoes which must be shipped long distances, first ripen on the vine. Instead, the ripening process, started before they are shipped, should be completed in the home. The problem is that people commonly put tomatoes into the refrigerator as soon as

they get home from the market. The tomatoes will not ripen at refrigerator temperatures, but they can ripen at room temperature.

Tomatoes naturally produce ethylene gas, which acts on the fruit like a ripening hormone. At temperatures between 65ºF and 75ºF they will ripen gradually. Thus, they can merely be set out on the kitchen counter. Ideally, however, they seem to do better in a humid environment. So, if they are prepacked in a container with air holes, simply leave them on the counter. Or, if you buy them in bulk, a paper bag with a few small air holes cut into the sides will also serve the purpose.

These tomatoes may not taste like the fruit you pick out of your own backyard or buy at the local farm stand, but following the above procedure should provide a somewhat more tasty winter tomato than you've had in the past.

Q. Recently I froze peaches for the first time. The directions I followed advised using a commercial antidarkening product made especially for the purpose. I did use it, adding it when I blanched the peaches in water. However, I was upset by the price, after an inspection of the label revealed that the first ingredient was sugar. I realize, of course, that the "active ingredient" listed was ascorbic acid. Could I add lemon juice to the light syrup to get the same effect?

A. By the time you use enough lemon juice to get the amount of ascorbic acid you need to prevent darkening, you may well go beyond the degree of tartness your family will accept. As an alternative, get a small amount of crystalline ascorbic acid at your local pharmacy. You will need to add about ½ teaspoon per quart of liquid.

Unfortunately, ascorbic acid pills which are readily available are not as satisfactory. They are more difficult to dissolve than the crystalline form, and the filler in the tablets may make the syrup cloudy. If you do use them, however, 1,500 milligrams of ascorbic acid in tablet form is equivalent to ½ teaspoon of the crystalline product.

Q. I really enjoy avocados and am willing to do without other things in order to continue to include them in my weight-reduction diet. In checking two calorie charts, however, I noticed two quite different caloric values for the same amount of fruit. Which one is right?

A. The difference in values can be explained by the fact that one was probably based either mainly or totally on California varieties and the other on avocados which come from Florida.

In this country, most avocados are from California. And, by law, California avocados cannot contain less than 8% fat. However, seasonal variations are considerable and fat content can run above 20%.

While the weight of California avocados can vary anywhere from under

4 ounces to more than 20 ounces, a typical fruit weighs about a half-pound. According to the latest figures available from the USDA, half of a California avocado of that size would contain about 3 ounces of edible fruit and would provide about 150 calories, most of them from 15 grams of oil.

The Florida varieties tend to be larger, so the ratio of edible fruit to waste is greater. A quarter of a 1-pound fruit would supply 85 calories and about 7 grams of oil. As in the California varieties, that oil contains mostly monounsaturated fatty acids. About 30% of the calories in the Florida varieties come from carbohydrate, while in the California varieties only about 16% come from that source.

Q. Can overripe bananas be frozen and used once they have been frozen?

A. Yes. They do darken and there are texture changes, but that is of little consequence when they are to be used in baking. The most efficient method for freezing bananas for use in baking is to mash them and freeze them in measured "recipe-specific" amounts. Not only will they be ready to use, but if freezer space is a problem, they will require less room.

Q. Most cookbooks seem to give directions for freezing fruits in sugar syrup. Is this really necessary to use sugar?

A. Some fruits like blueberries and cranberries can be washed and frozen "as is." Unfortunately, however, most fruits taste better and have a better texture if frozen with sugar. While the sugar provides extra calories, it does protect against oxidation which causes flavor and color changes and inactivates vitamins. Sugar also helps slow down undesirable changes produced by enzymes in the fruit during storage. As protection against browning during defrosting, ascorbic acid is usually mixed with the sugar or added to the syrup.

Q. I diced fresh pineapple and mixed it with cottage cheese early in the day. In the evening when I went to serve it, the texture of the cottage cheese had become quite runny and unpleasant. Can you tell me why?

A. The deterioration of the cottage cheese and pineapple mixture is the result of the activity of an enzyme in pineapple called bromelain. Because of the ability of bromelain to break down protein, fresh pineapple should be added to any protein-rich food only at the time it is served. Because the enzyme is inactivated by heat, canned pineapple does not have the same effect.

Q. How can you tell when a pineapple is ripe?

A. Fresh-looking leaves are a key to freshness, but there really is no way to judge ripeness. Color is not a key. Ripe pineapples can vary from green to quite yellow. And the notion that they are ripe if the leaves can be plucked easily from the center is a myth. In fact, pineapples are among the fruits which must be picked ripe. Further ripening does not occur during transport or as the fruit sits on your counter. So, once home, pineapple should be stored in the refrigerator.

Q. Do pickles have any nutritional value?

A. About the only thing that can be said in the nutritional defense of pickles is that most are low in calories. A medium sour or dill pickle, almost 4″ long and about 1¼″ in diameter provides just 7 calories. The notable exception are sweet gherkins, which contain considerable sugar. A large gherkin, about 3″ long and 1″ in diameter, provides about 50 calories, or as many as you would get from a half-cup of orange juice, a cup of cantaloupe balls, or a medium yellow peach, all of which provide considerably more generous amounts of several vitamins than pickles.

Many people enjoy the taste and crunch of a good pickle, its lack of nutrients notwithstanding. However, the process which converts cucumbers to pickles—holding them in a brine solution—turns a very low-sodium food into one which contains generous amounts, as much as 2 grams in a single large dill or sour pickle. In light of current recommendations to reduce sodium intake, it is probably better to eat pickles most often in their natural state, as cucumbers, and save moderate amounts of pickles for special treats.

Q. What causes the cut surfaces of some fruits to turn brown? Also, is it better to trim away browned areas?

A. The darkening which occurs when fruits are peeled, cut, and left exposed to air apparently results from the action of oxidizing enzymes on chemical compounds called phenols which are also present in the fruit. Lemon juice is often used to slow this browning process. The highly acid fruit apparently interferes with the activity of the oxidizing enzymes. Pineapple juice, which is much lower in acid, is effective, too. It is thought that a sulfur-containing compound in the juice acts as an antioxidant.

Browning may make the fruit appear less attractive, but it is not a harmful reaction.

Q. Why does broccoli turn a drab olive-green if cooked too long?

A. The color change in vegetables like broccoli is related to the effects of heat on chlorophyll.

Chlorophyll is the pigment which plays an essential role in converting carbon dioxide and water into carbohydrates. In nature, it is a fat-soluble compound tied to protein. When plant cells are killed as a result of aging, cooking, or other processing, the protein is altered and the chlorophyll may be released. It is then highly unstable and rapidly reacts with acid normally found in the plant to produce another compound called pheophytin. This reaction leads to the color change. The reaction proceeds more quickly in more acid environments, explaining, for example, what happens when lightly cooked, bright-green broccoli is tossed with vinaigrette dressing.

To prevent this color change it has sometimes been suggested that sodium bicarbonate be added to the water for cooking such vegetables as peas, spinach, and beans. However, the aesthetic trade-off is that the more alkaline solution causes the cellulose in these vegetables to soften, affecting the texture adversely. And from a nutritional point of view, it increases the losses of both vitamin C and thiamin during cooking.

Q. What causes potatoes to turn yellow after cooking?

A. The natural pigments that color a food can be changed by a variety of factors, including the relative acidity of the water in which the food is cooked.

A group of yellow compounds called anthoxanthins, which are found in both potatoes and apples, tend to become deeper yellow when cooked in an alkaline solution. And many water supplies are naturally somewhat alkaline. Acidifying the water with a little lemon juice would result in a whiter color.

These pigments, incidentally, belong to a class of compounds called flavonoids. Among other pigments in this group are the anthocyanins, responsible for the blue and red colors in grapes, berries, plums, and beets. These, too, are affected by the acidity of cooking water. Thus, the brilliant red color of beets will turn an even brighter color when they are cooked in vinegar. But in an alkaline solution fruits and vegetables containing anthocyanins tend to turn blue-gray or violet.

Q. I read an article advising against storing potatoes in the refrigerator, but it didn't explain why. If I don't keep them in the refrigerator, they sprout. Can you explain the reason for this recommendation and tell me whether it is really necessary?

A. At temperatures below 40°F, the starch in tubers is gradually converted to sugar. The increased sugar content can cause them to darken when cooked. It is generally suggested that a cool, moist (but not humid), and well-ventilated spot provides the ideal storage conditions for potatoes. Sprouting potatoes are safe to use. Just break off the sprouts before you cook them. You may also want to peel them before cooking.

While it is of relatively minor concern at home, temperature regulation to control the sugar content in potatoes is extremely important in commercial processing and it depends on the eventual use of the potatoes. For example, it is important to keep the sugar content in potatoes to be used in canned corned beef hash low, since high processing temperatures may result in off flavors and colors. If they are to be used in frozen French fries or hash browns, then the sugar content must be high enough to provide some color without prolonged heating. In making potato chips, the sugar content must be high enough to produce the desirable light brown color. If it is too high, the chips will burn or become black during heating.

In order to manipulate potatoes to the right sugar content for commercial processing, it is sometimes necessary to hold them under controlled conditions for anywhere from one to three weeks.

Q. My husband went to the supermarket and returned with a "bargain," a dozen avocados, reduced for quick sale because they were quite ripe. I managed to use them up before they spoiled. I would have preferred to have found a way to preserve them so we could have eaten them somewhat more leisurely. Is it possible to freeze avocados?

A. Indeed it is possible to spread out the enjoyment of your "bargain" by mashing the avocado and freezing it for later use. For guacamole and other unsweetened uses, add a tablespoon of lemon juice and a bit of salt to each cup of puree. But if you want to use it in a sweetened mixture, add 200 milligrams of crushed ascorbic acid tablets dissolved in a little water to each 2 cups of puree.

Q. What is the difference between green and black olives?

A. As picked, all olives are both green and bitter and must go through several processing steps before they are packed. First, a dilute alkaline solution is used to remove the bitterness. Then the olives are rinsed and put into a brine solution. At this point, for those which are to be black, air is bubbled through the solution to oxidize the fruit and an iron-containing compound, ferrous gluconate, is added to both fix and retain the color.

Nutritionally, both green and black olives provide little except calories. Just how many calories will, of course, depend on size, and there are no fewer than nine size categories. The smallest provide just 4 calories each, while at the other extreme, supercolossal olives provide 18 calories apiece. Olives also provide generous amounts of sodium—as many as 400 milligrams in just four of them. That is as much as you would get from an ounce-and-a-half of ham. And the sodium content of the imported varieties, commonly sold in bulk in ethnic groceries and specialty stores, varies greatly. Some apparently provide considerably more than those produced domestically. So if you are concerned about your sodium intake, save olives for special occasions and then use them only sparingly.

Q. In buying juice oranges, I have observed that sometimes the skin is quite green, but the flavor is unaffected. How does skin color relate to quality?

A. The old adage, "Beauty is only skin deep" just doesn't apply. In all likelihood the oranges you describe were from Florida, which has a law against selling unripe oranges. (Oranges, incidentally, don't ripen once they are picked.) In that state, cool nights can cause the chlorophyll in the skin to reappear. The green pigment competes with and sometimes overwhelms the orange pigment, causing the fruit to appear unripe. Brownish marks you may see on Florida oranges do not affect quality, either. "Wind scars," as they are called, occur as the ripening oranges are tossed around on the trees during storms.

Meat

Q. A friend recently told me that she has not bought extra-lean beef for several years, after reading that once the meat was cooked, regular beef, which is considerably higher in fat, contained no more fat. Is that true?
A. Those were the findings of a study conducted by food technologists at the United States Department of Agriculture's Meat Science Laboratory at the Agricultural Research Center in Beltsville, MD several years ago. After cooking, the weight of both types of patties was the same, but the explanation for the loss differed. Higher-fat beef patties, judged to be somewhat juicier and a bit tastier than the leaner beef, lost more fat, while the extra-lean patties lost larger amounts of water.

In this experiment, the ground beef was cooked in patties, so that the fat could easily be discarded. If you are concerned about both fat intake and cost, and use the higher-fat ground beef in mixed dishes, you will want to pay a little extra attention to technique. For example, make sure to cook and drain the beef before adding it to a mixture such as spaghetti sauce or chili con carne, precooking and draining small meat balls before adding them to a sauce, or periodically draining off the fat as a meat loaf cooks.
Q. Can ham be frozen?
A. Yes, although it does not hold up in the freezer as well as other meats. Cooked ham, if carefully wrapped in freezer foil can be stored for about two months at 0°F or below. If kept longer, it tends to lose both flavor and texture.

The USDA recommends, incidentally, that cooked ham be stored in the refrigerator for no more than four or five days. So, the next time you have a ham that you think will last beyond that, you may want to put part of the freshly cooked meat in the freezer while it is still at peak quality.
Q. Why is freezing cured meats not recommended?
A. Freezing causes the flavor of ingredients used in the curing process to get stronger, affecting both the taste and the texture of these foods adversely. In addition, seasonings used in the curing process actually increase the speed at which rancidity develops in these meats.

So top-quality cured meats should be eaten fresh. If you happen to find yourself with an excess that must be frozen to avoid spoilage, freeze corned beef and frankfurters just two weeks, bacon for a month, cured hams no more than two months, and fresh sausage for a maximum of three months. It is generally suggested that bologna and other luncheon meats, as well as smoked sausages, not be frozen.

Q. My supermarket carried large cuts of meat packaged in heavy plastic wrapping. The meat has a funny dark color and I wonder whether it's a different grade of beef or whether the color is the result of additives used in packaging. Can you tell me?
A. The dark color is related to neither of these things. Whole beef carcasses are usually cut into five large pieces, referred to as "primal cuts." These cuts are then further divided into what are called "subprimals." Indeed, most beef is now cut into subprimals at the packaging plant, vacuum-packed, and shipped to supermarkets in boxes. Subprimals available in the supermarket are usually the best parts of these cuts, with much of the bone and other waste already trimmed by the packer.

The reason the subprimals are a darker purplish color is because they are vacuum-packed right after they have been cut and are not exposed to air. Shortly after the package is opened, the meat will "bloom" and turn the bright red color you normally associate with fresh meat.

We should mention that when first opened, vacuum-packed meat has an odor sometimes described as "sour" or "off." This should disappear within an hour after opening.

Vacuum-packed meats have not been previously frozen. They can be frozen in their packaging or cut into family-size pieces, wrapped airtight, and then frozen. In the refrigerator, they will keep at least a week and probably longer.
Q. How long can I store ground beef safely in the refrigerator?
A. Assuming it is handled correctly—that is, brought home from the market promptly and then stored in the coldest part of the refrigerator—it may be kept for a couple of days. Beyond that, it is a good idea to store it in the freezer.

Two factors contribute to the increased perishability of ground beef over solid cuts. For one thing, it is often made from trimmings which have been handled more than other cuts. This adds to the bacterial count. In addition, grinding greatly increases the surface area exposed to bacteria naturally present in the environment. These microscopic organisms are not harmful, but they can cause both deterioration in quality and spoilage when ground meat is not handled properly.

If you do need to freeze ground beef, it is best thawed in the refrigerator. If that is not possible, the thawing process can be speeded up by placing the meat in a watertight bag in cold water. Be sure to use the meat as soon as it has thawed.
Q. When corn syrup is listed as an ingredient on frankfurters or bologna, how significant an amount do they contain?
A. Very little. Frankfurters, bologna, and similar types of cooked sausage

can contain no more than 2% corn syrup by weight. That translates to about a half-teaspoon in 3½ ounces of meat.

Q. What causes the warmed-over flavor of precooked meat?

A. Warmed-over flavor results from the oxidation of fat within the muscle tissue. Unlike other oxidation that gradually causes fat to develop off flavors, this process can occur quite rapidly. Turkey, beef, and pork are most susceptible to the development of WOF, as it is called by food technologists. Chicken, on the other hand, is fairly resistant, an asset thought to be linked to higher levels of vitamin E, which acts as an antioxidant in the tissues.

Warmed over flavor has limited the acceptability of precooked refrigerator meats. Considerable research has been done on the effectiveness of additives, sauces, and spices in preventing these oxidative changes, and there has been some progress. However, WOF, sometimes described as "cardboardy" or "painty," remains a problem for the refrigerated food industry. The USDA's Agricultural Research Service has recently reported on a promising new additive, a protein created by chemically treating chitin, found in the shells of lobster, crab, and shellfish. It bonds with the iron in ground beef, preventing the breakdown of fat. Researchers hope that it may also be effective in other meats and in poultry and fish.

Fish

Q. I live in an area where limited fresh fish is available, so I have to resort to frozen fish. I have noticed that it comes coated with a substantial layer of ice and wonder why am I paying for this extra water?

A. The ice coating on fish is put on by processors to protect against both damage to the surface caused by contact with oxygen in the air and freezer burn during storage. In glazing, as the process is called, the fish are frozen, dipped in water, and refrozen. Usually the process is repeated several times to build up a thick enough glaze.

The water added during glazing should not be included in the weight of fish sold to consumers. Unfortunately, however, there have been cases of overglazing, that is, coating with too much ice and including part of the weight of the ice in the net weight. It is the responsibility of the FDA to monitor frozen fish and identify violations of this type.

Q. Why does raw fish spoil so quickly?

A. There are four factors which explain why fresh fish deteriorates quickly. For one thing, the unsaturated fat it contains becomes rancid very quickly. For another, while the flesh of healthy fish is free of bacteria, once killed, fish quickly become vulnerable to microorganisms on the skin and in the digestive tract. These bacteria are adapted to living in cool water and can continue to grow even under refrigeration.

Third, fish store glycogen, or animal starch, in their tissues. The glycogen could potontially be broken down to lactic acid to act as a preservative once the fish are dead. But in the process of struggling against being caught, they use up these stores of glycogen.

Finally, combinations of fat and phosphates, or "phospholipids," are a rich source of a compound called trimethylamine. Once split from the phospholipids, both by bacteria and by enzymes in the fish, it has a strong fish odor. It is this compound which, in fact, accounts for much of the smell of fish.

Quality does begin to change as soon as fish are taken from the water. But the rate of change will depend on several factors, including the tissue composition of the particular species, the effect of season of the year on tissue composition, whether the fish are from fresh or salt water, and the catching and holding practices on fishing vessels.

Q. Is ice glazing the best method for freezing fish? If so, how does one do it?
A. Ice glazing is time consuming, but it is especially useful for protecting fish from drying out and spoiling during long-term storage—that is, more than a couple of months.

First, freeze the fish, unwrapped, on a tray covered with wax paper. Then dip it in ice water to coat it with ice. Put it back in the freezer for 20 minutes or so until the glaze is solid. Repeat the process up to six times, or until a thick coating has formed. Some authorities suggest that keeping quality is improved by adding commercially available anti-oxidants used to freeze fruit to the solution in amounts of 4 teaspoons per gallon of water. If you do use them, rinse the fish in cold water after you thaw it.

Once glazed, the fish should be tightly wrapped and stored in the coldest part of the freezer. The coating is fragile, however, so it is important to handle glazed fish carefully both during packing and storing.

Poultry

Q. I have noticed that there can be considerable variation in the color of chicken livers and have wondered whether color was a clue to safety. Can you tell me?
A. The U.S. Department of Agriculture's Food Safety and Inspection Service tells us that color variation in livers from healthy chickens is quite normal and can be explained by three factors. One is variation in the type of feed the birds have been given. A second is differences in the chickens' hemoglobin levels. And a final factor which may contribute is metabolic differences from one bird to another.

Q. In serving a broiler chicken which had been quartered and frozen for about three months, I noticed some discoloration and darkening in the flesh next to the bones. What causes this, and is it harmful?
A. The discoloration you noticed is not harmful. Freezing and thawing re-

lease hemoglobin from the red blood cells in the bone marrow. In young birds, the bone is quite porous and this hemoglobin can seep through to the flesh. Heating changes the pigment, which is then responsible for the darkening. This darkening does not occur in older birds that have been frozen because the bones are more dense and the hemoglobin cannot escape.

Q. How long can I keep leftover cooked chicken safely in the refrigerator once it has been cooked?

A. Cooked poultry will remain at top quality for three or four days. Beyond that, undesirable changes in flavor and texture begin to develop. To keep chicken even that long, it must be handled properly. That means storing it in the refrigerator as soon after it is cooked as possible in a shallow container that promotes rapid, even cooling. In the case of large roasting chickens and turkeys, the USDA's Food Safety and Inspection Service recommends removing the meat from the bones to shorten the cooling time.

Fats

Q. What is the difference between mayonnaise and mayonnaise-type salad dressing?

A. Nutritionally, the former contains 11 grams of fat and 100 calories per tablespoon while the latter contains slightly more than half that amount, 6 grams of fat and about 65 calories. That difference is accounted for by the fact that the Federal Standard of Identity, or official recipe for mayonnaise, specifies that it must contain at least 65% oil by weight compared to 30% of the weight of mayonnaise-type salad dressing.

Most ingredients, including oil and egg, acidifying agents such as vinegar, lemon, or lime juice, and citric acid, and seasonings such as salt, sugar, and spices like mustard or paprika are common to both products. However, mayonnaise depends entirely on the emulsifying properties of egg yolk for its thick texture, while salad dressing is thickened in part by a paste made either from food starch or from wheat, rye, or tapioca flour.

Q. What is "cold-pressed" oil? It is quite a bit more expensive than regular oil and I would like to know whether it is worth the additional cost?

A. "Cold-pressed" oils are oils that have been physically extracted from nuts or seeds in a way that does not require the use of chemical solvents or heat. True "cold-pressed" oils undergo no further processing, whereas in conventional processing both mechanical methods and solvents are used to extract the oil which then undergoes several additional refining steps.

Crude, unprocessed oils, like cold-pressed oil, contain impurities which may adversely affect the flavor, odor, performance, and even the safety of the oil. The refining process removes these impurities so that conventionally processed oils are usually lighter in color, have a milder flavor, hold up better and foam less during frying, and have a longer shelf life.

The refining process has no effect on the essential fatty acid content of the oil and only a small effect on the amount of vitamin E it contains. A leading oil producer tells us that, after refining, their oil retains at least three-fourths of its original vitamin E.

In short, we can see no reason to justify the additional expense of cold-pressed oil.

Q. Is it safe to continue to reuse oil for deep frying?

A. Yes, if it is handled properly. That means using the fat at the correct temperature to avoid overheating, smoking, and darkening. (A chart of correct temperatures for frying various types of foods is usually provided with frying appliances and correct frying temperatures are usually included in recipes for fried foods.) Used fats should be chilled if there is to be a long interval between uses. And finally, it is important to know when to throw out used fat and begin fresh. That point comes when excessive foaming occurs as the food is added to the kettle of hot fat and/or the fat develops strong flavors and odors.

Q. I am rather puzzled about two things. Why does regular mayonnaise contain 5 milligrams of cholesterol per tablespoon while the lite variety contains twice that amount.

A. The ingredients list suggests the answer to the cholesterol question. Whole eggs are used in regular mayonnaise, but only egg yolks, which contain the cholesterol, are used in the light variety. Apparently a bit more egg yolk is also used.

Q. At the top of the list of menu reforms in a local child-feeding program was the switch from commercial peanut butter "loaded with sugar" to natural peanut butter. Is commercial peanut butter heavily sweetened?

A. No. Peanut butter is among the group of foods for which there is a legally defined recipe, or Standard of Identity. According to that standard, at least 90% of the weight of peanut butter must be peanuts. That leaves little room for the other things manufacturers are allowed to add. These include hydrogenated or partially hydrogenated vegetable oils, which act as stabilizers to prevent the oil in the peanuts from separating from the solids and keep the butter spreadable, and "suitable seasonings." In terms of a serving of peanut butter, this is a very small amount. Two tablespoons of peanut butter, a reasonable amount for a sandwich, weighs about 32 grams, or a little over an ounce. Ten percent of that would be 3.2 grams, or about a half-teaspoon in all.

Q. Is 100% pure peanut butter preferable to those which contain partially hydrogenated vegetable fat?

A. No. As with sugar, the amount of additional saturated fat you would get by choosing commercial peanut butter over a locally prepared alternative is quite small.

And Also

Q. I have two questions about canned foods. While we commonly refer to "tin cans," is there really any tin in cans? Also, why is there a yellowish or white coating on the inside of some cans and not others?
A. Today's "tin can" contains little tin. The body of the can is 98% steel, plated with a thin tin coating to increase resistance to acid and to oxidation.

Enamel and lacquer coatings were first developed during the 1920s to prevent corrosion caused by the action of acids in fruit on tin plating. Today they are used in canning in a number of different foods, including beer, carbonated beverages, soft drinks, some vegetables, and seafood. In addition to preventing rust and corrosion, they serve several other purposes. They protect the contents of the can from metal contamination, help to preserve flavor and color, and allow longer storage. In some cases they reduce the amount of tin coating that must be used and thereby cut down on the cost of the can.

Q. What is the best way to keep frozen food when the power fails?
A. Once you discover that your freezer is not working, be sure to keep the door closed. Opening and closing it to check on the food will let warm air in and hasten thawing. If you expect prolonged power failure, you can maintain the temperature in your freezer for longer periods with dry ice. If added soon after the power fails, 25 pounds of dry ice will keep the temperature below freezing for three or four days in a fully loaded 10 cubic-foot refrigerator or for two to three days in one that is half-full. Dry ice should be handled carefully, however. Be sure the room is well-ventilated and wear heavy gloves while handling it. Put the dry ice on cardboards on top of the packages and open the freezer door only to add more.

Without dry ice how long your food will keep will depend on how much food is in the freezer. A fully loaded freezer will stay cold enough to keep food frozen for two days, while one that is only half-full will keep food frozen for only one day.

Q. How are so-called "freeze-dried" foods produced?
A. Freeze drying is a method of preserving foods in which two separate steps are used in the sequence implied in the name. Raw food is first frozen quickly and then put into a vacuum chamber where the moisture is removed by a process called sublimation. That is, in removing the water, ice crystals are converted directly to vapor without passing through a liquid stage.

Q. I had always believed that when wine is used in cooking, the calories it contains go up in smoke. But a friend, who like myself is trying to lose weight, tells me that it is not so. Which one of us is correct?

A. Your friend is. Alcohol in dilute solution evaporates very slowly, and wine is only about 12% alcohol to begin with. Add to that the fact that it is often combined with other liquids in a recipe, and the alcohol solution becomes even weaker.

But the simple fact is that even for the dieter, the amount of calories added by alcohol is probably of little significance. For example, a whole cup of wine, providing no more than 200 calories, might be used to make enough beef stew to serve eight people. That would add just 25 calories to each serving, and in return could help create a more interesting dish to satisfy the dieter.

Looked at another way, it is slightly over half as many calories as you would get by letting a single extra teaspoon of fat slip into your diet.

Q. I was just looking at a list of energy-saving tips. One of the recommendations was to avoid preheating the oven. Won't that ruin baked goods?

A. Not according to the results of studies reported recently. Researchers at the Consumer Nutrition Center of the USDA's Human Nutrition Information Service tested seven different items baked in four types of ovens: a standard gas oven with no built-in cleaning feature; a continuous-clean gas oven; a standard electric oven with no built-in cleaning feature; and a self-cleaning electric oven. Among the items tested were plain muffins, yellow cake, baked custard, and apple pie.

Researchers baked all dishes in each of the four types of ovens and under conditions of both preheating and nonpreheating. In addition to calculating differences in energy consumption, investigators performed objective tests of quality and used a taste panel to give palatability ratings.

Few significant differences were found in physical measurements or in eating quality either between preheated and nonpreheated ovens or among oven types. Products generally required five minutes or less extra baking time when cooked in nonpreheated ovens, but in general, this still meant that less energy was required to bake products without preheating. Savings averaged about 10%.

The overall conclusion confirmed that preheating ovens is not essential for good product quality and is an unnecessary use of energy. It is estimated that the elimination of preheating could save about 26 trillion BTU's of primary energy a year, or even more if people commonly preheat the oven for longer periods.

Q. I would like to buy a microwave oven, but remain skeptical about their safety. What is your opinion?

A. Concern about microwave ovens generally focuses both on the effects of microwaves on the food itself and on leakages from the ovens.

Microwaves are really quite harmless. In the oven, electromagnetic rays cause the molecules at the outer part of the food to vibrate. The vibration creates the heat necessary to do the task at hand, ranging from thawing, to thorough cooking, to simply reheating leftovers. Microwaves do not penetrate very thick foods. Instead, vibrating molecules near the surface agitate molecules in the interior, creating the friction necessary to heat the food.

As for safety, products now available have built-in safeguards to prevent any hazards as long as the products are in good repair. The FDA has set allowable leakage limits well below accepted danger levels. In addition, oven doors are required to have a double safety lock, so that no microwaves can be produced while the door is open. Other design features, including metallic screens on door windows, insure that microwaves remain inside the closed oven while it is operating.

Q. I make a large pot of soup, usually enough for one main course and a first course on a second night, nearly every week during the winter. I vary the ingredients, but usually it is a mixture of dried beans, meat or chicken, seasonings, and fresh or frozen vegetables. With the exception of seasoning vegetables, particularly onions and celery, I add the vegetables just before serving. Since I simmer the meat for a fairly extended period, are there any nutrients left in it by the time I serve it?

A. Yes. The common belief that by the time a piece of chicken or beef has cooked long enough to flavor a broth it is devoid of any nutrients is not true.

Some B vitamins are vulnerable to heat and will be destroyed with prolonged cooking. Much of the thiamin originally present would have disappeared by serving time. That cannot be avoided. Other water-soluble B vitamins may leach out in the broth. That is of little nutritional consequences, since the broth will be consumed anyway. Beyond that, most of the protein and iron and some of the B vitamins remain in the meat or chicken.

There are a number of strengths to both your methods and your general recipe outline. Adding vegetables just before serving is a key factor in minimizing losses of both heat-labile B vitamins and vitamin C. The combination of beans, pasta, and vegetables with just a small amount of meat or chicken improves the usefulness of the nonmeat proteins to the body. Finally, the presence of both animal protein and some vitamin C remaining in briefly cooked vegetables increases the absorption of iron, found particularly in the dried beans.

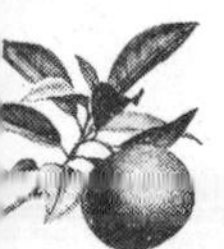

A NUTRITIONAL GLOSSARY OF FOOD

Alfalfa. A native European leguminous plant, grown in this country as a forage crop. It is also widely available in tablet form in health food stores and has been promoted as a treatment for arthritis for some time, even though there really is no basis for that or any other health claim for alfalfa.

Alfalfa sprouts. Sprouted alfalfa seeds. Low in calories (there are only 60 calories in 4 cups of them), the amount in a salad or sandwich will not provide appreciable amounts of any nutrients.

Alginates. Gelling agents extracted from brown seaweed. Because of their excellent stabilizing and thickening properties they are added to sauces and gravies, milk drinks, and bakery fillings of all types. They are also used in ultrapasteurized cream to give it stability, allowing it to whip properly and to act as it would if it had been pasteurized by the standard method. The fact that alginates form a heat-stable gel also makes them particularly desirable in many fabricated foods. Propylene glycol alginate is also used at low levels to provide stability to beer foam.

Annato extract. Natural food coloring derived from the brick-red seeds of the annato tree, native to tropical America. The extract, a compound called bixin, is a member of carotenoid family, responsible for the yellow and orange hues of many fruits and vegetables. Annato extract has been used as a coloring for centuries. The

Spanish found the Mexicans reddening their chocolate beverages with it during the sixteenth century. And annato extract has been used to color hard cheeses for over 200 years. It is sometimes added to cream to deepen the yellow hue of butter, to color margarine, and to lend a yellow tint to frozen desserts.

Arginine. An amino acid the body uses to build proteins. Manufacturers of arginine have claimed that it, along with ornithine, another amino acid, stimulate growth hormone and "burn fat" overnight. While some preliminary studies did show that these amino acids may stimulate growth hormone, the relationship to weight loss is unclear. Besides, if they do have this capacity, they may stimulate other hormones, thereby altering internal functioning in potentially dangerous ways.

Arrowroot. A starch obtained from the root of a West Indian plant called *Maranta arundinacea,* and considered especially useful when a delicate texture is desired. Unlike flour and cornstarch, it does not need to be cooked to remove the "rawness," and it thickens at lower temperatures than either of them. That makes it particularly useful in egg or other sauces which should not boil. On the other hand, it does not hold up well on standing, and sauces thickened with arrowroot cannot be reheated. Arrowroot provides a sauce-thickening option for individuals with wheat allergies, but as wheat-sensitive individuals know, the first ingredient in so-called "arrowroot cookies" available in the supermarket is wheat flour.

Artichokes, French or globe. The most highly prized vegetable of the ancient Romans, who raised their plants in the dark to keep them white and tender. The edible portion of the species they grew included the young leaves and underdeveloped stalks. The number of calories an artichoke provides may depend on how long it has been stored. The reason appears to lie in the fact that much of the carbohydrate in freshly harvested artichokes is thought to be inulin, a polysaccharide the body cannot digest. During storage, inulin is converted to simple sugars the body can use quite readily. A fairly large, cooked artichoke weighing about 3½ ounces could contain anywhere from 10 to 45 calories, depending on how long it has been stored. A far greater number of calories may come from the sauce with which it is served.

Artichokes, Jerusalem. The edible tuber of a species of sunflower native to North America, observed by Samuel de Champlain growing in Indian gardens on Cape Cod in the early 1600s. They bear little physical resemblance to the globe artichoke and grow quite differently, but Champlain and others after him observed a similarity of taste. That explains the "artichoke" part of the name, but nobody is quite sure of the origin of "Jerusalem." Like the globe variety, freshly dug Jerusalem artichokes also contain inulin. On standing, much of the inulin is converted to fructose which the body can absorb. (In fact until fairly recently, Jerusalem artichokes were used commercially as a source of fructose.) Four small, freshly dug Jerusalem artichokes may provide as few as 7 calories, but after long storage, about 75 calories. While most recipes suggest boiling Jerusalem artichokes and seasoning them with lemon juice, pepper, salt, and possibly some chives, they can also be baked like a potato, or peeled, thinly sliced, and added raw to green salad.

Arugola. A leafy green, resembling radish leaves in appearance, with quite a peppery flavor. It can be used by itself or as one of several greens in a mixed salad. It is also the key ingredient in a wonderful Italian soup, where the main ingredients are stale bread and potato, and it is used in chilled summer soups and even in a souffle, along with goat cheese.

Bioflavonoids. Once known as vitamin P, they are a group of naturally occurring compounds, the first of which was isolated from citrus rind about 50 years ago. Results of studies conducted at the time suggested that they might be useful in reducing hemorrhages which occur in various diseases. The findings were never confirmed, but bioflavonoids have remained on health food store shelves as supplements of unproven value.

Bok choy. Also called Chinese cabbage, this is one of the milder members of the cabbage family. It has long, smooth, and very white stems with large, crinkly dark green leaves. Sometimes the tender heart, which has yellow florets, is sold separately. Bok choy cooks quite quickly, and it can be either stir-fried or sliced and cooked in soup. It is quite low in calories, just 10 in a whole cup of cooked, shredded vegetable. It is also high in calcium, providing about 160 milligrams per cup, about as much as a half-cup of milk. It provides small amounts of B vitamins and appreciable vitamin C. The dark green leaves are an excellent source of beta carotene.

Breadfruit. A large round fruit native to Polynesia. It was, of course, the cause of the mutiny aboard Captain Bligh's infamous ship *Bounty* nearly 200 years ago. Noting that it was extraordinarily prolific (a single tree produced enough fruit to last a good-sized family for a year), British planters in the West Indies thought it would be the ideal food to feed slaves on the sugar plantations. At their request, George III sent Captain Bligh to pick up young trees and take them to the West Indies. In his zeal to find 1,000 of the best saplings, Bligh lingered well beyond what the crew, who wanted to get back to England, found reasonable. As a final and disastrous insult to his already enraged men, he reduced their drinking water ration to keep the trees alive on the trip back to the West Indies. The crew mutinied. Bligh was set adrift in an open boat, and the trees were tossed overboard. On a second mission six years later in 1793, he brought what has been described as a floating forest into Jamaica. Ironically, however, the breadfruit did not become an instant dietary staple among the slaves. They preferred the plaintains they knew. Nonetheless, over the years, breadfruit did eventually become an important food all over the Caribbean. Trees now grow on the mainland everywhere from Mexico south to Brazil. When baked or roasted, breadfruit has the texture of bread, which explains the origin of its name. Descriptions of its taste vary. Alexandre Dumas, the great French writer and an authority on food, thought it tasted like a combination of trimmed bread, with a slight suggestion of globe and Jerusalem artichoke. Obviously, it takes a bit of imagination to figure out from that description exactly what the flavor is. Beyond question, however, it is bland.

Brassica vegetables. A subgroup of the larger category of cruciferae (See *cruciferae)*. Also called the "mustard family," brassicas produce four-petal flowers suggesting a cross. Brassicas include cabbage, Chinese cabbage, Brussels sprouts, broccoli, kale, kohlrabi, collards, mustards, and cauliflower. In recent years some evidence suggests that increased intake of cruciferae are associated with decreased risk of certain cancers.

Bulgur. A lightly processed form of whole wheat in which whole-wheat kernels are parboiled, dried, and then broken up. It is a rather versatile grain which can be prepared in several ways. To produce the excellent Middle Eastern dish called tabbouleh, the uncooked kernels are soaked and then seasoned with mint, lemon juice, and oil. Bulgur can also be baked with broth and served as a pilaf, and it may be mixed with other grains. As a cereal, it can be served with dried fruits, yogurt, or nuts. And it's particularly good when soaked and mixed with ground lamb in another Middle Eastern dish called kibbe. When cooked, a cup of bulgur contains about 200 calories.

Calcium chloride. A calcium compound used in canning tomatoes. It binds with pectin in the tomatoes to produce an insoluble compound called calcium pectate which increases structural rigidity and helps maintain the desired firm texture.

Capers. The unopened flower buds of a trailing shrub known to humans since ancient times. While it is not completely clear exactly where capers originated, the late Waverley Root, in a delightful volume called, quite simply, *Food* (Simon and Schuster, 1980) theorizes that they came from the Sahara, pointing out that the plant, *Capparis spinosa,* is clearly designed for desert existence and that it is still popularly known in North

Africa as the Sahara caper tree. Capers were introduced into France by the Greeks as early as 600 B.C., and today the finest capers come from the Department of Var in France, where the plants are picked over every couple of days to find only the tiniest edible buds.

Cardoon. A member of the thistle family, native to the Mediterranean, it looks like an enormous, spiny bunch of very pale celery. The tough outer stems and leaves must be stripped away to get to the inner stalks and hearts. To be eaten raw, perhaps with a vinaigrette, the strings and inner skin must be stripped away. Or it can be cooked and served plain, simmered in broth to give it additional flavor, combined with onions and other vegetables, or served in any way you might choose to prepare braised celery.

Carnitine. A nutrient essential for transporting long-chain fatty acids into the part of the cell where energy is produced. Carnitine is produced in the liver and kidneys and is widely available in the diet. The best sources include animal flesh and dairy products. Because it is made in the body and is so widely available, a deficiency was discovered only recently and is a rare phenomenon. There is no need for healthy individuals to take it as a supplement.

Carob. Also known as St. John's bread, because it was believed to be the locusts eaten by St. John the Baptist in the desert. It is the fruit of an evergreen native to the Mediterranean coast. The sweet, fleshy pods, anywhere from 4 to 8 inches in length and 1½ inches in width, are filled with several hard seeds. They are harvested in early fall, dried, and chewed like candy. The pods, not widely available in this country, are also used for animal feed and fermented into alcohol. Flour made from carob is used in this country as a chocolate substitute to produce cookies, candy, cakes, and ice cream for those who wish to avoid the caffeine family of compounds. The relationship between its sweet, bland flavor and chocolate is questionable.

Casein. Extracted commercially from skim milk, it is the main protein in milk, accounting for as much as ⅘ of the total. Casein has certain properties which make it particularly useful as a food additive. Its ability to act as a binder has been used since the 1970s in imitation cheese production. That accounts for nearly half of all casein used in food manufacture in this country today—about 42 million pounds. Because it can also emulsify, or hold in suspension, fats and other compounds, it is used in cream substitutes to prevent the fat from separating and rising to the top. Finally, it is used in many convenience foods and bakery products. Casein has been recognized as a binder for centuries, long before it was used in commercial food processing. It has been identified as the glue in ancient artifacts and in wooden frames of the Renaissance era. Even today, many of its uses are unrelated to food for humans. In addition to being used in animal feeds, it may be added to such things as glues and adhesives and paper coatings. It is used in a variety of medical and pharmaceutical products, as well as in an assortment of other industrial products.

Cassava. A starchy, edible root, shaped like a sweet potato. Cassava, also known as manioc, is calorically quite dense, with 3½ ounces providing 120 calories. It is an important dietary staple in many developing countries, since it can be cultivated on marginal land. Unfortunately, it is a poor source of essential nutrients. Tapioca is a starch extracted from cassava.

Celeriac. Celeriac, long popular in Europe and in recent years more widely available in this country, is a member of the same family as stalk celery and is grown especially for the root. Also called celery root or celery knob, a half-cup raw provides 30 calories and considerable potassium. In addition to serving it raw in salads, it can be cubed, boiled, and served with cheese sauce, or braised in meat stock. Because it has a stronger flavor than stalk celery, it is sometimes pureed and combined with mashed potato, or used with potatoes in cream soup. Once peeled, it darkens quickly, so if prepared ahead of time, it should be held in water made acidic with vinegar or lemon juice.

Cheese, process. This is a blend which usually contains a mixture of cheese that has not fully ripened, so-called "green cheese," together with some aged cheese, such as Swiss, cheddar, or Roquefort. Emulsifiers are added for smoothness and texture and to prevent the fat from separating. Sorbic acid may be used to prevent mold growth. Nutritionally, it is similar to cheddar, providing 105 calories per ounce.

Cheese food, process. A similar blend to process cheese, it contains more moisture and less fat. It provides 90 calories per ounce.

Chestnuts. Imported from Italy, these nuts are popular in Europe where they are used in everything from soups to dessert. They have also been part of Chinese cuisine for centuries. They are relatively lower in calories than other nuts, providing 310 calories per cup. Most of the calories come from carbohydrate rather than fat. Unlike other nuts, chestnuts have a porous skin and lose moisture rapidly. They should, therefore, be kept in a refrigerator and used promptly—within a couple of weeks.

Cider, apple. Nutritionally the same as apple juice. Cider is usually made from a blend of juice from two or more apple varieties, selected for their flavor. The juice is simply strained and allowed to sit for several hours so that large particles and seeds not removed during pressing settle out. The particles which remain give cider its cloudy appearance, and the uptake of oxygen from the air impart the dark color and characteristic flavor. Small amounts of benzoate of soda may be added to extend shelf life by a few days. Because there is no Standard of Identity for cider, manufacturers can decide to produce a clearer drink, to pasteurize it, and to label the resulting beverage, indistinguishable from apple juice, as cider.

Citric acid. A natural compound found in vegetables and fruits, especially citrus fruits. As an additive, it is used to prevent fruits from turning brown during processing, to provide acidity in beverages and desserts, and to maintain color, control acidity, and enhance the flavor of tomatoes and certain other vegetables during canning. It may also be used in processed cheese to tie up metals that cause off flavors. Because it is also used in recipes for "sweet and sour" dishes, you are likely to find it on your supermarket shelf in the seasoning section. A recent investigation of taste preference confirmed the results of 20-year-old studies which demonstrated that citric acid also enhances saltiness. While the highest taste preference was for juice as normally salted during commercial processing, neither palatability nor perceived saltiness was significantly different when half of the salt was replaced with citric acid.

Cocoa, Dutch process. "Dutching" is a process in which cocoa beans are soaked in alkali to improve flavor and color. Hydroxide, sodium carbonate, and sodium bicarbonate are used in the process and add a little to the sodium content of the finished product. While regular cocoa contains negligible sodium, Dutch process contains about 40 milligrams per tablespoon.

Cornmeal, unbolted. Whole grain cornmeal. "Bolting" is a sifting process used to separate coarse particles of hull and some of the germ from the endosperm, or starchy portion of the corn kernel. Because fat in unbolted cornmeal makes it more vulnerable to rancidity, it should be stored in the refrigerator and used within a reasonably short period of time.

Corn syrup, regular. A viscous sweetener containing glucose molecules of different chain lengths, it was first produced in the 1920s by treating a watery cornstarch mixture with acids, heat, and/or enzymes. It is less sweet than sucrose.

Corn syrup, high fructose. Produced by an enzyme method developed during the 1970s, it contains between 40% and 100% fructose. Because it is sweeter than sucrose, less can be used to achieve the desired sweetness level.

Couscous. The term is used either for the tiny balls of semolina flour or to the stewlike mixture, which is the national dish of Morocco. It usually contains meat or chicken, vegetables, perhaps some dried fruit, and spices, as well as the couscous itself. How many calories and what other nutrients are in a stew will depend on the ingredients. However, ⅓ cup of the dry grain will provide about 200 calories.

Cruciferae. A family of vegetables, which includes the brassicas as well as cress, radishes, and horseradish.

Currants, zante. Unrelated to fresh currants, which are widely available in Europe in blue, red, and white, but are rare in this country, dried currants are produced from Black Corinth grapes. They provide 400 calories per cup. If eaten in large enough amounts they can contribute to iron intake. For example, ½ cup would provide 13% of the U.S. RDA for iron.

Daikon. Also called icicle radishes or winter radishes, they are shaped somewhat like turnips and may be black, violet, or red on the outside. They are frequently cut into very thin slices and perhaps into fancy shapes and eaten raw. The Japanese may also pickle them. In Oriental cooking they may be boiled or made into soup. They can also be grated and served with a more Westernized salad dressing, such as a vinaigrette with Dijon-style mustard. Nutritionally they are most notable for the fact that, like the radishes with which we are more familiar, they are very low in calories.

EDTA. Ethylene diaminetetraacetic acid, one of a number of so-called chelating agents. It ties up metal ions to stabilize processed foods. Many metals in foods, like magnesium in chlorophyll and iron in hemoglobin, exist in a chelated state. When released, as they might be in food processing, they can participate in reactions that can lead to undesirable changes, including discoloration, oxidative rancidity, turbidity, and alterations of flavor. Chelating agents are sometimes added to tie up these metals and prevent these reactions. EDTA is particularly effective in preventing oxidative changes in emulsified foods such as salad dressing, mayonnaise, and margarine. Because it is such an effective chelator, there have been questions about whether excessive use in foods could lead to the depletion of calcium and other minerals from the body. While it appears that this should not be a problem, measures have been taken to regulate the amount allowed and the types of uses to which it can be put. In some cases, to further reduce any possibility of excess chelation of minerals in food, EDTA is chemically modified by adding sodium and calcium.

Emulsifiers. Compounds which alter the surface properties of ingredients, thereby lowering their resistance to combine with other ingredients. While perhaps used most widely when it is necessary to mix oil and water, they are also used in other ways. In bakery products they improve volume, moisture retention, uniformity, and fineness of grain, retard staling and increase the strength of the dough. They improve the texture of pasta and inhibit clumping, a particular problem in commercially produced canned and frozen foods. In both dairy products and nondairy substitutes, like coffee whiteners, they provide stability to the existing emulsion and help maintain the starch and protein complexes in these foods. In ice cream, emulsifiers are used to insure proper texture. In processed cheese, they are responsible for keeping the fat, which holds the flavor, evenly dispersed, and for preventing the cheese from "weeping" as it melts.

Fennel. Popular in both France and Italy, fennel's overall appearance is similar to celery. Although the base or bulb is somewhat fatter and the leaves are feathery and fernlike, the tender stalks may be eaten raw like celery and both the stalks and the bulb, which are mildly anise-flavored, may be used in salads and cooked with celery. Fennel can also be braised and served plain or with a sauce, or it may be cooked together with a mixture of other vegetables.

Feta. A cheese made from the milk of cows, sheep, or goats, or from a mixture of sheep's milk and milk from either of these other animals. Native to Greece, it is now produced in a number of countries, including Denmark, Bulgaria, and the United States. Increasing amounts of French feta also appear to be making their way into the U.S. market. Feta's tart and tangy flavor comes in part from acid-forming bacteria which are used in separating the curds from the whey. An ounce of feta provides about 75 calories and about 6 grams of fat, making it somewhat lower in fat than many hard cheeses. Since it is packed and held in a brine solution, feta is among the saltier cheeses, containing on average more than 300 milligrams of sodium per ounce. Tastings of different batches indicate that some may contain considerably more.

Flour, bleached. Bleaching is a commercial "aging" process. When freshly milled, flour has a rather yellowish color and produces baked products of relatively low volume and coarse texture. If allowed to stand for several months, natural oxidation whitens the flour. The texture becomes finer and baking quality improves. Natural aging is somewhat impractical, requiring both time and large amounts of space. The flour must also be carefully protected against insects and vermin. Moreover, oxidation does not proceed evenly throughout the sack. At the beginning of the twentieth century, food technologists found that bleaching and maturing agents could quickly achieve the same effect as natural aging. Some of the additives used do destroy vitamin E, but white flour is not an important source of vitamin E anyway. Both bleached and unbleached flours are readily available, and if a flour has been bleached it must say so on the label.

Flour, instantized or instant-blending flour. Regular all-purpose flour, to which a little mashed barley flour may have been added. It is processed by moistening and redrying. As a result of this processing, the flour forms small particles of similar size which stick together to form larger particles with somewhat different properties than regular flour. The advantages claimed for instantized flour are that it does not pack, requires no sifting, flows freely, creating no dust, and measures easily. The resulting granules, which have a porous structure similar to that of nonfat dry milk particles, blend more easily with liquids than regular flour. Because it doesn't lump, instantized flour is of some benefit in making gravies and sauces. However, the cost of the convenience is considerable.

Fruit spreads. These "substitutes" for jam and jelly, made from juice concentrate, contain 14 calories per teaspoon, compared to 16 and 18 for jam and jelly, respectively. They do not provide appreciable amounts of vitamins and minerals.

Ginseng. A root used in Oriental folk medicine for its curative and preventative properties, as well as for aphrodisiac powers. Popular literature in this country has promoted using the root in tea or as a liquid extract to boost energy, and in capsule form for disease resistance. Ginseng does contain certain compounds which have been shown to produce physiological effects in laboratory animals. But no controlled studies have demonstrated benefit to humans. Moreover, a variety of symptoms in people who have taken large amounts over long periods have been reported. Finally, analyses of "ginseng" products have found that many of those available contained very little or no ginseng at all.

Gjetost. Pronounced "yay-toast," it has a sweet, caramel-like flavor. It is native to Norway, where it has been the national cheese for over 100 years. It is one of the few cheeses made from whey rather from the casein-rich curds. Gjetost may be made solely from goat's milk or from a mixture of 10% goat's-milk whey and 90% cow's-milk whey. A similar cheese, Mysost, is made from 100%-cow's milk whey. Nutritionally these cheeses are somewhat different than other cheeses. In addition to the lactose naturally present in whey, more is added during production. So an ounce of cheese contains as much carbohydrate as a glass of milk, but less than half the protein in the milk or in an ounce of other hard cheeses. The fat content, 8 grams per ounce, is comparable to that in other common cheeses, including Edam, fontina, or Swiss. If wrapped tightly, it will keep quite a long time in the refrigerator.

Granola. There is no true definition of the term. The first granola, or "granula," as it was called, was produced by Dr. James C. Jackson of Dansville, N.Y. in the late nineteenth century. A heavy whole-wheat dough was baked into loaves until dry, broken into pieces, baked again, and ground into smaller pieces. The pieces were soaked overnight to be eaten as breakfast cereal. Today, granola recipes vary greatly. Many of the commercial varieties contain considerable amounts of sweeteners as well as fat, which may be highly saturated. The only way to learn about the nutrient composition of a particular granola is to check the labeling information.

Guar gum. Actually a mucilage, it is extracted from the endosperm, or starchy portion of leguminous guar seeds. In the plant, it protects the seed against drying. Commercially, it is of value because of its thickening and jelling properties. Another common source of mucilage is locust bean or carob seeds. Common gums you're likely to see on ingredients lists include gum arabic, karaya gum, and gum tragacanth.

Guava. A fruit native to Mexico and South America, now being cultivated in Hawaii, southern California, and Florida. The color of the fruit, which has a rather pearlike shape and a somewhat tangy flavor, depends on the variety. Those available in the U.S. are usually green to yellow. Usually served raw, either alone or in fruit cup, it may also be used in fruit ices. A 3½-ounce fruit provides 45 calories, along with very generous amounts of vitamin C, some beta carotene, and some B vitamins. It is also a good source of potassium.

Gum arabic. A water-soluble polysaccharide made up of many single units of glucose which exudes in teardrop-shaped globules from bark wounds to acacia trees. In use for over 2,000 years, it is of particular value when a highly soluble gum is needed. In sweets it prevents sugar from crystallizing, prevents moisture absorption in icing and glazes on baked goods, and is used either as an emulsifier or foam stabilizer in some beverages. It may be used in ice cream and other dairy products to help form and maintain small ice crystals.

Gum tragacanth. A water-soluble polysaccharide collected from a low, bushy shrub called astragalus, which grows in the Middle East. Because it is stable in heat and acid, gum tragacanth is especially useful in salad dressings and sauces. It may also provide body and texture in frozen desserts and improve quality in frozen fruit pie fillings.

Jicama. A very common root vegetable in Mexico, jicama gets its name from the Aztec word *xicamatl* and is also known as yambean. It can be cooked by first peeling away the skin and tough layer immediately underneath, and then boiling, steaming, or frying it as you would a potato.

Make sure to cook it only until it is tender. Smaller roots can be eaten raw, either sliced into salad or served with a dunking sauce. A whole cup of raw slices provides 50 calories, mainly from carbohydrate. Both the raw and cooked varieties provide some vitamin C and small amounts of B vitamins.

Kefir. A sour-milk product, which originated in the Caucasus. The rather chalky-textured product is produced by adding two types of bacteria, lactobacilli and streptococci, and a lactose-fermenting yeast to fresh milk. Kefir, available in supermarkets, is commonly jazzed up by the addition of a variety of sweeteners—raspberries, honey, or raspberry and apple concentrate. There appears to be no particular health benefit to drinking kefir, and if made with whole milk, it is a relatively generous source of saturated fat.

Kiwi. A relatively new fruit to Americans, kiwi have apparently grown in the Yangtze valley in China since time immemorial, and has been in cultivation in China for about 300 years. In China, the fruit is known as yangtao. At the turn of this century, horticulturalists in New Zealand began to cultivate them and renamed the fruit the Chinese gooseberry. (The more exotic name, kiwi, was chosen to tempt Americans who are not familir with the gooseberry.) In 1953, New Zealand first exported the fruit to London. An average kiwi contains about 55 calories, putting it into the ball park with a grapefruit half or a small orange. It also provides over 1½ times the Recommended Dietary Allowance for vitamin C, and it is a good source of potassium.

Kohlrabi. Sometimes called "turnip cabbage," it gets its name from the German word *kohl* (cabbage) and the Latin word *rapa* (turnip). Although the name of the vegetable certainly does not have an Oriental ring, you are quite likely to find it in Chinese markets. That's because kohlrabi was brought to China from Europe during the early seventh century and has been part of the Chinese diet ever since. Botanically a member of the cabbage family, it has a pale green round stem growing just above the ground. While the young leaves are edible, the turniplike root is generally considered the better part of the vegetable. Kohlrabi can be prepared by slicing or dicing it and cooking until tender in boiling water. Or it may also be served *au gratin* or with a cream sauce. Sometimes it is even stuffed. Cold, it can be served with a vinaigrette dressing. A cup of cooked kohlrabi contains about 40 calories, some B vitamins, and considerable vitamin C. It is also an excellent source of potassium.

Leek. One of the oldest vegetables cultivated by man. The ancient Sumerians, whose Farmer's Almanac dating back to 2500 B.C. is one of the earliest surviving reference works, included leeks, along with garlic and onions, among the staples of their diet. Nutritionally, their contribution is modest. Three-and-a-half ounces (about 3 fairly small leeks trimmed to a length of 5 inches) provide about 50 calories and a little calcium, as well as some B vitamins and iron. The raw vegetable also contains a significant amount of vitamin C, but much of that is probably destroyed when the leeks are cooked. The dark green portions of the leaves undoubtedly contain vitamin A, and it is a pity they are often discarded. Gently braised with the rest of the leek, they lose their toughness.

Mahi-mahi. Native to Hawaii, it is also called dolphin fish. It is quite lean, with 3 ounces providing only 95 calories.

Mango. Sometimes called the apple of the tropics, it is the most widely eaten and favorite tropical fruit. Mangoes have been under cultivation since before recorded history, so there is no way to know for sure where they originated. It is believed that they are native to India and were originally grown from eastern India through Burma. Even today, India is the world's most important producer of the many varieties of mangoes, which range in size from a plum to a football, and weigh 4 or 5 pounds. In this country, mangoes are grown most successfully in southern Florida. Nutritionally, they are most notable as a source of carotene, the vegetable form of vitamin A. Half of a medium mango, or about a cup of the diced fruit, provides about 110 calories and supplies over one-and-a-half times the U.S. RDA for vitamin A, as well as enough ascorbic acid to more than meet the day's need. Mangoes are also an excellent source of potassium and fiber, and they contain some B vitamins. Mangoes should ripen at room temperature until just soft to the touch.

Mayonnaise. According to the Standard of Identity, or legal recipe for mayonnaise, it must contain at least 65% oil as well as egg yolk, acidifying agents, like vinegar or lemon juice, and seasonings, including salt, sugar, and spices such as mustard and paprika. It contains 100 calories per tablespoon. While mayonnaise depends entirely on the emulsifying properties of egg yolk for thickening, mayonnaise-type salad dressing is thickened in part by a paste made either from food starch or from wheat, rye, or tapioca flour. It contains 65 calories per tablespoon.

Milk, buttermilk. Originally, buttermilk was the liquid left in the churn after the butter was removed. It was, therefore, low in fat. Most of today's buttermilk is similarly low in fat, but for a different reason. While it may be made from whole milk, it is most commonly produced from skim milk to which a specially prepared bacterial culture is added. Two factors contribute to the smooth, heavy texture. One is the result of bacterial action. The other is that buttermilk is pasteurized at a higher temperature and for a longer period of time than regular milk. It is now available in fat-free form, providing 90 calories per cup, or with 1% fat, providing 100 calories per cup. If salt is added, as it commonly is, sodium content may be as high as 250 milligrams, almost double that in a cup of regular milk.

Milk, evaporated. Milk in which a little more than half the water has been removed from fresh whole or skim milk. Nutritionally, the only difference between fresh milk and evaporated milk is that if used undiluted, evaporated milk contains twice as many calories and other nutrients per ounce as the milk from which it was made. Evaporated whole milk contains roughly 40 calories per ounce and evaporated skim milk about 20 calories per ounce. Under current federal regulations, if shipped in interstate commerce, it must be fortified with Vitamin D. Evaporated milk, which costs less than whole milk, can be diluted with an equal amount of water and used in any recipe which calls for whole milk.

Milk, sweet acidophilus. Milk to which lactobacillus acidophilus bacteria are added. While growing the bacteria in the milk produces an undesirable tart flavor, adding them directly preserves the natural milk flavor, as long as the milk is kept cold. Studies have failed to demonstrate that sweet acidophilus milk is of benefit to individuals with lactose intolerance.

Milk, sweetened condensed. Milk prepared by first adding 15% sugar to fresh whole milk and then removing two-thirds of the water. The resulting product contains over 40% sugar and about 120 calories an ounce. Because of its high sugar content, it is generally used only in certain types of baked products. Even when diluted as directed, it provides more than twice as many calories per ounce as regular whole milk.

Milk, UHT. Introduced in Europe over 20 years ago, UHT (ultra high-temperature milk) was first marketed in this country in 1980. It was expected to provide some relief from the traditional problems associated with marketing fresh milk, especially perishability and sharp seasonal variability in supply and demand. But consumer acceptance did not grow as expected. One major drawback is that while the flavor is superior to that of canned milk, it is not comparable to fresh milk. The very high temperatures used to process it as a sterile product, and slight increases in temperature or holding time, cause significant flavor problems. Moreover, higher production costs are not offset by lower handling and storing costs. It, therefore, costs the consumer more for a product they will find less acceptable. So, while UHT milk now accounts for more than 20% of the milk sold in France, Germany, Italy, and Switzerland, use in this country is expected to be limited.

Millet. A staple cereal food for humans in much of the world, including India, Africa, China, and even parts of Russia. One of its advantages is that it will grow in poorer soils and can withstand extremes of weather better than other, generally more popular, cereals. Thought to have originated in Asia or Africa during the Neolithic era, it was probably the first cereal to be cultivated. In Europe, during the Middle Ages, more millet was grown than wheat. Millet flour has no gluten and, therefore, it cannot be used by itself in leavened bread. It may be baked into a flatbread, but it is usually used as a gruel or cereal. A half-cup of cooked millet cereal or porridge contains about 55 calories, mostly from carbohydrate. It also provides some iron and small amounts of B vitamins.

Miso. A centuries-old Oriental sauce made from fermenting a mixture of soybeans, sometimes a cereal grain, salt, and a mixture of microorganisms which is allowed to ferment. Miso has a texture similar to peanut butter and varies in color from yellow-brown to almost black.

Modified food starch (MFS). Starches produced by changing the carbohydrate chain. The process of making modified food starch involves chemical treatment and may include bleaching, the addition of oxygen to the starch, partial splitting of starch chains or restructuring the chains by adding other compounds. The raw materials from which MFS may be derived include tapioca, potatoes, or one of several cereals such as wheat, rice, or corn. The variety of sources and different modifications provide food processors with additives containing different properties. MFS can affect clarity, acid tolerance, gel permanence, and even blandness of flavor. They are used to increase the viscosity or thickness of a solution, to keep ingredients from separating, and to prevent caking of powdered sugar and baking powder. Despite its widespread use, it was estimated several years ago that a man weighing 150 pounds consumes on average, 1 gram or a quarter of a teaspoon a day.

Molasses. The residue remaining after most of the sucrose crystals are removed from the concentrated juices of either sugar cane or sugar beets. By weight, it contains 70% sugars, including sucrose, glucose, and fructose, about 25% water, and a maximum of 5% mineral ash. Not all molasses commercially available is a "by-product" of sugar production. One form is produced directly from sun-ripened sugar cane and is generally sold as "unsulphured molasses." (The sulfur remaining in some molasses is present as a residue left behind when a sulfur-containing compound is used in the production of sugar from sugar beets.) Blackstrap molasses, an unpalatable component of many folk remedies, is what remains after the sugar concentration in the syrup is too low to make further extraction feasible. Most is used in rum production. Molasses does contain some nutrients other than calories, most notably iron and some calcium.

Just how much depends on the concentration of the sweetener. Light molasses provides less than a milligram of iron per tablespoon, while the blackstrap variety contains over 3 milligrams or 16% of the Recommended Dietary Allowance. Similarly, there are just 33 milligrams of calcium in a tablespoon of the former; the latter contains 137 milligrams, an amount comparable to that in a half-cup of milk.

Monoglycerides and diglycerides. Molecules in which glycerol is linked to just one or two fatty acids. They occur naturally and can be formed during cooking. Commercially they are produced by heating fats and oils. The chemical configuration of these glycerides allows them to act very effectively as emulsifiers and to improve the texture and consistency of many different products. They are used to prevent the oil and peanuts in peanut butter from separating, to keep margarine from splattering when heated, and to improve the incorporation of air into commercial cake mixes, thereby increasing their volume. Mono-and diglycerides are also produced in the body during the digestion of fats and, unlike triglycerides, which must be broken down into these smaller units, both can be absorbed.

Oil, "winterized." Oil that has been processed to prevent certain fatty acids in it from crystallizing and thus giving it a cloudy appearance as it sits on the shelf. Commonly, drums of oil are put in rooms at temperatures lower than that to which they will be exposed later. The crystals which form are then removed.

Okra. A member of the hibiscus, or mallow, family of plants, the same group which provided the gummy juice from which the French made the first marshmallowlike candy called *paté de Guimauve.* Gastronomically, okra, which the British call lady's fingers, is prized by those who like gumbo for the gelatinous quality it imparts to the dish. To avoid the gummy texture which many people find objectionable, okra can be sautéed slowly in a little oil, a method commonly used in Indian cooking. A cup of cooked okra provides 50 calories, as well as considerable ascorbic acid, some beta carotene and protein, and small amounts of B vitamins.

Orange roughy. Available in this country only since 1982, it is one of a group of fish from New Zealand being marketed here in increasing numbers. The fish, as you would expect, is orange. It has a large head and weighs about 3½ pounds. The pale white flesh has a relatively firm and flaky texture, similar to haddock or cusk. It is very low in calories, only 76 in a 3½-ounce portion, and virtually all of these calories come from protein.

Ornithine. An amino acid from which the body builds proteins. It is often sold at health food stores in combination with arginine.

Palmitate. A long-chain fatty acid found in palm oil often attached to vitamin A when that nutrient is added to food. While it is highly saturated, the amount present is too small to be of any consequence.

Papain. An enzyme, the "active ingredient" in meat tenderizer. It is readily destroyed at relatively low temperatures, and in the unlikely event that any papain remains in cooked meat, it is quickly destroyed by stomach acid. There are critical temperatures at which papain works best. Remaining inactive in the refrigerator, it works slowly at room temperature, and becomes increasingly effective at temperatures of up to 150°F. Above that, it is destroyed. Meat tenderizer, then, has its greatest impact when the meat is first put in the oven. There is really no reason to apply it several hours in advance while the meat is still sitting in the refrigerator. Natives of Mexico, South America, and the South Sea Islands have long tenderized their meat by wrapping it in papaya leaves. The leaves, like the underripe fruit from which papain is extracted commercially, also contain the enzyme.

Papaya. A rather bland fruit with a slightly sweet taste. It is grown only in limited areas in this country—in Hawaii, Florida and southern California. Health food manufacturers have produced a wide variety of "digestive aids" containing papaya, papaya leaves, or papain. All are ineffective. Papain is destroyed by stomach acid and therefore is useless as a digestive aid.

Parsnips. Hardly regarded as nutritional powerhouses, medieval physicians believed them to have remarkable powers, including an ability to cure toothaches, treat stomachaches, and even to keep snakes away. The origin of the root, which was a dietary staple in Europe during the Middle Ages and an especially important food during Lent and on other fast days, remains a mystery. A half-cup serving of mashed parsnip provides about 80 calories, nearly all from carbohydrate. It also provides some vitamin C and folic acid, small amounts of other B vitamins, and it is a good source of fiber.

Passion fruit. Also called a purple granadilla, from a Spanish word meaning little pomegranate. There is, however, also a yellow variety. It belongs to the same group of plants as the well-known passionflower associated with the Signs of the Passion. The flower, native to Brazil, was especially prized by Spanish Jesuit missionaries who believed it had been thoughtfully arranged by the creator and planted in the New World to help in the conversion of the Indians. Most species are grown for their ornamental flowers rather than for the fruit. The flowers of the fruit-bearing varieties are not especially impressive. A one-ounce fruit provides only 18 calories. It also provides some vitamin C and amounts of both vitamin A and B vitamins.

Pear apple. Tottori, or twentieth-century pears, as they are called, were found growing wild on the northern coast of Western Japan at the turn of the century. Also known as the "King of the Japanese pears," they are grown with great care. Blossoms are hand pollinated, and once the fruit begins to mature, they are wrapped in wax-treated bags as protection against insects and disease. They are quite mildly flavored, and have a more pronounced grittiness than other pears. That is because they contain more lignin, a so-called nonpolysaccharide fraction of fiber. A 3½-ounce serving provides about 40 calories.

Persimmon. Also called Japanese persimmon, it is actually native to China and remains popular in both countries. Early colonists in this country used a different variety, a native persimmon, to make a fermented beer-like beverage. A piece of fruit weighing about 7 ounces contains 130 calories. It is perhaps most notable as a good source of beta carotene, which the body converts to vitamin A, but it also contains some B vitamins and vitamin C and is a good source of potassium.

Pine nuts. The naked seeds of pine trees, which until recently came to us mainly from Italy and Spain. The pine nuts we now get come from Portugal and China. An ounce of nuts, about ¼ cup, provides about 155 calories, more than 70% of them from fat. Data with respect to other nutrients is limited. But they do provide some iron and small amounts of several B vitamins.

Plantains. Similar to bananas, they are calorically more dense, with 3½ ounces (⅔ cup) providing 120 calories compared to 90 in a banana. While frying is a common method of preparing them, they can be diced and added raw to soups, stews, or omelets. They can also be diced and cooked in boiling water until tender. Plantains are apparently native to India and Malaya, and were introduced to Africa at around 500 A.D., and to the Americas by Spanish and Portuguese explorers during the fifteenth and sixteenth centuries.

Pretzels. A type of cracker. Made with enriched flour, they provide some B vitamins and iron as well as a little protein. An ounce of pretzels, whether consumed as two long rods or 30 thin sticks, contributes about 115 calories. Our real reservation about pretzels has to do with the amount of salt they contain. The very thinnest rods are really little more than a vehicle for salt. The fatter the pretzel, the higher the ratio of cracker to salt and, to our mind, the more desirable the pretzel. With increased emphasis on cutting down on salt, unsalted pretzels are widely available and the preferred choice.

Prickly pear. This fruit, native to North America and introduced to Europe by the Spanish in the sixteenth century, grows on the prickly pear cactus. It is also known by several other names, including Indian pear and

Indian, Barbary, or tuna fig. A whole fruit, peeled and eaten as is, contains about 500 calories, small amounts of B vitamins, minerals, and considerable vitamin C.

Propionate, sodium (or calcium). So-called "salts" of propionic acid, they retard mold growth and help prevent "ropiness," which can occur in nonacid bread stored in a damp environment. Ropiness is caused by a bacteria called *Bacillus mesentericus.* The spores, which can be present in the flour or other ingredients used to make bread, are not destroyed by baking. Within a few days, the growing bacteria cause the interior of the bread to develop a sticky texture which can be pulled into syrupy "ropes." An unpleasant odor, sometimes described as that of "overripe melon" develops at the same time. Propionic acid, the basic compound in these additives, is also the result of bacterial action. It is produced naturally in Swiss cheese by bacteria acting on lactic acid. It is responsible for the characteristic "eyes," and contributes to the nutty flavor of the cheese. It is believed that while man has no trouble in metabolizing this fatty acid compound, bacteria and mold cannot break it down and it is, therefore, toxic to them.

Pyrophosphate. An additive that can effectively prevent crystal formation in canned fish. Not too many years ago, it was not uncommon to find clear crystals that might have been mistaken for glass in canned fish, including both tuna and shrimp. The crystals were actually a chemical compound called magnesium ammonium sulfate. Struvite, as it was called, which formed naturally during processing, is not harmful.

Quince. A round yellow fruit which resembles a yellow delicious apple. They are the original fruit for marmalade which gets its name from the Portuguese word for quince, *marmelo.* Because it contains considerable pectin and acid, quince is a good fruit for making preserves. Some varieties can be eaten raw if very ripe. However, a small amount of cooking, either baking or stewing with little or no sweetener, is more usual. Since they bruise easily, it is best to buy them underripe and let them ripen in a brown bag. A whole quince, weighing about 5 ounces, provides 55 calories and small amounts of vitamins and minerals. Native to central Asia, they occupied an important spot in ancient Greek and Roman mythology as the fruit of love, marriage, and fertility.

Rice, brown. Rice containing most of the whole grain, with just a small part of the bran removed, making it a somewhat better source of fiber than white rice. It also contains some minerals that are stripped away during the milling process and not added back during enrichment. Because the bran layer of brown rice contains some oil, it does not keep as well as white rice, which will stay on the shelf for years.

Rice, converted. Rice treated by soaking whole brown rice kernels, steaming them under pressure, and drying them. This process forces the water-soluble vitamins and minerals from the bran and germ into the endosperm, preserving as much as 90% of the water-soluble vitamins in the whole grain. Converted rice is sometimes supplemented with B vitamins and iron, however.

Rice, enriched. Rice to which iron and the vitamins thiamin, niacin, and riboflavin are added back after the milling process.

Rice, wild. Not a true rice, but the seed of a plant called *zivania aquatica,* or "water grass." It was first harvested several hundred years ago from boats by the Chippewa Indians in the shallow lakes and streams that dot northern Minnesota and Canada. During the 1800s, the Indians used it as a food to barter with traders. Nutritionally, wild rice is generally comparable to regular white rice, although it does contain a little more protein and a few less calories. Like regular rice, it also provides some B vitamins and iron.

Rose fish. A particularly good variety of ocean perch. Because it has a firm texture and delicate flavor, it lends itself to almost any cooking method. Exact analyses for rose fish are not available. But you can assume that, nutritionally, it closely resembles other types of ocean perch. That is, 4 ounces of raw fish contain about 120 calories, over 20 grams of protein, and a small amount of fat.

Rutabaga. A variety of turnip which apparently originated in Bohemia in the seventeenth century, and was later introduced to Sweden, where it is, in fact, called "swede." The name we give it comes from a Swedish dialect word, *rotbagga,* or ram's root, which we Anglicize to rutabaga. Eaten raw, it is quite low in calories. A half-cup, rather a lot to eat raw, provides just 30 calories as well as some B vitamins and vitamin A. Cooked and mashed, a half-cup provides just 40 calories, unless you add margarine or butter to it.

Sablefish. Also named black cod, because of its greenish to slate-black skin on the top, or butterfish. It typically weighs about 8 pounds, but can grow up to 40 pounds. Its high fat content makes it particularly desirable for smoking. Three-and-a-half ounces contain 185 calories.

Salsify. For reasons which remain unclear since it has neither the taste nor the texture of the mollusk, it is commonly but mistakenly called oyster plant. In fact, we think it most closely resembles a mild parsnip in flavor. A tuberous vegetable, which freshly grows in a long, rather parsniplike shape, it provides just 16 calories per cup when freshly dug. During storage, the calorie content climbs to as much as 95 per cup as the indigestible carbohydrate called inulin is converted to simple sugars the body can use. Salsify also contains some B vitamins and iron, and it's an excellent source of potassium. Most of the "salsify" available in local markets is not true salsify, which has a white skin, but its cousin, called "scorzonera," or black oyster plant. The two taste almost the same.

Scrod. A term most often used to describe a young cod, weighing between 1½ and 2½ pounds. Other young fish, including haddock and sometimes even pollock, may also be labeled "scrod." Nutritionally there is very little difference among these fish. A whole pound of raw cod or haddock provides about 355 calories, nearly all of them from protein. The cod contains less than 1½ grams of fat per pound and the haddock less than a half-gram. Pollock is a bit more dense and slightly fattier, but not enough to make a big difference. It contains about 4 grams of fat and about 75 calories more than either cod or haddock per pound.

Sea salt. Usually promoted on the grounds that it is more "natural," sea salt contains mainly the same sodium chloride found in ordinary table salt. In fact, sodium chloride accounts for 95% of the weight of sea salt. The other 5% is made up mainly of compounds of magnesium and calcium. While both of these minerals are essential, the amounts you would get from sea salt are of little consequence nutritionally. Moreover, the iodine in sea salt is lost during the drying process.

Semolina. The milled endosperm, or starch portion, of the durum wheat kernel. Because of the structural relationship between the protein and starch and because of the higher ratio of protein to starch in the flour, durum wheat is the grain of choice for making pasta.

Sodium benzoate. An additive which both prevents microorganisms from utilizing the energy-rich compounds they need to live and interferes with the growth of spores. In the presence of benzoate, microbial spores may take up water and germinate to the point of bursting the spore wall, but then are unable to enlarge and grow into cells which can divide and multiply. The many foods in which benzoates, and their chemical cousins, parabenzoates, are used include fruit juice, pickled vegetables, relishes, cheeses, carbonated beverages, and syrups, especially chocolate syrup. Benzoic acid, from which sodium benzoate is derived, occurs naturally in cranberry concentrations as high as 4% to 5%, many times the amount which is used as an additive in food processing.

Sorbitol. A sugar alcohol often used in low calorie foods. It is absorbed more slowly than regular sugar, but it provides just as many calories. Excessive amounts can cause gastrointestinal discomfort, including diarrhea.

Sorrel. Sometimes called dock. It is used quite widely in France and in many other countries, but it tends to be available in this country only in a limited number of stores, usually those that carry specialty produce items. It does grow wild in some places, if you know where to look, and apparently is quite easy to cultivate. Sorrel is a rich source of vitamin A. It contains some vitamin C and it is, of course, low in calories. It is used raw in salads, as a filling in omelettes, or as a major seasoning in soups and sauces for fish, veal, and eggs. It can be served as a vegetable by itself, either braised or pureed, but because of its strong flavor, it is more commonly mixed with other greens, like spinach or chard.

Squid. A mollusk, whose shell has evolved into an internal cartilage, which, because of its shape is called a "pen" or "quill." Squid is high in protein and low in fat and calories, with just 95 in a 4-ounce serving. It is among the more generous sources of dietary cholesterol, however.

Stabilizers. Additives used in situations where a solid, liquid, or foam is dispersed in a liquid medium, and there is a tendency for the dispersed substance to become unstable, or separate out. Stabilizers minimize this tendency.

Sugar, beet. Sucrose was first extracted from bees during the mid-eighteenth century by Andreas Morgraf, a German chemist. It took the Napoleonic Wars, some 60 years later, to spark the commercial development of the sugar beet industry. The advantage of sugar beets, a white root much larger than the familiar red vegetable, is that, unlike sugar cane, they can be grown in a temperate climate. When the English blockades of European ports threatened a cutoff of West Indian cane sugar, Napoleon ordered the commercial planting of sugar beets and factories to process them. Waterloo and the lifting of the blockades dampened the development of the sugar beet industry. In fact, it did not become firmly established in Europe until the mid-ninteenth century and somewhat later in this country. At present, about 40% of the world's sucrose comes from beets.

Sugar, cane. Apparently native to India, it is known to have been used as early as 400 B.C. The cultivation of sugar spread quite slowly at first, reaching China around the first century B.C. It came to the Mediterranean much later, possibly in the sixth century A.D. The Crusaders, who tasted what they called "honey from the reeds," brought cane sugar back to central and western Europe. The development of sugar plantations in tropical and semitropical countries which began in the sixteenth century made sugar far more plentiful (though still an expensive luxury) and spurred the tragic expansion of the slave trade.

Sugar, invert. A mixture of two simple sugars, glucose and fructose, it has several properties which make it useful to the confectionary industry. It decreases the rate of crystallization as syrup cools and retards the development of larger crystals during storage. It also attracts water, which helps to prevent chewy candy from drying out. It is produced commercially for the confectionary industry, but it forms naturally during cooking when an acid like cream of tartar is present.

Sugar, raw. Varying in color from tan to brown, it is a coarse, granulated solid obtained by evaporating the juice expressed out of sugar cane. According to FDA regulations, raw sugar may be sold only if dirt and other impurities are removed.

Sugar, turbinado. Erroneously called raw sugar sometimes, it is produced by separating raw sugar crystals and washing them with steam. Refining eliminates the impurities and most of the molasses. Neither turbinado nor raw sugar differs significantly from ordinary sucrose or table sugar.

Superoxide dismutase (SOD). An enzyme that acts as a free radical scavenger, helping to break down the products of body metabolism as well as harmful substances taken in from the environment. It is found not only in human cells but in all life forms that use oxygen. While the superoxide dismutase produced by our bodies is certainly essential to health, taking it by mouth to forestall aging, promote good looks, or for any other reasons is useless. Not only is SOD not a wonder supplement, but when it is taken by mouth, it will not reach the cells intact. The reason is that it is a protein. Therefore, if taken orally, it will be digested like any other protein.

Surimi. The basic ingredient for making imitation crab legs and other seafood look-alikes. First produced by Japanese fishermen about 1100 A.D. as a means of keeping fish, the process involves several steps. Mechanically deboned fish, usually Pacific pollock, is washed with cold water to remove all taste and odor, and then drained and strained. The resulting pulp is mixed with sugar, water, sorbitol, salt, and polysorbates. It is then shaped and frozen. If surimi is to be made into imitation seafoods, it is thawed, mixed with other ingredients, and shaped.

Sweet potatoes. Native to tropical America, the flesh is usually yellow to orange, but there are red and purple varieties. Calorically more dense than white potatoes, a 3½-ounce potato provides 140 calories. They are an excellent source of carotene and provide considerable vitamin C, as well as B vitamins, iron, and other minerals, especially potassium.

Tannins. Colorless compounds in tea which combine with minerals such as calcium and magnesium as the tea cools to form dark brown tannin complexes. Adding lemon juice, and thereby making the solution more acid, reverses the reaction, dissolving the particles and lightening the color. It is the release of large amounts of tannins during prolonged brewing of tea leaves which causes the excessive astringency and puckery feeling in the mouth.

Tapioca. A starchy product made from the cassava or manioc root. In the U.S., it is sold either in coarse granular form or in pearls of varying size and is used mainly as a thickening agent. Two tablespoons, enough to thicken four servings of pudding, contains about 60 calories, virtually all of them from carbohydrate. Tapioca is of some value as a thickening for sauces and gravies for individuals who are allergic to wheat or who have gluten-sensitive enteropathy and must avoid wheat, rye, oats, and barley. Two teaspoons of quick-cooking tapioca replace 1 tablespoon of wheat flour.

Tempeh. Originally from Indonesia, it is produced by adding spores of a microorganism called *Rhizopus oligosporus* to soybeans which have been soaked, boiled, dehulled, drained, and dehydrated. The mixture is then wrapped in banana leaves or placed in perforated containers and held at a warm temperature for 24 hours. During that time, the spores produce a network of branching filaments or "mycelia," which hold the soybeans together in a cakelike form. Tempeh is usually sliced and fried.

Tilefish. A lean, white-fleshed fish, of which there are several varieties from both Atlantic and Pacific waters. Tilefish has a mild, shellfishlike flavor. A 6-ounce serving provides just 135 calories.

Tripe. The lining of the first two stomachs of ruminant animals. The first and largest of these, the rumen, provides honeycomb tripe, so-called because of its appearance. Among food authorities, it has received less than rave reviews. Waverly Root, the late food historian, says "it is an ideal carrier for other tastes since it has virtually none of its own to compete with them, once it has been cooked long enough to rid itself of its boiling-laundry odor." It provides just 28 calories per ounce and is low in fat and cholesterol, so long as you do not add a lot of fat in preparing it.

Triticale. A cereal grain first found growing in Scotland more than 100 years ago. It is a cross between wheat and rye and gets its name from the Latin word for wheat, *triticum,* and secale for rye. It contains more protein and protein of higher quality than other grains, and some varieties may be more resistant to cold and drought than wheat. With the recent development of better strains, it is now being grown in the U.S., Canada, and other countries.

Turkey ham. Cured turkey thigh meat, low in fat and high in protein. The addition of moisture makes it lower in calories than dark-meat turkey, providing 37 per ounce compared to 53 per ounce. However, considerable sodium is added in processing. So while regular turkey provides 25 illigrams of sodium per ounce, the same amount of cured meat contains 280 milligrams.

Water, club soda. Water to which minerals are added for flavoring. These may include sodium bicarbonate, sodium phosphate, salt, and potassium sulfate. The addition of these compounds means that the amount of sodium they contain varies. Some brands are labeled, but some are not.

Water, seltzer. Drinking water that has been filtered and carbonated. Those we have found were labeled "sodium free," but it is possible that if they were prepared in an area where the sodium content of the water was high, they would contain more. For that reason, it is a good idea to check the label for sodium information.

Wheat berries. A fancy name for whole-wheat kernels.

Wheat germ. The sprouting portion of the wheat kernel. Wheat germ contains B vitamins, especially thiamin, a little protein, and some minerals. It is where all of the fat in the wheat kernel is found, and with that fat there is some vitamin E. In fact, largely because it contains vitamin E, wheat germ has gained a reputation as a "special" food. While it is a good source of vitamin E, it is hardly the only one. Vitamin E is also found in vegetable oils and margarines, as well as in whole-grain breads and cereals, green leafy vegetables, nuts, and seeds.

Wheat, sprouted. Whole-wheat kernels that have been sprouted. Wheat kernel sprouts can be grown at home using the same method as for growing other types of sprouts.

Xanthan gum. A polysaccharide food additive and the only one which comes from microbes. A variety of characteristics make it particularly useful in salad dressings, where it allows the liquid to flow easily from the bottle, then to cling to the vegetables or other foods on which it is used. Since it disperses readily in hot or cold water, it is used to control viscosity in dry mixes for milk shakes, sauces, bakery fillings, and desserts. It is also combined with other additives to modify texture. In some cases it is effective as a flavor improver. And small amounts may be added to starch-thickened frozen foods to improve their stability.

Xylitol. A sugar alcohol which occurs naturally in small amounts in strawberries, raspberries, and other fruits and vegetables. In Finland, where it is widely used, it is produced both from birch chips and berries. Although xylitol is about as sweet as sugar and provides a comparable number of calories, insulin is not needed for its metabolism. For this reason it has been used as a sweetener by diabetics in some European countries. When taken in large amounts, however, it causes flatulence and diarrhea.

Yams. Botanically unrelated to sweet potatoes, true yams, whose flesh may range from white to yellow, generally weigh between 2 and 8 pounds, but can reach 100 pounds or more. Native to Africa and probably introduced to this country by slaves, yams are calorically quite dense, providing 80 calories per half-cup serving. In terms of vitamins and minerals they are quite unremarkable, with one exception. They are a potent source of potassium.

Yeast, brewer's "debittered". Brewer's yeast supplements are produced from yeast that has been used in beer production. The yeast is washed in an alkaline solution to remove bitter-tasting compounds, including hop resins and tannins that collected on the surface of microorganisms during processing.

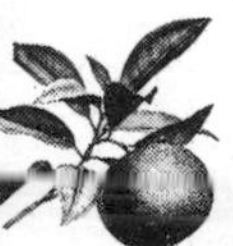

28-DAY MENU PLAN WITH RECIPES

The four weeks of menus which follow have been planned with a particular emphasis on current recommendations with respect to fat, saturated fat, cholesterol, and sodium. Believing that it is easier for nondieters to increase portions to meet their caloric requirements, we have specified portions for 1,200 calories, with suggestions about how to add more calories without adding excessive amounts of salt, fat, and sugar. We have tried to ensure that each day's menus meet the Recommended Dietary Allowances for all essential nutrients. But to maximize variety on a 1,200-calorie diet and adhere to dietary guidelines for chronic disease risk reduction is not always possible to ensure the recommended quantities for all nutrients. We suggest that as an extra measure of nutritional insurance, individuals using the 1,200-calorie version of these menus take a multivitamin and multimineral supplement which provides no more than 100% of the Recommended Dietary Allowances for essential nutrients.

How to Add Calories to the 1,200-Calorie Diet

To add 200 or 400 calories per day to the 1,200-calorie diet, foods can be added as a snack between meals, mealtime serving sizes can be enlarged, or extra foods can be added to breakfast, lunch, or dinner. Other foods can be added as well. Keep in mind that the starred choices are higher in fat than the other foods. Choose only one of these foods per day if you are adding 200 calories, or two if you are adding 400 calories per day. Use the list below to help guide your selections.

FOOD	PORTION	CALORIES
Grains		
Bread	1 slice	60-100
Pita Bread	½ pocket	100-150
Bagel	1 bagel	175-200
Raisin bread	1 small slice	70
Muffins	small	125
	large	300-350
Pancake	1-4″ diameter	60
Waffle	¼-9″ square	135
French toast	1 slice	90
Cereal	¾ cup (unsweetened)	110
Cheese crackers	½ cup	130
Saltine crackers	½ cup	85
Popcorn	1 cup (plain)	25
	*1 cup (buttered)	55
Pretzels	1 cup	175
Rice cakes	2 cakes	75
***Meat, lean only**	1 oz. (no fat/oil added)	
Beef		70
Veal		60
Pork		100
Ham		50
Poultry	1 oz. (skin removed)	
Chicken		65
Turkey		45
Fish	1 oz. (no fat/oil added)	
Haddock/cod/ any lean white fish		35
Salmon		45
Tuna (water-pack)		40
Swordfish		45
Dairy Foods		
*Hard cheese		
Cheddar/Swiss	1 oz.	110
Grated parmesan	2 tbsp.	60
Yogurt	8-oz. container	
(plain)		145
(plain/lowfat)		125
(fruit/lowfat)		225
(frozen dessert)		215
*Ice cream,	½ cup	
premium		250-325
regular		130-150

FOOD	PORTION	CALORIES
Fruits	1 medium piece	
Apple		105
Banana		110
Kiwi		50
Plum		35
Nectarine/peach		60-90
Orange		70-100
Pomegranate		105
Blueberries	1 cup	90
Strawberries		45
Raspberries		60
Cherries		80
Fresh fruit cup		95
Watermelon		50
Pineapple (fresh)		75
Melon	1 wedge	50
Raisins	3 tbsp.	80
Fruit Juice	1-cup serving	
Apple		110
Grape		130
Grapefruit		95
Orange		110
Pineapple		130
Tomato		40
V-8		55
Vegetables, cooked	1-cup serving	
Green beans		40
Kidney beans		265
Broccoli		40
Carrots		45
Corn		175
Peas		105
Potatoes		100
Spinach		40
Summer Squash		30
Sweet potato		160
Vegetables, raw		
Alfalfa sprouts	½ cup	10
*Avocado	1 medium	325
Carrots	5 stalks	25
Cauliflower	1 stalk	10
Celery	1 cup, diced	20
Lettuce	1 cup	10
Onion	3 tb	10
Peas	¾ cup	85
Green pepper	1 large	20
Spinach	1 cup	10

MENUS:
Week 1—Day 1

Breakfast	Calories
¾ cup fresh orange sections	70
Poached egg on 1 slice whole-wheat toast	70
Coffee with skim milk	15
	225
Lunch	
1 cup vegetable soup	85
1 small roll	75
¼ small avocado with 3 oz. low-fat spiced cottage cheese	100
Tomato wedges, broccoli florets, vegetable sticks	40
Apple or ½ small cantaloupe	60
Hot or iced tea with lemon	10
	370
Dinner	
Noodles Alfredo (¼ recipe)	330
Wilted spinach with garlic	110
Bibb lettuce	75
Low-cal dressing	
Frozen apricot ice (¼ recipe)	115
	630
Total:	**1,225**

% of Total Calories: Carbohydrate = 59%; protein = 18%; fat = 23% (saturated fat = 7%)
Cholesterol: 263 mg.
Sodium: 2,048 mg.

RECIPES:
Week 1—Day 1

■ Noodles Alfredo

5 cups noodles, cooked
2 cups part-skim yogurt
½ cup Parmesan cheese, grated
Freshly ground black pepper
¼ cup chopped parsley

1. Toss noodles with yogurt. Season with black pepper.
2. Top each serving with 2 tbsp. Parmesan cheese and minced parsley.

NOTE: If desired, lightly cooked mushrooms may be added with the yogurt.

4 servings/330 calories per serving

■ Wilted Spinach with Garlic

3 cloves garlic, sliced
1 10-oz. package fresh spinach, cleaned and trimmed
1 tbsp. olive oil
Salt and pepper
Freshly grated nutmeg

1. Heat oil in skillet. Add garlic and brown.
2. Add spinach, and salt briefly.
3. Cover and cook until spinach is barely wilted.

4 servings/110 calories per serving

■ Frozen Apricot Ice

1 can (1#) dietetic canned apricots
¼ cup superfine sugar
1 tbsp. lemon juice
Grated rind of one lemon
1 egg white
Two drops almond extract

1. Drain and pit apricots, reserving liquid.
2. Put apricots, sugar, and lemon juice in blender or food processor and puree.
3. Add reserved liquid, if necessary, to make 1 cup puree.
4. Beat egg white until stiff, but not dry. Add to apricot puree and mix to blend. Add almond extract.
5. Pour into freezer tray and let freeze until just set. Remove from freezer and beat vigorously. Return to freezer. Repeat this process once more and pour into individual serving dishes for final freezing.

4 servings/115 calories per serving

MENUS:
Week 1—Day 2

Breakfast	Calories
½ cup grapefruit juice	50

½ cup part-skim yogurt with ½ cup blueberries or	
½ cup water-packed sliced peaches	45
1 slice whole-wheat toast	70
Coffee with 1 tbsp. skim milk	5
	295

Lunch

Scallops a la Greque (¼ recipe)	245
Assorted raw vegetables on lettuce	
17 fresh cherries or a medium apple	80
Hot or iced tea with lemon	10
	335

Dinner

Baked manicotti with tomato sauce (⅕ recipe)	415
Tossed salad with 2 tbsp. low-calorie dressing	50
¾ cup sliced kiwi and orange slices	45
Hot tea or coffee with skim milk	5
	515
Total:	**1,145**

% of Total Calories: Carbohydrate = 55%; protein = 19%; fat = 26% (saturated fat = 5%)
Cholesterol: 89 mg.
Sodium: 1,748 mg.

RECIPES:
Week 1—Day 2

■ Scallops a la Greque

1 lb. bay scallops
2 tbsp. olive oil
¼ cup lemon juice
Salt and pepper
¼ tsp. thyme
2 tbsp. chopped parsley
¼ tsp. fennel seeds
½ bay leaf
1 clove garlic, minced
½ tsp. rosemary
2 cups cooked and diced potatoes

1. Poach scallops in water seasoned with salt, pepper, and lemon juice until barely done (about 5 minutes).
2. Combine all seasonings; blend well.

3. Combine scallops and cooked potatoes. Pour dressing mixture over them and marinate several hours or overnight.

4 servings/245 calories per serving

■ Baked Manicotti with Tomato and Mushroom Sauce

Tomato and Mushroom Sauce

1 cup onions, chopped
2 cloves garlic, minced
2 tbsp. oil
1 lb. mushrooms, sliced
1 medium can Italian tomatoes
1 small can tomato paste
1 10-oz. beef broth
½ tsp. salt
Freshly ground black pepper
½ tsp. oregano
½ tsp. basil

1. In a pot large enough to hold the sauce, cook onion and garlic in oil until brown. Remove and lightly cook mushrooms.
2. Return onions and garlic to pot. Add all ingredients except oregano and basil. Stir thoroughly and bring to a boil. Reduce heat and simmer about one hour.
3. Add oregano and basil and cook 45 minutes longer.

Yield: 1 Qt. Sauce, enough for manicotti recipe before.

Manicotti

½ pkg. (½ lb. lasagna noodles)
1 lb. part-skim ricotta cheese
¼ lb. part-skim mozzarella cheese, grated
¼ cup chopped parsley
1 tsp. basil
¼ tsp. thyme
1 egg, lightly beaten
Salt and pepper to taste
3 cups tomato sauce
¼ cup bread crumbs

1. Cook lasagna noodles in boiling water for 5 minutes. Drain. Cut noodles in half.
2. Mix together cheeses, seasonings, and bread crumbs.
3. Divide the filling evenly among the noodles, and roll them up.
4. Spread 1 cup of sauce over bottom of glass baking dish.
5. Arrange manicotti rolls over sauce. Pour remaining sauce on top.
6. Bake at 350°F for 30 minutes.

5 servings/415 calories per serving

MENUS:
Week 1—Day 3

Breakfast	Calories
½ cup grapefruit juice	50
2 oz. low-fat cottage cheese	40
Small bran muffin	105
Hot coffee with skim milk	5
	200
Lunch	
Curried Zucchini Soup (⅙ recipe)	130
3 oz. white meat chicken (½ small breast without skin)	90
Sliced raw mushrooms, water chestnuts, bean sprouts, and spinach with teriyaki dunking sauce	55
1 piece French bread (2″ x 2½″ x ¾″ thick)	55
1 slice fresh pineapple	40
Hot or iced tea with lemon	10
	380
Dinner	
Mongolian beef with asparagus or green beans (¼ recipe)	270
¾ cup steamed rice	145
Cucumber and yogurt salad (⅙ recipe)	45
½ cup mint sherbet layered with ¾ cup fresh strawberries	170
Hot tea or coffee with skim milk	5
	635
Total:	**1,215**

% of Total Calories: Carbohydrate = 54%; protein = 24%; fat = 22% (saturated fat = 8%)
Cholesterol: 138 mg.
Sodium: 3,360 mg.

RECIPES:
Week 1—Day 3

■ Curried Zucchini Soup

2 lb. zucchini, trimmed, cleaned, and cubed
2 tbsp. butter
1 tbsp. curry powder
4 tsp. ground cumin
½ cup watercress, chopped
2 cups chicken broth
3 cups buttermilk
Salt and pepper
1 carrot, minced
2 radishes, minced
¼ cup parsley, minced

1. Cook zucchini and scallions in butter over a low flame until tender, about 15 minutes.
2. Add curry, cumin, and chicken broth and bring to a boil. Let cool.
3. Puree soup mixture in food processor. Beat in buttermilk. Chill.
4. Combine parsley, watercress, radishes, and parsley.
5. Top each serving of soup with this mixture.

6 servings/
130 calories per serving

■ Mongolian Beef with Asparagus or Green Beans

1 lb. flank steak, sliced very thin and cut in strips about 2″ wide
2 tbsp. light soy sauce
3 tbsp. hoisin sauce
1 tbsp. sake or rice wine
1 tbsp. cornstarch
1 tsp. sugar
1½ lbs. asparagus or green beans cut into 2″ pieces
2 tbsp. peanut oil
1 clove garlic, minced
1 slice fresh ginger, minced
⅛ tsp. red pepper seeds

1. Marinate flank steak in mixture of soy sauce, rice wine, cornstarch, and sugar for about one hour.
2. Blanch asparagus or green beans until just tender, about 5 minutes.
3. Heat 2 tbsp. oil and stir-fry the asparagus or green beans for 2 minutes.
4. Remove from pan and add 2 tbsp. more oil. Add garlic, ginger, and pepper seeds, and stir-fry a minute or so. Add meat and cook for three minutes, or until it is cooked on the outside and pink inside.
5. Arrange on platter with vegetable and serve.

4 servings/
270 calories per serving

■ Cucumber and Yogurt Salad

3 large cucumbers, peeled and sliced very thin
1 cup part-skim yogurt
Salt and pepper
1 tbsp. salt
2 tbsp. white vinegar
Chopped dill

1. Salt cucumbers and let stand 20 minutes to remove moisture. Drain and rinse.
2. Combine with vinegar and yogurt and season with salt, pepper, and dill.

6 servings/
45 calories per serving

MENUS:
Week 1—Day 4

Breakfast	**Calories**
¾ cup fresh orange sections	70
1 slice cinnamon French toast with 1 tbsp. syrup or jam	100
Hot coffee with skim milk	5
	175
Lunch	
Salade Niçoise with flaked tuna, hard-boiled egg, anchovies, black olives, and assorted vegetables on crisp lettuce	315
Small bunch green grapes	110
Hot or iced tea with lemon	10
	435
Dinner	
3 oz. medallions of veal in white wine with mushrooms	265
¾ cup rice pilaf	145
1 med. stalk fresh broccoli with lemon	30
Belgian endive and watercress salad with 1½ tbsp. Dijon vinaigrette dressing	80
1 cup fresh melon balls	90
Hot tea or coffee with skim milk	10
	620
Total:	**1,230**

% of Total Calories: Carbohydrate = 53%; protein = 16%; fat = 31%; (saturated fat = 7%)
Cholesterol: 200 mg.
Sodium: 1,462 mg.

RECIPES:
Week 1—Day 4

■ Salade Niçoise

4 medium boiled potatoes, sliced thin
1 7-oz. can tuna (water-pack), drained and flaked
2 ripe tomatoes, peeled and cut into wedges
½ lb. cooked, whole green beans
3 hard-boiled eggs, sliced
1 green pepper, cut in rings
Lettuce
Radishes
2 anchovy fillets
2 black olives
¼ cup olive oil
¼ cup wine vinegar
2 tbsp. capers
1 tsp. dried basil
1 tbsp. Dijon mustard
¼ tsp. salt
⅛ tsp. pepper

1. Mix oil, wine vinegar, capers, basil, mustard, salt, and pepper.
2. Place potatoes, tuna, and green beans in bowl.
3. Pour on dressing and let stand 30 minutes or more.
4. Shred lettuce into individual bowls.
5. Add tuna-potato-bean mixture.
6. Garnish with tomato wedges, egg slices, radishes, black olives, and anchovy fillets.

6 servings/315 calories per serving

■ Medallions of Veal in White Wine

1 lb. veal scallops
¼ cup milk
2 tbsp. flour
Salt and pepper
1½ tbsp. oil
½ cup white wine
1 cup mushrooms, sliced
Lemon wedges
Chopped parsley

1. Using a cleaver, pound veal slices between two pieces of waxed paper.
2. Dip the veal scallops in milk and coat lightly with flour.
3. Brown quickly on both sides in hot oil.
4. Season with salt and pepper and a little lemon juice.
5. Remove veal from pan and place in a warm oven.
6. Quickly sauté the mushrooms; remove from pan and sprinkle over veal.
7. Add the wine and reduce the cooking liquid rapidly until only about ¼ cup remains.

8. Pour over veal; sprinkle with chopped parsley, garnish with lemon wedges, and serve.

4 servings/
215 calories per serving

■ Rice Pilaf

1 cup rice
2½ cups chicken broth
1 onion, finely chopped
1 tbsp. fresh, or 1 tsp. dried, chervil

1. Bring chicken broth to a boil. Add finely chopped onion.
2. Add rice. Cover tightly and bake at 350°F for about 30 minutes.
3. Season to taste with salt and pepper, and garnish with chopped chervil.

4 servings/
125 calories per serving

■ Belgian Endive and Watercress Salad with Dijon-Style Mustard

2 small heads Belgian endive
½ bunch watercress
3 tbsp. oil
2 tbsp. lemon juice
1 tbsp. wine vinegar
1 tbsp. light cream
¼ tsp. salt
⅛ tsp. freshly ground black pepper
2–3 tbsp. dijon-style mustard
1 shallot, minced

1. Wash watercress, picking off stems. Dry carefully and cut into small pieces.
2. Slice Belgian endive very thin. Mix the greens together.
3. Combine oil, vinegar, lemon juice, light cream, and seasonings and blend.
4. Pour over salad greens and toss lightly.

4 servings/
80 calories per serving

MENUS:
Week 1—Day 5

Breakfast	**Calories**
½ cup grapefruit juice	50

½ cup part-skim yogurt with small sliced peach or ½ cup dietetic canned peaches	125
1 slice whole-wheat toast	60
Coffee with skim milk	5
	240

Lunch

1 cup hot or chilled borscht	40
Spinach and mushroom salad (¼ recipe) with 2 tbsp. parmesan cheese and 2 tbsp. sesame-seed dressing	160
Small hard roll	80
1 Medium apple or 17 fresh cherries	80
Hot or iced tea with lemon	5
	365

Dinner

Gruyère cheese soufflé (¼ recipe)	280
2 small parslied new potatoes	110
5 large fresh or frozen asparagus spears	15
Sliced marinated cucumbers in vinegar	20
¾ cup fresh pineapple chunks with ¼ cup lemon sherbet	125
Hot tea or coffee with skim milk	5
	555
Total:	**1,160**

% of Total Calories: Carbohydrate = 56%; protein = 15%; fat = 29% (saturated fat = 9%)

Cholesterol: 283 mg.
Sodium: 2,406 mg.

RECIPES:
Week 1—Day 5

■ Spinach and Mushroom Salad with Sesame-Seed Dressing

1 lb. spinach, cleaned and trimmed
¼ lb. mushrooms, cleaned and sliced
1 small clove garlic, minced
1 tbsp. sesame seeds
3 tbsp. lemon juice
1 tbsp. wine vinegar
¼ tsp. salt
Pepper
1 tsp. dried basil, if desired
4 tbsp. parmesan cheese
3 tbsp. olive oil

1. Brown garlic and sesame seed in 1 tbsp. oil. Let cool.
2. Combine with salt, pepper, oil, vinegar, and lemon juice. Shake well.
3. Pour over spinach and mushrooms.

4 servings/160 calories per serving

■ Gruyère Cheese Soufflé

2 tbsp. butter or margarine
2 tbsp. minced onion
3 tbsp. flour
1 cup skim milk, scalded
1 cup (4 oz.) Gruyère cheese, shredded
4 eggs (at room temperature) plus
1 egg white
¼ tsp. dry mustard
¼ tsp. salt
Black pepper to taste

1. Grease a 2-quart straight sided soufflé dish.
2. Melt butter or margarine. Add onion and cook until tender.
3. Add flour and stir over low heat 3 minutes.
4. Remove from heat; beat in milk.
5. Return to stove and cook, stirring until mixture is thick. Add cheese and seasonings.
6. Separate eggs and beat in yolks, one at a time.
7. Beat egg white until stiff but not dry. Fold into cheese mixture.
8. Pour into souffle dish and bake at 375ºF for about 30 minutes or until puffed and brown.

4 servings/
280 calories per serving

MENUS:
Week 1—Day 6

Breakfast	Calories
½ cup orange juice	55
1 cup oatmeal	140
½ cup skim milk	50
½ tsp. brown sugar	25
Coffee with skim milk	5
	270

Lunch	
Onion soup gratin (⅙ of recipe)	100
Tossed salad with 2 tbsp. low-calorie dressing	60

Small piece French bread (3/4″ thick x 2½″ wide x 2″ high) toasted with ½ tsp. oil and minced garlic	90
1 tangerine or 2 fresh apricots	85
Hot or iced tea with lemon	10
	345

Dinner

Chicken Provencale (¼ of recipe)	205
½ cup noodles	100
1 cup julienne carrots and zucchini	20
Marinated pea pods	135
2 small fresh poached plums with cinnamon or ¾ cup fresh fruit cup	95
Hot tea or coffee with skim milk	5
	580
Total:	**1,175**

% of Total Calories: Carbohydrate = 52%; protein = 18%; fat = 30% (saturated fat = 5%)
Cholesterol: 99 mg.
Sodium: 1,886 mg.

RECIPES:
Week 1—Day 6

■ Onion Soup Gratin

4 cups onions, sliced
2 tbsp. margarine
6 cups beef stock or canned beef bouillon
6 tbsp. grated Parmesan cheese
6 tbsp. grated Gruyère cheese
1 tsp. flour

1. Sauté the onions very slowly in the melted butter or margarine, stirring occasionally for about 30 minutes, or until they are tender.
2. Add flour and stir for about 2 minutes, until it coats the onions and is lightly colored.
3. Add the beef stock and season with salt and pepper. Simmer about 30 minutes longer.
4. To serve, put 1 tbsp. Parmesan cheese and 1 tbsp. Gruyère cheese in the bottom of each soup bowl. Pour soup over the cheese.

6 servings/100 calories per serving

■ Low-Calorie Vinaigrette Dressing

¼ cup vegetable oil
¼ cup wine vinegar
¼ cup lemon juice
¼ cup tomato juice
1 clove garlic, minced
⅛ tsp. dry mustard
⅛ tsp. black pepper
¼ tsp. crushed thyme
¼ tsp. salt
2 tsp. chopped parsley
¼ tsp. oregano
1 shallot, crushed

Mix all ingredients and store in the refrigerator.

16 tablespoons
30 calories per tablespoon

■ Chicken Provencale

One 3½ lb. chicken, cut into 8 pieces
1 tbsp. oil
1 tbsp. chopped parsley
1 clove garlic, minced
5 chopped green onions
2 ripe tomatoes, peeled, seeded, and chopped
½ tsp. basil
½ cup white wine
Salt and pepper to taste

1. Wash chicken and pat dry with paper towels.
2. Heat oil, add garlic, and brown chicken. Season to taste with salt and pepper.
3. Reduce heat, cover, and simmer for about 8 minutes. Pour off the oil.
4. Add half the wine and continue cooking for 10 minutes.
5. Add green onions, mushrooms, tomatoes, and basil, and continue cooking until tender (15 to 20 minutes longer).
6. Sprinkle with chopped parsley.

4 servings/
205 calories per serving

■ Marinated Pea Pods

10 oz. fresh pea pods lightly steamed or 1 10 oz. pkg. frozen pea pods, cooked according to package directions
¼ cup olive oil
3 tbsp. lemon juice
1 tbsp. wine vinegar
1 tbsp. crushed capers
1 tsp. Dijon mustard
½ tsp. crushed thyme
Salt and pepper
1 hard-boiled egg, chopped
Pimiento strips

1. Mix oil, vinegar, lemon juice, and seasonings.
2. Pour on pea pods and let marinate several hours.
3. Drain and serve on crisp greens, garnished with pimiento strips and chopped egg.

4 servings/
135 calories per serving

MENUS
Week 1—Day 7

Breakfast	**Calories**
1 cup blueberries or ½ cup orange juice	90
1 cup dry cereal	175
½ cup skim milk	45
Coffee or tea with skim milk	5
	315
Lunch	
3 oz. turkey breast	130
2 slices cracked-wheat bread	130
2 tsp. mustard	10
1 fresh peach	65
Iced tea with lemon	10
	345
Dinner	
Mediterranean fish stew with diced potatoes	305
1 cup tossed salad	40
2 tbsp. low-calorie dressing	
½ cup lemon granite	200
	545
Total:	**1,205**

% of Total Calories: Carbohydrate = 59%; protein = 23%; fat = 18% (Saturated fat = 2%)
Cholesterol: 121 mg.
Sodium: 2,048 mg.

RECIPES:
Week 1—Day 7

Mediterranean Fish Stew

2 medium onions, chopped fine
¼ cup olive oil
2 cloves garlic, minced
1 15-oz. can tomatoes, drained
2 cups water
1 bay leaf
2 tbsp. dried parsley or ¼ cup fresh, chopped
Salt and pepper
1 tsp. basil
3 cups potatoes, cubed
1 lb. white fish fillets, cut into pieces

1. Cooked onions and garlic in oil until tender.
2. Add tomatoes and cook over moderately high heat for 4 or 5 minutes.
3. Add water, clam juice, and seasonings and simmer 20 minutes. Add potatoes and cook until tender.
4. Add fish fillets and simmer until fish flakes easily, about 8 to 10 minutes.

NOTE: If desired, omit potatoes and serve ¾ cup linguine with each portion of fish.

4 servings/
305 calories per serving

Lemon Granite

1 cup sugar
2 cups water
½ cup freshly squeezed lemon juice
Grated rind of one lemon

1. Heat sugar and water until dissolved. Add lemon rind and bring to a boil. Boil for five minutes. Cool.
2. Add lemon juice. Freeze in electric freezer, or proceed to next step.
3. Pour into refrigerator tray. In about 1 hour, as the mixture begins to freeze, remove and beat thoroughly.
4. Return to freezer and beat again in 30 minutes. Repeat once more or until granite is thoroughly frozen.

6 servings/
200 calories per serving

MENUS:
Week 2—Day 1

Breakfast	Calories
½ cup grapefruit juice	50
3 Puffy Apple Pancakes	195
Hot coffee with skim milk	10
	255

Lunch	
1 oz. smoked whitefish or smoked salmon on 1 bagel with 2 tbsp. cream cheese	385
Cold marinated beets (⅙ recipe), served with raw cauliflower, celery sticks, and cucumber slices	140
2 fresh or water-packed canned plums	35
Hot or iced tea with lemon	10
	570

Dinner	
Steak au Poivre Vert (⅙ recipe)	220
Grilled tomato with herbs	20
Celery hearts braised in beef stock	25
Sliced cucumbers in tarragon wine vinegar	5
1 cup melon balls with lime	60
Hot tea or coffee with skim milk	10
	340
Total:	**1,165**

% of Total Calories: Carbohydrate = 48%; protein = 22%; fat = 30% (saturated fat = 10%)
Cholesterol: 180 mg.
Sodium: 1,322 mg.

RECIPES:
Week 2—Day 1

■ Puffy Apple Pancakes

2 eggs
¼ cup sugar
⅔ cup flour
½ tsp. cinnamon
⅛ tsp. salt
1½ cups apples, peeled and chopped
1½ tbsp. butter or margarine

1. Beat eggs and sugar together until the mixture is pale and thick and forms a ribbon as it leaves the beater.
2. Sift dry ingredients together and blend into egg mixture.
3. Stir in chopped apples.
4. Heat a skillet or griddle; melt butter or margarine and drop pancake batter, by tablespoonfuls onto griddle. When brown on one side, flip to brown on the other.

16 pancakes
70 calories each

■ Cold Beets Marinated

12 medium beets, cooked until tender and peeled
1 minced shallot
½ tsp. dried oregano
Salt and pepper
⅛ tsp. dried mustard
¼ tsp. dried thyme
3 tbsp. wine vinegar
1 tbsp. olive oil

1. Mix seasonings together with wine vinegar and oil. Pour over beets while they are still warm.
2. Let the mixture sit in the refrigerator overnight. Drain well to serve.

6 servings/
99 calories per serving

■ Steak au Poivre Vert

Six 4-oz. portions lean sirloin steak, about ¾″ thick
2 tbsp. minced shallots
½ cup canned beef bouillon
¼ cup cognac
2 tbsp. green peppercorns
1 tbsp. oil
2 tbsp. butter or margarine

1. Place the peppercorns in a bowl and crush thoroughly.
2. Dry steak thoroughly and rub crushed peppercorns onto both sides of the meat. Press pepper in thoroughly. Cover with waxed paper. Let stand for at least 3 hours.
3. Heat butter and oil until very hot. Brown the steak thoroughly for 3 or 4 minutes. Turn and brown on the other side. Remove to a warm platter and keep warm.
4. Add shallots to pan and cook slowly for a minute or two. Pour in beef bouillon and boil down rapidly, scraping up juices. Add cognac and boil

off rapidly. Pour sauce over meat and serve. (Carefully trim excess fat from meat for dieters.)

6 servings/
220 calories per serving

MENUS:
Week 2—Day 2

Breakfast	Calories
½ banana sliced in ½ cup orange juice	110
1 small bran muffin	105
Hot coffee with skim milk	10
	235

Lunch	
½ cup apple juice	60
Open-faced Swiss cheese (2 oz. cheese) and tomato sandwich with Dijon mustard and oregano on 1 slice pumpernickel bread	295
Dill pickle spears	5
Carrot sticks	10
Small bunch green grapes	110
	480

Dinner	
Chinese vegetable soup (¼ recipe)	45
Vegetable Cashew Curry (¼ recipe)	290
¾ cup steamed rice	140
½ cup fresh pineapple	40
Hot tea or coffee with skim milk	10
	525
Total:	**1,240**

% of Total Calories: Carbohydrate = 57%; protein = 15%; fat = 28% (saturated fat = 9%)
Cholesterol: 53 mg.
Sodium: 2,876 mg.

RECIPES:
Week 2—Day 2

■ Chinese Vegetable Soup

½ cup fresh mushrooms sliced
½ cup cabbage, shredded
½ cup celery, sliced
¼ cup water chestnuts, sliced
½ cup carrots, sliced
2 scallions, sliced
1 tbsp. oil
6 cups water
4 tsp. soy sauce
1 tbsp. sherry
Salt and pepper to taste

1. Heat oil in a 2½-qt. saucepan. Add vegetables and stir only until they begin to soften. Add soy sauce and sherry.
2. Add water. Bring to a boil, cover, and cook for 10 minutes.
3. Top with sliced scallions and if desired, a fluted mushroom cap.

4 servings/
45 calories per serving

■ Vegetable Cashew Curry

¾ cup soybeans, cooked
2 carrots, diced
2 onions, sliced
½ cup celery, diced
1 cup cauliflower, broken into small pieces and blanched
¼ cup raw cashews
1 tbsp. curry powder
1 tbsp. mango chutney
1 tbsp. oil
2 tbsp. flour
¼ cup water
½ cup frozen peas

1. Heat oil. Add onions, carrots, and celery and cook 2 minutes.
2. Add 1 cup water and simmer 10 minutes.
3. Add cauliflower, cashews, soybeans, curry powder, and chutney, and cook five minutes longer. Add peas.
4. Mix flour and ¼ cup water to a paste.
5. Add to vegetables, bring to a boil, and stir until lightly thickened. Serve over rice.

4 servings/
290 calories per serving

MENUS:
Week 2—Day 3

Breakfast	Calories
½ cup pineapple juice	70

2 oz. low-fat cottage cheese	40
2 slices raisin bread	140
Coffee with skim milk	10
	260

Lunch

1 cup hot consomme with carrot and turnip	70
Spinach and mushroom salad with bacon (1/4 recipe)	160
1 piece French bread (2½″ long x 2″ wide x ¾″ thick)	70
1 tangerine	40
Hot or iced tea with lemon	10
	350

Dinner

Shrimp and Scallop Casserole Gratin (1/6 recipe)	265
1 cup string beans steamed with 1/8 tsp. chili pepper	35
2 medium boiled red skin potatoes	110
Watercress and radish salad on Bibb lettuce	75
¾ cup chilled pineapple chunks with	55
¼ cup lemon sherbet	65
Coffee or tea with skim milk	10
	615

Total: 1,225

% of Total Calories: Carbohydrate = 51%; protein = 20%; fat = 29% (saturated fat = 6%)
Cholesterol: 83 mg.
Sodium: 2,047 mg.

RECIPES:
Week 2—Day 3

■ Hot Consomme with Carrot and Turnip

6 cups chicken stock
1½ cups raw turnip, halved and sliced
1½ cups raw carrots, halved and sliced

1. Heat chicken stock.
2. Add vegetables and simmer until tender, about 6 to 8 minutes.

6 servings/
70 calories per serving

■ Spinach and Mushroom Salad

1 lb. spinach, trimmed and cleaned
¼ lb. mushrooms, sliced
6 strips bacon, cooked crisp and drained well
2 tbsp. olive oil
¼ cup Parmesan cheese
¼ cup lemon juice
Pepper

1. Dry spinach thoroughly.
2. Crumble bacon and add to spinach. Add mushrooms and toss to blend.
3. Add olive oil and freshly ground black pepper. Toss.
4. Add lemon juice and Parmesan cheese and toss again.

4 servings/
160 calories per serving

■ Shrimp and Scallop Casserole Gratin

1 lb. large shrimp
1 lb. bay scallops
2 tbsp. sherry
½ cup parsley, chopped
2 cloves garlic, crushed
1 tbsp. shallot, minced
¼ tsp. dried oregano
½ cup dry white bread crumbs
⅛ tsp. pepper
2 tbsp. butter, melted

1. Arrange shrimp and scallops in 6 individual serving dishes.
2. Mix seasonings and bread crumbs together and sprinkle over shellfish.
3. Pour on butter.
4. Bake at 375°F for about 12 to 15 minutes, until the crumbs are toasted.

6 servings/265 calories per serving

■ Watercress and Radish Salad

1 bunch watercress, cleaned and trimmed
8 radishes, sliced thin
2 tbsp. oil
1 head bibb lettuce, cleaned and dried
¼ cup red wine vinegar
1 tbsp. Dijon mustard
Salt and pepper

1. Toss watercress and radishes together.
2. Beat oil and vinegar together. Pour over vegetables. Season.
3. Serve on Bibb lettuce.

4 servings/
75 calories per serving

MENUS:
Week 2—Day 4

Breakfast	Calories
½ cup orange juice or other fruit juice	55
¾ cup whole-grain cereal	110
½ cup skim milk	45
½ cup fresh peaches, sliced	40
Coffee with skim milk	10
	260
Lunch	
½ cup flaked tuna with lemon wedge	120
1 slice rye bread	70
Green salad with low-calorie dressing	40
½ cup grapefruit sections or strawberries	45
Hot or iced tea	10
	185
Dinner	
Roast Pork a l'Orange (4 oz.)	390
¾ cup wild rice	90
5 asparagus spears poached in white wine	40
Celeriac on crisp romaine lettuce	55
1 cup Kiwi and raspberries or oranges	90
Hot tea or coffee with skim milk	10
	675
Total:	**1,220**

% of Total Calories: Carbohydrate = 48%; protein = 25%; fat = 27% (saturated fat = 8%)
Cholesterol: 156 mg.
Sodium: 1,207 mg.

RECIPES:
Week 2 —Day 4

■ Roast Pork a l'Orange

4 lb. pork loin roast, boneless
Salt and pepper
1 small onion, sliced
1 orange cut into sections
1 cup orange juice
½ cup celery
¼ tsp. oregano
2 tbsp. red wine vinegar

1. Combine onion, celery, oregano, wine vinegar, orange sections, and juice.
2. Season pork roast with salt and pepper.
3. Pour sauce into bottom of roasting pan.
4. Place roast on rack, put in pan.
5. Roast at 350°F for about 25 minutes per pound (or until meat thermometer reaches 170° F), basting with pan juice about every 20 minutes.

Approximately 7 servings, 4 oz. each
390 calories per 4 ounce serving of trimmed pork

■ Celeriac on Crisp Romaine

- 2 celery roots, cooked in boiling water until just tender
- 1 tbsp. shallot, chopped fine
- 2 tbsp. olive oil
- 1 tbsp. chopped parsley
- ¼ cup lemon juice
- Salt and pepper
- ¼ tsp. dried mustard
- ¼ tsp. thyme
- Romaine lettuce

1. Peel the celeriac and cut into julienne strips.
2. Mix oil, shallots, lemon juice, and seasonings and toss with celeriac.
3. Let marinate several hours or overnight.
4. Serve on crisp romaine lettuce.

6 servings/
55 calories per serving

MENUS
Week 2—Day 5

Breakfast	Calories
½ cup cranberry juice	75
⅔ cup whole-wheat cereal	90
3 tbsp. dried apricot pieces	45
½ cup skim milk	45
Coffee or tea with skim milk	10
	265
Lunch	
½ cup tomato juice	25
2 oz. Swiss cheese	185
Marinated red pepper and mushroom salad on lettuce (¼ recipe)	145

1 slice pumpernickel bread	60
1 Granny Smith apple	105
Hot or iced tea with lemon	10
	530

Dinner

1½ cups ziti with	310
fresh zucchini sauce (¼ recipe)	75
2 tbsp. grated Parmesan cheese	55
Tossed salad with low-calorie dressing	40
1 wedge melon with fresh mint, if available	60
Hot tea or coffee with skim milk	10
	475
Total:	**1,270**

% of Total Calories: Carbohydrate = 58%; protein = 15%; fat = 27% (saturated fat = 10%)
Cholesterol: 63 mg.
Sodium: 3,005 mg.

RECIPES:
Week 2—Day 5

■ Marinated Red Pepper and Mushroom Salad

1½ cups water
2 tbsp. olive oil
¼ cup white wine vinegar
Cheesecloth bag containing:
3 scallions, chopped
1 stalk celery, chopped
4 sprigs parsley
2 cloves garlic
¼ tsp. thyme
¼ tsp. coriander
8 peppercorns
¾ lb. mushrooms, quartered
4 large red peppers
12 large black olives
½ tsp. salt

1. Combine water, oil, vinegar, and spices, bring to a boil, and simmer for 15 minutes. Add mushrooms and simmer, covered, for 5 minutes.
2. Remove mushrooms with a slotted spoon. Reduce marinade to ½ cup and save.
3. Discard spice bag.
4. Broil red peppers under broiler for 3 minutes on each side about 4″ from flame. Skins should be charred.

5. Remove stems and peel peppers while still warm. Remove seeds and ribs and cut into strips. Combine peppers and mushrooms and pour marinade on them. Grate fresh black pepper over the mixture and chill for at least 4 hours.
6. Serve on lettuce with black peppers.

Note: Cheese may be sliced and put into dish to marinate with the vegetables if desired.

4 servings/
145 calories per serving

■ Fresh Zucchini Sauce

1 lb. zucchini
1 tbsp. butter or margarine
1 large clove garlic, minced
Black pepper and grated nutmeg
2 tbsp. olive oil
1 small onion, chopped

1. Scrub zucchini and cut into fine julienne strips. Sprinkle with coarse salt and set in a colander to drain for about one hour.
2. Gently squeeze out excess moisture and dry on paper towels.
3. In a skillet, sauté onion and garlic until lightly browned. Add zucchini and cook until tender, about 4 minutes.
4. Season with black pepper and nutmeg. Serve over ziti or shells. Top each serving with 2 tbsp. Parmesan cheese.

6 servings/75 calories per serving

MENUS:
Week 2—Day 6

Breakfast	**Calories**
½ cup orange juice	55
1 slice whole-grain toast	70
2 oz. low-fat cottage cheese with fruit	60
Coffee with skim milk	10
	195
Lunch	
Lean corned beef (2 oz.)	210
Large pita bread	195
1 tbsp. mustard	25
Vegetable sticks	30

1 fresh peach	65
Hot or iced tea with lemon	10
	545

Dinner

1 small chicken breast with 2 tbsp. barbeque sauce	185
1 large ear corn on the cob with 1 tbsp. margarine	145
Tossed salad with low-calorie dressing	40
1 cup fresh strawberries	45
Coffee with skim milk	10
	425
Total:	**1,165**

% of Total Calories: Carbohydrate = 51%; protein = 21%; fat = 28% (saturated fat = 8%)
Cholesterol: 125 mg.
Sodium: 1,923 mg.

MENUS: Week 2—Day 7

Breakfast	**Calories**
Two 4½″ square waffles	275
1½ tbsp. maple syrup	50
½ cup blueberries	45
Coffee with skim milk	10
	380

Lunch

1 cup bulgur wheat tabouleh, with 2 tbsp. green onion, 1 tsp. oil, and 2 tbsp. lemon juice served on lettuce and raw spinach	300
1 cup bing cherries	80
Hot or iced tea with lemon	10
	390

Dinner

Fish and Potato Salad (¼ recipe) served on romaine-lettuce with mustard mayonnaise and cherry tomatoes, zucchini slices, and green pepper	365
Assorted fresh fruits	70

Hot coffee or tea with skim milk	10
	445
Total:	**1,215**

% of Total Calories: Carbohydrate = 60%; protein = 16%; fat = 24% (saturated fat = 4%)
Cholesterol: 161 mg.
Sodium: 2,056 mg.

RECIPES:
Week 2—Day 7

■ Fish and Potato Salad

1 lb. poached whitefish fillets
3 gherkin pickles, sliced thin
2 tbsp. capers, mashed
2 tbsp. chopped parsley
1 tsp. chopped tarragon
2 cups cooked potatoes, diced
1 cup cooked peas
3 tbsp. mayonnaise
½ cup part-skim yogurt
2 tbsp. Dijon mustard
2 tbsp. lemon juice
Romaine lettuce
Zucchini slices
Green pepper rings
Cherry Tomatoes

1. Mix all ingredients except raw vegetables together and chill.
2. Serve on crisp romaine lettuce with zucchini slices, cherry tomatoes, and green pepper rings.

4 servings/
365 calories per serving

■ Tabooli

1 cup bulgur wheat
¾ cup chopped green onion
1¼ cups parsley
¼ cup dried mint
Fresh ground pepper
1 tbsp. olive oil
¼ cup lemon juice

1. Cover bulgur with cold water and drain after two hours.
2. Mix in the rest of ingredients.

3. Chill and serve.

Makes two 1-cup servings (285 calories) or four ½ cup servings (140 calories)

MENUS:
Week 3—Day 1

Breakfast	**Calories**
¾ cup cranberry juice	75
¼ cup low-fat cottage cheese	165
1 whole-wheat English muffin	60
Coffee or tea with skim milk	10
	310

Lunch	
Large tossed salad with 1 tbsp. peanuts and 2 tbsp. sunflower seeds	180
1 tbsp. low-calorie dressing	30
2 rice cakes	70
½ grapefruit	45
Hot or iced tea with lemon	10
	335

Dinner	
Mixed bean casserole with yogurt topping (⅛ recipe)	315
1 cup whole green beans with dill and lemon	35
Grated daikon with mustard vinaigrette on watercress (2 tbsp. dressing)	145
¾ cup strawberries, bananas, and kiwi	35
Hot coffee or tea with skim milk	10
	540
Total:	**1,185**

% of Total Calories: Carbohydrate = 62%; protein = 16%; fat = 22% (saturated fat = 4%)
Cholesterol: 5 mg.
Sodium: 607 mg.

RECIPES:
Week 3—Day 1

■ Grated Daikon with Mustard Vinaigrette Dressing

2 cups grated daikon (Chinese white radish)
1 bunch watercress, cleaned and trimmed
4 tbsp. olive oil
4 tbsp. yogurt
2 tbsp. wine vinegar
1 shallot, minced
1½ tsp. Dijon-style mustard
Salt and pepper to taste

1. Combine oil, yogurt, vinegar, mustard, and seasonings and mix well.
2. Toss with shredded daikon and chill for an hour or more.
3. Serve on watercress.

4 servings/
145 calories per serving

■ Mixed Bean Casserole with Yogurt Topping

1 cup dried white beans
1 cup dried black beans
2 onions stuck with a whole clove
2 carrots, peeled and sliced
2 stalks celery
2 large sprigs parsley
2 bay leaves
2 tsp. thyme
Salt and pepper
1 cup canned chick-peas, drained and rinsed
3 cloves garlic, minced
1 tsp. oil
4 tbsp. tomato paste
1½ tsp. dried oregano
2 cups canned tomatoes, drained
½ cup dry red wine
1 cup part-skim yogurt

1. Put white beans and black beans in separate pots. Cover with plenty of water. Bring to a boil and remove from heat. Let soak one hour or longer.
2. To each pot, add one onion, one carrot, one stalk of celery, one sprig of parsley, one tsp. thyme, one bay leaf, and salt and pepper.
3. Bake at 325°F until the beans are tender. Discard onions, celery, parsley, and bay leaves and drain. Combine with chick peas.
4. Saute garlic in oil. Add tomato paste, oregano, tomatoes, and red wine.
5. Pour this mixture over the beans. Return to oven. Bake at 325°F for about 45 minutes. Serve topped with yogurt seasoned with minced garlic.

8 servings/
315 calories per serving

MENUS: WEEK 3—DAY 2

Breakfast	Calories
½ cup apple juice	60
¾ cup bran cereal	130
½ cup skim milk	50
Coffee with skim milk	10
	250
Lunch	
1 cup hot or cold beef consommé with lemon	20
Cold shrimp and artichoke salad	185
1 slice Italian bread	75
¾ cup green grapes	85
Hot or iced tea with lemon	10
	375
Dinner	
Spanish Beef Stew with Potatoes	440
½ cup broccoli with lemon	25
Marinated zucchini on Bibb lettuce	70
1 cup watermelon balls	50
Coffee with skim milk	10
	595
Total:	**1,220**

% of Total Calories: Carbohydrate = 50%; protein = 20%; fat = 30% (saturated fat = 7%)
Cholesterol: 140 mg.
Sodium: 1,460 mg.

RECIPES: Week 3—Day 2

■ Cold Shrimp and Artichoke Salad

10 canned artichoke hearts, quartered
4 tbsp. mayonnaise
2 tbsp. lemon juice
1 tbsp. Dijon mustard
2 capers, chopped
6 large black olives, sliced
16 large shrimp, cooked and cleaned
Assorted raw vegetables:
Tomato, Sliced zucchini, Endive

1. Mix mayonnaise with lemon juice, mustard, capers, and olives. Toss with sliced artichokes.
2. Arrange Bibb lettuce on four salad plates; divide artichoke mixture and place in the center of the plates.
3. Arrange four shrimp and cold vegetables around artichokes.

4 servings/185 calories per serving

■ Spanish Beef Stew with Potatoes

1¼ lbs. very lean stewing beef
1 medium onion, sliced
1 large tomato, cut into wedges
2 cloves garlic, unpeeled
2 tbsp. olive oil
½ cup dry white wine
2 tbsp. cognac
2 tbsp. flour
½ tsp. paprika
1 small bay leaf
½ tsp. dried thyme
⅛ tsp. cinnamon
4 medium potatoes
Salt and pepper to taste

1. Heat oil in a pot large enough to hold the stew. Brown meat well, a few pieces at a time, on all sides. Remove from pot.
2. Add onion and garlic, salt and pepper, thyme, and bay leaf. Cook, covered, until onion and garlic soften (about 5 minutes). Add tomato and continue cooking until juice is nearly evaporated.
3. Add wine and cognac, raise heat, and cook until liquid is reduced a bit.
4. Lower heat, add flour, and stir until blended. Return meat to the pot. Add cinnamon and paprika and enough boiling water to just cover the meat.
5. Place in the oven at 350°F for about 2 hours, adding more liquid if necessary.
6. About 30 minutes before meat is finished, cook potatoes until done. Add to stew immediately before serving.

4 servings, 3½ oz. beef per serving/440 calories per serving

■ Marinated Zucchini on Bibb Lettuce

2 lb. zucchini, washed, trimmed, and sliced into sticks about 1″ long
1 tbsp. olive oil
¾ cup wine vinegar
¼ cup olive oil
1 small garlic, crushed
1 tbsp. dried basil
Salt and pepper
⅛ tsp. dried thyme
1 tbsp. chopped parsley

1. Sauté zucchini quickly in hot olive oil until lightly cooked. Drain on towels.

2. Combine ¼ cup olive oil, wine vinegar, and seasonings, except parsley, and simmer for about 5 minutes.
3. Put zucchini in glass bowl, pour on marinade, and let chill for 3 or 4 hours.
4. Serve on Bibb lettuce and garnish with chopped parsley and lemon wedges.

8 servings/
70 calories per serving

MENUS:
Week 3—Day 3

Breakfast	**Calories**
½ cup orange juice	55
1 slice whole-wheat toast with	110
1 thin slice mozzarella cheese (½ oz)	
Coffee or tea with skim milk	10
	175
Lunch	
Bagel with 1 tbsp. cashew or peanut butter	275
Raw cauliflower, radishes, and green pepper rings	
1 small apple or ½ small cantaloupe	60
Hot or iced tea with lemon	10
	345
Dinner	
Grilled or broiled marinated swordfish or halibut steaks	220
Tossed salad with	
2 tbsp. low-calorie dressing	40
¾ cup brown rice with red pepper slices	175
5 large asparagus spears	20
½ cup sherbet with ¾ cup fresh raspberries	180
	635
Total:	**1,155**

% of Total Calories: Carbohydrate = 60%; protein = 19%; fat = 21% (saturated fat = 4%)
Cholesterol: 18 mg.
Sodium: 800 mg.

RECIPES:
Week 3—Day 3

■ Steak of Halibut or Swordfish

1 5-oz. halibut or swordfish steak per person
½ tsp. olive oil
1 tsp. lemon juice per steak
1 tsp. capers (crushed)

1. Marinate for 30 minutes in lemon juice, oil, and crushed capers. Drain, and broil or grill.

220 calories per serving

MENUS:
Week 3—Day 4

Breakfast	**Calories**
½ cup tomato juice	20
1 tsp. fruit jam	20
1 small bran muffin	105
Hot coffee with skim milk	10
	155
Lunch	
¾ cup lentil soup with lemon wedge	105
Greek salad bowl with 1 oz. feta cheese	85
and low-calorie dressing	30
1 oz. wedge Syrian bread	105
2 fresh apricots or tangerine	40
Hot or iced tea with lemon	10
	375
Dinner	
Veal Rollatini (1/6 of recipe)	295
Polenta (1/6 of recipe)	215
1 cup fresh spinach	55
Mushroom salad	90
¾ cup orange and grapefruit sections	60
Hot tea or coffee with skim milk	10
	725
Total:	**1,255**

% of Total Calories: Carbohydrate = 53%; protein = 18%; fat = 29% (saturated fat = 9%)
Cholesterol: 105 mg.
Sodium: 3,055 mg.

RECIPES:
Week 3—Day 4

■ Veal Rollatini

1½ lbs. veal scallops, pounded flat
¾ cup prosciutto, finely chopped
2 tbsp. parsley, chopped
1 clove garlic, minced
Salt and pepper to taste
1 onion, chopped
1 stalk celery, chopped
¼ cup flour
2 tbsp. margarine
½ cup white wine
2 cups chicken stock
1 carrot minced
½ tsp. rosemary

1. Combine prosciutto, garlic, parsley, and salt and pepper. Stuff 1 tsp. of this mixture into each piece of veal, roll the meat, and fasten with a toothpick.
2. Dredge each roll in flour and brown them in margarine.
3. Add chicken stock, wine, carrots, celery, onion, and seasonings. Bring to a simmer.
4. Cook for about 20–25 minutes, or until veal is tender.

6 servings/
295 calories per serving

■ Polenta

4½ cups water
1½ cups cornmeal
1 tsp. salt
1½ tbsp. margarine

1. Bring water to a boil. Add salt and stir in cornmeal very gradually.
2. Cook over direct heat for about 5 minutes. Transfer to a double boiler and cook for about 30 minutes, stirring occasionally.
3. Beat in margarine.

6 servings/
215 calories per serving

■ Mushroom Salad

1 lb. mushrooms, sliced
1 medium onion, chopped
Lettuce
¼ cup chopped watercress
½ cup chopped parsley
1 clove garlic, minced
3 tbsp. olive oil
2 tbsp. lemon juice
½ tsp. tarragon
Salt and freshly ground black pepper

1. Simmer mushrooms and onions, covered, for 5 minutes in a small amount of water. Drain and chill.
2. Combine the rest of the ingredients, except lettuce, pour over mushrooms and onions and toss.
3. Serve on lettuce.

6 servings/
90 calories per serving

MENUS:
Week 3—Day 5

Breakfast	**Calories**
Small wedge honeydew melon	30
¾ cup oatmeal with 1 tbsp. raisins	160
½ cup skim milk	50
Coffee with skim milk	10
	250
Lunch	
2 oz. Swiss cheese and sliced tomato on 2 slices rye bread	235
Sliced cucumber, carrots, and green pepper with 1 tbsp. low-calorie dressing	70
1 small banana	85
Hot or iced tea with lemon	10
	400
Dinner	
1½ cups linguine	235
3 tbsp. pesto sauce	210
Tossed salad with 1 tbsp. low-calorie dressing	30
1 fresh pear, sliced	95
Hot tea or coffee with skim milk	10
	580
Total:	**1,220**

% of Total Calories: Carbohydrate = 60%; protein = 13%; fat = 27% (saturated fat = 7%)
Cholesterol: 35 mg.
Sodium: 1,100 mg.

RECIPES:
Week 3—Day 5

■ Pesto Sauce

½ cup olive oil
2 tbsp. dried basil
Black pepper
1 large clove garlic
10 large spinach leaves, trimmed and shredded
½ cup walnuts
½ cup Parmesan or sardo cheese, grated

1. Put oil into a blender or food processor. Add garlic and spices and blend.
2. Add spinach leaves and chop.
3. Add nuts and let run until finely chopped.
4. Add cheese and blend until all ingredients are well mixed.

Makes about 1¼ cups
70 calories per tablespoon

NOTE: When fresh basil is in season, omit spinach leaves and use 1 cup fresh basil leaves.

■ Low-Calorie Vinaigrette Dressing

¼ cup vegetable oil
¼ cup wine vinegar
¼ cup lemon juice
¼ cup tomato juice
1 clove garlic, minced
⅛ tsp. ground pepper
¼ tsp. crushed thyme
¼ tsp. salt
2 tsp. chopped parsley

Mix all ingredients well. Store in refrigerator.
1 cup dressing=30 calories per tablespoon

MENUS:
Week 3—Day 6

Breakfast	Calories
½ cup orange juice	55
1 cup dry cereal with ½ cup skim milk	225
Hot coffee with skim milk	10
	290

Lunch

Portugese Kale Soup with Linguicia (1/10 recipe)	170
Small corn muffin	65
Green salad with	
2 tbsp. low-calorie vinaigrette dressing (see #2 **Lunch**)	40
Fresh plum	35
Hot or iced tea with lemon	10
	320

Dinner

Chicken with Egg and Lemon Sauce (1/4 recipe)	255
3/4 cup rice	145
1 cup steamed spinach with chopped green onions	45
Sliced cucumbers in dill-flavored yogurt and wine vinegar	40
3/4 cup fresh fruit cup	70
Hot tea or coffee with skim milk	10
	565
Total:	**1,175**

% of Total Calories: Carbohydrate = 53%; protein = 19%; fat = 28% (saturated fat = 7%)
Cholesterol: 160 mg.
Sodium: 1,750 mg.

RECIPES:
Week 3—Day 6

■ Portugese Kale Soup

1 lb. kale
4 large potatoes
2 tbsp. olive oil
Salt and pepper
1/2 lb. linguica or Portugese sausage, cooked, well drained, and sliced thin

1. Wash and dry kale and chop fine.
2. Peel 4 large potatoes. Boil in 2 1/2 quarts of water with 2 tbsp. olive oil.
3. When potatoes are tender, drain, reserving cooking liquid.
4. Mash potatoes and whisk back into cooking liquid.
5. Simmer for 30 minutes more.
6. Add chopped kale, linguica, and salt and pepper to taste. Simmer for 10 minutes, or until kale is tender.

10 servings/
170 calories per serving

■ Chicken with Egg and Lemon Sauce

3 lb. chicken cut into quarters and skinned
1½ tbsp. olive oil
1 tbsp. flour
Salt and pepper
1 cup chicken broth
1 egg, lightly beaten
2 tbsp. lemon juice

1. Heat oil and sauté chicken on both sides until golden brown (about 6-10 minutes).
2. Sprinkle on flour, season with salt and pepper and cook 3 or 4 minutes longer.
3. Pour chicken stock over chicken, bring to a boil. Reduce heat and simmer for about 30 minutes or until chicken is tender.
4. Beat egg and lemon together.
5. Remove chicken from pan and put in a warm oven.
6. Whisk the egg and lemon mixture into cooking liquid and cook over very low heat, beating vigorously as you pour. Continue stirring over low heat until mixture thickens. Do not let it boil or it will curdle.
7. When thick, pour sauce over chicken and serve.

4 servings/
255 calories per serving

MENUS:
Week 3—Day 7

Breakfast	**Calories**
½ cup cranberry juice	75
1 slice whole-grain currant quick bread	165
¼ cup low-fat cottage cheese	40
Coffee with skim milk	10
	290
Lunch	
Large tossed salad with 3 tbsp. low-calorie dressing	65
2 tbsp. humus spread on pita bread	175
¾ cup fresh melon or kiwi	55
Hot or iced tea with lemon	10
	305
Dinner	
Barley and Mushroom Casserole with pearl onions and cheddar cheese topping (⅙ recipe)	325
½ cup fiddle head ferns, if available, with lemon, or 1 cup green beans	35

Baked Stuffed Cucumbers	80
Poached whole pear with 2 tbsp. raspberry sauce	105
Hot tea or coffee with skim milk	10
	555
Total:	**1,170**

% of Total Calories: Carbohydrate = 66%; protein = 12%; fat = 22% (saturated fat = 3%)
Cholesterol: 90 mg.
Sodium: 1,050 mg.

RECIPES: Week 3—Day 7

■ Whole-Grain Currant Quick Bread

1 cup rolled oats
½ cup brown sugar, firmly packed
1 cup whole-wheat flour
½ tsp. cloves
1 tsp. salt
5½ tsp. oil
1 cup buttermilk
1 egg, beaten
1 tsp. cinnamon
1 tsp. baking powder
½ tsp. baking soda
½ cup currants

1. Soak oats in buttermilk for an hour or longer.
2. Mix with egg and brown sugar.
3. Combine the rest of the dry ingredients and stir into oat mixture.
4. Add oil and currants.
5. Pour into greased baking dish. Bake at 400ºF for 35 to 45 minutes.

18 slices
165 calories per slice

■ Barley and Mushroom Casserole

2 cups pearl barley
1 large onion, chopped
½ lb. mushrooms
1 tbsp. oil
Salt and pepper
1 qt. liquid (water or vegetable stock)
3 oz. cheddar cheese, grated
12 pearl onions, lightly cooked
Chopped parsley

1. Sauté onion and mushrooms in oil until tender. Add barley and brown lightly.
2. Transfer mixture to oven-proof casserole with cover.
3. Season with salt and pepper. Pour on half the cooking liquid and bake at 350ºF for 30 minutes.
4. Add the rest of the liquid and cook until all the broth is absorbed and barley is tender. Fold in pearl onions, top with cheddar cheese, sprinkle on parsley, and bake 15 minutes longer.

6 servings/
325 calories per serving

■ Baked Stuffed Cucumbers

6 cucumbers, peeled and seeded
2 tomatoes, peeled, seeded, and chopped
1 small onion, chopped fine
1 tbsp. oil
1 tsp. dried basil
Salt and pepper
1 clove garlic, minced

1. Brown onion and garlic in oil. Add tomato and seasonings. Cook over moderate heat until liquid evaporates.
2. Stuff cucumbers with this mixture.
3. Bake at 350ºF about 35 minutes, or until cucumbers are tender.

6 servings/
80 calories per serving

■ Raspberry Sauce

Drain syrup, after thawing, from one 10-ounce package of frozen raspberries. Put raspberries into a blender jar or food processor and blend on high speed until thick. If necessary, add a little syrup to thin. Force through a fine sieve to remove seeds.

8 tablespoons sauce
15 calories per tablespoon

MENUS:
Week 4—Day 1

Breakfast	**Calories**
½ grapefruit	40
6 oz.-container low-fat fruit yogurt	85

1 slice whole-wheat toast with 1 tsp. jam	80
Coffee or tea with skim milk	10
	315
Lunch	
½ cup flaked tuna with lemon	120
1 slice French bread	80
Raw vegetable sticks	25
1 cup grapes	115
Hot or iced tea with lemon	10
	350
Dinner	
Lamb shish-kebab (3 oz. lamb)	205
Mushrooms and green pepper chunks	35
½ cup tabooli salad	115
1 cup steamed zucchini	30
Tossed salad with 2 tbsp. low-calorie dressing	40
1 medium apple	60
Tea or coffee with skim milk	10
	495
Total:	**1,150**

% of Total Calories: Carbohydrate = 55% protein = 24%; fat = 21% (saturated fat = 3%)
Cholesterol: 137 mg.
Sodium: 1,325 mg.

RECIPES:
Week 4—Day 1

■ Lamb Shish-kebab

2 lbs. lean leg of lamb, trimmed and cut into 1½″ cubes
¾ cup red wine
1 tbsp. oil
¼ cup lemon juice
2 cloves garlic, crushed
½ tsp. oregano
¼ tsp. black pepper

1. Soak meat in marinade made from wine, spices, seasonings, and ¼ cup oil.
2. Drain and dry the meat on paper towels.

3. Place meat cubes on skewers alternating with mushrooms and green pepper sections.
4. Brush with small amount of oil.
5. Cook on charcoal grill or under the broiler until desired doneness.

6 servings/
205 calories per serving

MENUS:
Week 4—Day 2

Breakfast	**Calories**
½ cup orange juice	60
⅔ cup hominy with skim milk	150
Hot coffee with skim milk	10
	220
Lunch	
Chef's salad with ½ oz. turkey, ½ oz. ham, 1 oz. cheese, and 3 tbsp. low-calorie dressing	220
Breadsticks	95
1 cup strawberries or grapefruit half	45
Hot or iced tea with lemon	10
	370
Dinner	
Baked shrimp with feta cheese (¼ of recipe)	240
¾ cup steamed rice with parsley	140
Medium stalk broccoli with lemon wedge	25
Green salad with 2 tbsp. low-calorie dressing	40
¾ cup pineapple chunks with ¼ cup orange sherbet	130
Tea or coffee with skim milk	10
	585
Total:	**1,175**

% of Total Calories: Carbohydrate = 55%; protein = 20%; fat = 25% (saturated fat = 6%)
Cholesterol: 70 mg.
Sodium: 2,250 mg.

RECIPES:
Week 4—DAY 2

■ Baked Shrimp with Feta Cheese

4 tbsp. olive oil
3 medium tomatoes, peeled, seeded, and chopped
1 medium onion, sliced
1 lb. shrimp, shelled and deveined
2 cloves garlic, minced
1 bay leaf
½ cup dry white wine
Salt and pepper
4 oz. feta cheese

1. Heat oil in skillet and cook onion and garlic until tender.
2. Add tomatoes and seasonings, including salt and pepper to taste.
3. Add wine and bring mixture to a boil. Simmer, uncovered, for about 20 minutes. Cool.
4. Put shrimp in oven-proof casserole, add liquid, and crumble feta cheese over the mixture.
5. Bake at 400°F for about 15 minutes until the cheese is melted.

4 servings/
240 calories per serving

MENUS:
Week 4—Day 3

Breakfast	**Calories**
½ cup cranberry juice	75
½ cup blueberries or ½ sliced small banana	70
¾ cup dry cereal with ½ cup skim milk	180
Hot coffee with skim milk	10
	335
Lunch	
Hot or chilled gazpacho (⅛ recipe)	115
Smoked salmon, 1 oz.	45
3 rye wafers	50
Celery and carrot sticks	25
17 fresh cherries or small bunch black grapes with 1 oz. blue or other dessert cheese	180
Hot or iced tea with lemon	10
	425
Dinner	
Baked Stuffed Artichokes	215
1 cup whole green beans with tarragon	35

Broiled tomato half	20
Romaine salad with marinated cauliflower, cucumbers, sliced black olives, and 2 tbsp. green herb dressing	130
¾ cup sliced peaches with 1 tbsp. kirsch	95
Hot tea or coffee with skim milk	10
	505
Total:	**1,265**

% of Total Calories: Carbohydrate = 53%; protein = 15%; fat = 32% (saturated fat = 9%)
Cholesterol: 135 mg.
Sodium: 1,250 mg.

RECIPES:
Week 4—Day 3

■ Gazpacho

1 clove garlic
6 large tomatoes, peeled, seeded and finely chopped
½ cup minced green pepper
½ cup onion, minced
2 cucumbers, peeled, seeded, and finely chopped
2 cups tomato juice
3 tbsp. lemon juice
¼ cup oil
Salt and pepper to taste
Dash tabasco

1. Rub glass bowl with garlic.
2. Add chopped vegetables.
3. Pour tomato juice and oil over the vegetables.
4. Season to taste with lemon juice, salt, pepper, and tabasco.
5. Chill, or if desired, warm, and serve.

8 servings/
15 calories per serving

■ Baked Stuffed Artichokes

6 large or 12 small globe artichokes
Vinegar and lemon juice
3 oz. part-skim mozzarella cheese, grated
1 cup part-skim ricotta cheese
¼ cup grated Parmesan cheese
One 10-oz. pkg. chopped spinach, cooked and drained well
2 eggs
¼ cup bread crumbs
Salt and pepper
Freshly grated nutmeg
2 tbsp. olive oil

1. Prepare artichokes: cut stem, trim leaves. Place prepared artichokes in water to cover, containing one tablespoon vinegar or lemon juice per quart (this prevents darkening).
2. Boil prepared artichokes in salted water for 20 minutes or until stem end can be gently pierced with a knife. Remove and place upside down on a rack to drain. When cool, gently peel back the inner leaves and remove the hairy choke (or "heart") in the center of the vegetable.
3. Mix cheese, spinach, eggs, and bread crumbs. Season with salt, pepper and nutmeg.
4. Stuff artichokes. Place in a greased pan just large enough to hold them. Fill pan with water to come one-third of the way up the vegetables. Add oil.
5. Cover tightly. Bake at 350°F for 20 minutes. Remove cover and bake 15 minutes longer, basting occasionally.

6 servings/
215 calories per serving

■ Green Herb Dressing

½ cup mayonnaise
1 tbsp. chives, chopped
1 tsp. dried chervil
¼ tsp. white pepper
½ cup low-fat yogurt
1 tbsp. parsley, minced
1 tbsp. fresh, or ½ tsp. dried, dill weed

Combine all ingredients and blend thoroughly. Chill.

16 tablespoons
60 calories per tablespoon

MENUS:
Week 4—Day 4

Breakfast	Calories
½ cup pineapple juice	70
1 slice cinnamon French toast made with 1 pat margarine	125
Coffee with skim milk	10
	205
Lunch	
Scallop, cauliflower, and snow pea salad with sesame oil dressing	290
1 small piece French bread	40
1 fresh plum	35

Hot or iced tea with lemon	10
	375
Dinner	
Pasta Carbonara (1/6 recipe)	435
Tossed salad with	
2 tbsp. low calorie dressing	40
3/4 sliced bananas and oranges	165
Hot tea or coffee with skim milk	10
	650
Total:	**1,230**

% of Total Calories: Carbohydrate = 51%; protein = 18%; fat = 31% (saturated fat = 7%)
Cholesterol: 25 mg.
Sodium: 1,400 mg.

RECIPES:
Week 4—Day 4

■ Scallop, Cauliflower and Snow Pea Salad

2 lb. fresh scallops
1 small onion
1 bay leaf
1/2 lemon
1 head cauliflower, blanched 1 min. and drained
3/4 lb. snow peas, blanched 1 min. and drained
1 bunch watercress
1/3 cup rice wine vinegar
2 tbsp. green onion, minced
1 tsp. chervil, minced
1/4 cup peanut oil
1 tbsp. sesame oil
Romaine lettuce
1/2 tsp. dried tarragon
5 peppercorns

1. Put enough water to cover scallops in a saucepan with onion, bay leaf, lemon, and peppercorns. Bring to a boil, and simmer 5 minutes.
2. Add scallops and simmer until just done, about 5 minutes. Drain and cool.
3. Combine wine vinegar, seasonings, peanut oil, and sesame oil.
4. Pour half of dressing mixture over scallops. Divide the rest between the snow peas and cauliflower. Let marinate 45 minutes.
5. Arrange scallops on romaine with watercress, cauliflower, and snow peas and whatever other cold vegetables are desired. Top with minced greem onion.

6 servings/290 calories per serving

■ Pasta Carbonara

4 slices (4 oz.) lean Smithfield-type ham
2 tbsp. oil
4 eggs
¾ cup grated Parmesan cheese
Black pepper
1 cup lightly cooked green peas
9 cups freshly cooked hot pasta

1. Dice ham and cook lightly in ½ tbsp. oil.
2. Combine eggs and cheese.
3. Put 1 tbsp. oil into a large frying pan over low heat. Add the hot pasta and pour on the egg and cheese mixture. Toss.
4. Add ham and continue tossing until the egg has coagulated with the cheese and sticks to the pasta.
5. Pour into a serving dish. Pour on the peas and serve.

6 servings/435 calories per serving

MENUS:
Week 4—Day 5

Breakfast	**Calories**
½ cup orange juice	55
1 small bagel with 1 tbsp. cream cheese	235
Hot coffee with skim milk	10
	300
Lunch	
Chinese noodle salad with tilefish (1⁄6 recipe) on lettuce with sliced tomatoes, green pepper strips, carrot sticks, and bean sprouts	290
¾ c. honeydew cubes or grapefruit half	45
Hot or iced tea with lemon	10
	345
Dinner	
Stir-fry chicken with mushrooms (¼ recipe)	205
1 cup steamed rice	190
¾ cup asparagus tips	25
Radishes, tomato wedges, and lettuce with 2 tbsp. low-calorie dressing	40
½ cup ginger ice cream	135

Hot tea or coffee with skim milk	10
	605
Total:	**1,250**

% of Total Calories: Carbohydrate = 52%; protein = 18%; fat = 30% (saturated fat = 8%)
Cholesterol: 130 mg.
Sodium: 2,325 mg.

RECIPES:
Week 4—Day 5

■ Chinese Noodle Salad with Tilefish

1 lb. tilefish or other white fish
¼ cup lemon juice
1 tbsp. peanut oil
1 tbsp. sesame oil
¼ cup canned chicken broth
1½ tsp. sugar
1 clove garlic, mashed
Dash tabasco
4½ cups cooked fresh Chinese noodles (if available) or fine egg noodles
2 tbsp. soy sauce
1½ tbsp. smooth peanut butter
1 tbsp. white vinegar
1 scallion, chopped

1. Poach fish in lemon juice and water, using just enough water to cover fish. Cook about 5 minutes and let cool in broth. Skin and flake fish.
2. Toss noodles with 1 tbsp. peanut oil and 1 tsp. sesame oil.
3. Combine chicken broth, soy sauce, vinegar, peanut butter, sugar, ginger root, garlic, and tabasco. Mix well.
4. Arrange fish on top of noodles and pour sauce over fish. Top with chopped scallions and arrange raw vegetables around platter.

6 servings/290 calories per serving

■ Stir-Fry Chicken with Mushrooms

2 whole chicken breasts, skinned and boned
2 tbsp. cornstarch
½ tsp. salt and ¼ tsp. pepper
3 cloves garlic, minced
1 tbsp. light soy sauce
½ lb. mushrooms, sliced
6 water chestnuts, sliced
24 snow peas, if available, or sugar snap peas
3 slices fresh ginger root, minced
2 tbsp. oil
¼ cup chicken broth

1. Cube chicken. Coat with 1 tbsp. cornstarch seasoned with salt and pepper.
2. Heat oil in large skillet. Add ginger and garlic and cook until lightly colored.
3. Add chicken and cook, stirring until brown.
4. Add mushrooms and cook a minute or two.
5. Add soy sauce, water chestnuts and optional snow peas.
6. Combine 1 tbsp. cornstarch with ¼ cup cold chicken broth or water. Add to skillet and stir until lightly thickened.

4 servings/205 calories per serving

MENUS:
Week 4—Day 6

Breakfast	**Calories**
½ cup grapefruit juice	60
Poached egg on whole-wheat toast with 2 tsp. butter	135
Hot coffee with skim milk	10
	205
Lunch	
Braised spinach with mozzarella cheese (¼ recipe)	280
Small hard roll	80
Sliced tomato with chopped basil and fresh black pepper, vinegar, 2 tsp. of olive oil	25
1 fresh tangerine or 2 fresh apricots	40
Hot or iced tea with lemon	10
	435
Dinner	
Veal Marsala (¼ recipe)	240
¾ cup noodles	155
1 cup julienne carrots, summer squash, and turnip lightly cooked, seasoned with 1½ tsp. margarine per serving and grated nutmeg	120
¾ cup sliced strawberries, banana, and green grapes	35
Hot tea or coffee with skim milk	10
	560
Total:	**1,200**

% of Total Calories: Carbohydrate = 46%; protein = 21% fat = 33% (saturated fat = 11%)

Cholesterol: 225 mg.
Sodium: 1,200 mg.

RECIPES:
Week 4—Day 6

■ Braised Spinach and Mozzarella

2 lb. spinach, cleaned and trimmed
1 medium onion, chopped
2 tbsp. margarine
1 cup grated low-fat mozzarella cheese
1 cup grated Parmesan cheese
Freshly grated nutmeg
Salt and pepper
2 hard-boiled eggs, chopped
2 scallions, chopped

1. Blanch spinach in boiling water for two minutes. Drain and run under cold water to stop cooking. Press moisture out thoroughly.
2. Chop spinach in food processor.
3. Heat margarine in a skillet, add onion, and cook until tender.
4. Add spinach and heat through. Add cheeses and stir until they are melted. Season to taste with salt, pepper, and nutmeg.
5. Serve individual portions topped with chopped egg and scallions.

4 servings/280 calories per serving

■ Veal Marsala

1 lb. veal scallopini, cut thin and pounded
2 tbsp. olive oil
¾ lb. fresh mushrooms, sliced
2 cloves garlic, minced
Salt and pepper to taste
½ cup Marsala wine
½ cup scallions, sliced

1. Dry veal scallops. Heat skillet with 1 tbsp. oil and brown veal quickly on both sides, cooking for two minutes in all. Remove to a hot platter and place in warm oven.
2. Add 1 tbsp. oil to skillet, add garlic, and cook until brown. Add mushrooms and cook until they are tender. Season with salt and pepper. Pour over veal scallops.
3. Add Marsala wine to skillet and boil quickly until it is reduced to half. Pour over veal. Sprinkle scallions on the veal and serve.

4 servings/
240 calories per serving

MENUS:
Week 4—Day 7

Breakfast	Calories
1 cup oatmeal	140
1 cup blueberries	90
½ cup skim milk	50
Hot coffee with skim milk	10
	290
Lunch	
2 oz. lean roast beef	135
2 slices rye bread	185
Mustard, lettuce	5
Tossed salad with	
2 tbsp. low-calorie dressing	40
1 cup mixed fresh fruits	95
Hot or iced tea with lemon	10
	470
Dinner	
Broiled salmon steak (4-oz. steak) with	210
1 tsp. olive oil and dill weed	40
½ cup coleslaw	115
Grilled tomatoes	25
1 slice watermelon	100
Hot tea or coffee with skim milk	10
	460
Total:	**1,220**

% of Total Calories: Carbohydrate = 51%; protein = 18%; fat = 31% (saturated fat = 4%)
Cholesterol: 85 mg.
Sodium: 1,350 mg.

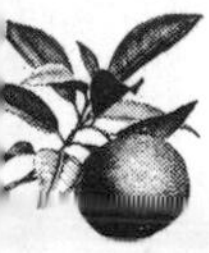

FAST FOOD: THE NUTRITIONAL PICTURE

Abbreviations

Cals.—Calories
Pro.—Protein (grams)
Car.—Carbohydrate (grams)
% Cals. Fat—The percentage of calories in that food coming from fat
Fat.—Fat (grams)
SF—Saturated Fat (grams)
Chol.—Cholesterol (milligrams)
Sod.—Sodium (milligrams)
Dash(-)—No information provided by the company
The Value of 0—None, or trace amount present

Calories, cholesterol, and sodium are rounded to the nearest 5. Protein, carbohydrate, fat, and saturated fat are rounded to the nearest 1.

Hardees

BREAKFAST	CALS.	PRO.	CAR.	%CALS. FAT	FAT	SF	CHOL.	SOD.
Rise 'n' Shine Biscuit	320	5	34	53	19	4	0	722
Cinnamon 'n' Raisin Biscuit	315	4	37	49	17	5	9	515
Sausage Biscuit	450	12	35	60	30	9	20	1,055

Hardees (cont.)

BREAKFAST	CALS.	PRO.	CAR.	%CALS. FAT	FAT	SF	CHOL.	SOD.
Sausage & Egg Biscuit	530	16	33	63	37	11	140	1,125
Bacon Biscuit	315	7	34	49	17	5	5	850
Bacon & Egg Biscuit	450	15	43	48	24	7	90	985
Bacon, Egg & Cheese Biscuit	490	17	47	50	27	9	125	1,050
Ham Biscuit	320	12	34	42	15	4	10	1,075
Ham & Egg Biscuit	405	17	34	49	22	5	160	1,130
Country Ham Biscuit	348	12	35	47	18	3	15	1,280
Country Ham & Egg Biscuit	405	16	37	49	22	6	105	1,435
Canadian Rise 'n' Shine Biscuit	480	20	36	53	28	6	185	1,550
Steak Biscuit	520	14	48	52	30	6	20	1,375
Steak & Egg Biscuit	565	22	42	54	34	10	103	1,425
Chicken Biscuit	450	15	41	50	25	5	10	1,310
Big Country Breakfast (Saus.)	1,005	32	55	65	73	16	280	1,950
Big Country Breakfast (Bac.)	755	23	45	64	54	9	350	1,660
Big Country Breakfast (Ham)	770	28	59	55	47	12	265	2,020
Hash Rounds	230	3	24	55	14	3	0	560
Biscuits 'n' Gravy	420	9	48	45	21	3	0	1,380
Orange Juice								
(6 oz.)	83	1	20	0	-	-	0	5
(10 oz.)	138	2	34	0	-	-	0	10

(carbohydrate information not provided by Pizza Hut. It is estimated.)

Hardees (cont.)

HAMBURGERS AND SANDWICHES	CALS.	PRO.	CAR.	%CALS. FAT	FAT	SF	CHOL.	SOD.
Hamburger	265	14	39	34	10	4	25	500
Cheeseburger	310	17	32	38	13	6	30	680
Quarter-Pound Cheeseburger	510	32	29	51	29	14	60	1,075
Big Deluxe Burger	495	27	33	49	27	12	60	825
Bacon Cheeseburger	610	32	33	58	39	16	60	975
Mushroom & Swiss Burger	515	29	36	49	28	13	55	1,030
Regular Roast Beef	340	21	31	40	15	6	35	965
Big Roast Beef	395	27	31	41	18	8	50	1,275
Hot Ham 'n' Cheese	315	21	35	31	11	4	40	1,495
Turkey Club	375	28	33	34	14	4	45	1,295
Fisherman's Filet	510	27	44	44	25	7	40	860
All-Beef Hot Dog	305	12	29	47	16	7	23	775

SALADS (WITHOUT DRESSING)	CALS.	PRO.	CAR.	%CALS. FAT	FAT	SF	CHOL.	SOD.
Side Salad	20	2	1	45	1	-	-	15
Garden Salad	208	14	3	61	14	8	100	265
Chef Salad	250	28	1	54	15	9	115	930
Chicken Fiesta Salad	285	24	6	44	14	9	130	535
Chicken Stix Salads								
(6-piece)	210	19	13	39	9	2	35	680
(9-piece)	315	28	20	40	14	3	55	1,055

SIDE DISHES	CALS.	PRO.	CAR.	%CALS. FAT	FAT	SF	CHOL.	SOD.
Regular French Fries	225	3	30	44	11	2	0	85

Hardees (cont.)

SIDE DISHES	CALS.	PRO.	CAR.	%CALS. FAT	FAT	SF	CHOL.	SOD.
Large French Fries	360	4	48	43	17	3	0	135
Big French Fries	495	6	66	42	23	5	0	180
Cheese Slice	45	2	1	80	4	3	5	225

DRINKS	CALS.	PRO.	CAR.	%CALS. FAT	FAT	SF	CHOL.	SOD.
2% Milk	145	9	12	31	5	3	20	150
Vanilla Shake	280	9	46	19	6	4	20	225
Chocolate Shake	445	11	83	16	8	5	25	340
Strawberry Shake	410	10	76	15	7	5	25	275

DESSERTS	CALS.	PRO.	CAR.	%CALS. FAT	FAT	SF	CHOL.	SOD.
Vanilla Cool Twist Cone	190	5	30	28	6	4	15	80
Chocolate Cool Twist Cone	210	6	32	26	6	4	18	80
Van/Choc Cool Twist Cone	205	5	31	26	6	4	20	85
Hot Fudge Cool Twist Sundae	245	6	37	29	8	6	15	145
Caramel Cool Twist Sundae	270	5	47	23	7	4	20	175
Strawberry Twist Sundae	240	5	43	23	6	4	15	85
Apple Turnover	270	3	38	40	12	4	0	245
Big Cookie	250	3	31	47	13	4	0	240

Burger King

SANDWICHES AND FRENCH FRIES	CALS.	PRO.	CAR.	%CALS. FAT	FAT	SF	CHOL.	SOD.
Whopper	628	27	46	52	36	12	90	880
with Cheese	711	32	47	54	43	17	115	1,165
Hamburger	275	15	29	39	12	5	35	510
Cheeseburger	317	17	30	43	15	8	50	650

(carbohydrate information not provided by Pizza Hut. It is estimated.)

Burger King (cont).

SANDWICHES AND FRENCH FRIES	CALS.	PRO.	CAR.	%CALS. FAT	FAT	SF	CHOL.	SOD.
Bacon Double Cheeseburger	510	33	27	55	31	15	105	730
Whopper Junior	320	15	30	48	17	6	40	485
with Cheese	365	17	31	49	20	9	50	630
Whaler Fish Sandwich	490	19	45	50	27	6	75	590
Ham & Cheese Specialty Sandwich	470	24	44	44	23	9	70	1,535
Chicken Specialty Sandwich	690	26	56	52	40	8	80	1,425
Chicken Tenders (6 pieces)	205	20	10	44	10	2	44	635
Onion Rings	275	4	28	52	16	3	0	665
French Fries	225	3	24	52	13	7	15	160

BREAKFAST ITEMS	CALS.	PRO.	CAR.	%CALS. FAT	FAT	SF	CHOL.	SOD.
Breakfast Croissan'wich	305	11	20	56	19	6	245	635
Bacon Croissan'wich	355	14	20	61	24	8	250	760
Sausage Croissan'wich	540	20	20	68	41	14	295	1,040
Ham Croissan'wich	335	17	20	54	20	-	260	985
Breakfast Bagel Sandwich	385	17	46	33	14	5	270	780
Bacon Bagel Sandwich	440	20	46	39	19	7	275	905
Sausage Bagel Sandwich	620	26	46	52	36	13	320	1,185
Ham Bagel Sandwich	420	23	46	32	15	5	285	1,130
Scrambled Egg Platter	470	15	33	57	30	-	370	810

Burger King (cont).

BREAKFAST ITEMS	CALS.	PRO.	CAR.	%CALS. FAT	FAT	SF	CHOL.	SOD.
with Sausage	700	24	33	67	52	-	420	1,215
with Bacon	535	19	33	61	36	-	380	975
French Toast Sticks	500	9	49	42	29	5	75	500
Great Danish	500	5	40	65	36	23	5	290

DRINKS (REGULAR SIZE)	CALS.	PRO.	CAR.	%CALS. FAT	FAT	SF	CHOL.	SOD.
Milk 2%	120	8	12	38	5	3	20	120
Milk Whole	155	8	11	52	9	6	35	120
Orange Juice	80	1	20	0	0	0	0	0
Coffee	2	0	0	0	0	0	0	0
Shakes								
Vanilla (regular)	320	9	49	28	10	-	-	205
Chocolate (regular)	320	8	46	34	12	-	-	200
Vanilla (syrup added)	335	9	51	27	10	-	-	215
Chocolate (syrup added)	375	8	60	26	11	-	-	225
Pepsi	160	0	40	0	0	0	0	-
Diet-Pepsi	1	0	0	0	0	0	0	-
7-UP	145	0	38	0	0	0	0	-

DESSERTS	CALS.	PRO.	CAR.	%CALS. FAT	FAT	SF	CHOL.	SOD.
Apple Pie	305	3	44	35	12	4	5	410

SALADS (WITHOUT DRESSING)	CALS.	PRO.	CAR.	%CALS. FAT	FAT	SF	CHOL.	SOD.
Chicken Salad	140	20	8	26	4	-	50	440
Chef Salad	180	17	7	45	9	-	120	570
Garden Salad	90	6	7	50	5	3	15	125
Side Salad	20	1	4	0	0	0	0	20

Burger King (cont).

DRESSING (1 PACKET)	CALS.	PRO.	CAR.	%CALS. FAT	FAT	SF	CHOL.	SOD.
1,000 Island	240	1	7	86	23	4	35	470
Bleu Cheese	300	2	3	93	31	5	40	600
House	260	2	5	90	26	4	20	530
Reduced-Calorie Italian	30	0	4	60	2	0	0	870
French	280	0	17	74	23	4	0	690
Bacon Bits	16	1	0	56	1	-	-	1
Croutons	30	1	5	30	1	-	-	88

McDonalds

BREAKFAST ITEMS	CALS.	PRO.	CAR.	%CALS. FAT	FAT	SF	CHOL.	SOD.
Egg McMuffin	295	18	28	37	12	4	300	740
Hotcakes/Butter, Syrup	415	8	74	20	9	4	20	640
Scrambled Eggs	155	12	1	64	11	3	545	290
Pork Sausage	180	8	0	80	16	6	50	350
English Muffin/ Butter	170	5	27	26	5	2	10	270
Hash-brown Potatoes	130	1	15	49	7	3	10	330
Biscuit with Spread	260	5	32	45	13	3	1	730
with Sausage	440	13	32	59	29	9	50	1,080
with Sausage and Egg	530	20	33	59	35	11	360	1,250
with Bacon, Egg, and Cheese	450	17	33	54	27	8	335	1,230
Sausage McMuffin	370	17	27	54	22	8	65	830
with Egg	450	23	28	54	27	10	335	980
Apple Danish	390	6	51	42	18	4	25	370
Iced Cheese Danish	395	7	42	50	22	6	45	420
Cinnamon Raisin Danish	445	6	58	43	21	4	35	430
Raspberry Danish	415	6	62	35	16	3	25	310

McDonalds (cont.)

SANDWICHES AND FRENCH FRIES	CALS.	PRO.	CAR.	%CALS. FAT	FAT	SF	CHOL.	SOD.
Hamburger	255	12	31	35	10	4	35	460
Cheeseburger	310	15	31	41	14	5	55	750
Quarter-Pounder	415	23	34	46	21	8	85	660
with Cheese	515	29	35	51	29	11	120	1,150
Big Mac	560	25	43	51	32	10	105	950
Filet-O-Fish	440	14	38	53	26	5	50	1,030
McDlt	675	28	46	56	42	12	110	1,170
Chicken McNuggets	290	19	17	50	16	4	65	520
McNugget Sauce								
Hot Mustard	65	1	8	55	4	1	5	250
Barbeque	55	0	12	16	1	0	0	340
Sweet & Sour	55	0	14	0	0	0	0	190
Honey	45	0	12	0	0	0	0	0
Regular French Fries	220	3	26	49	12	5	10	110
Large French Fries	310	4	37	47	16	7	10	155

DESSERTS	CALS.	PRO.	CAR.	%CALS. FAT	FAT	SF	CHOL.	SOD.
Soft Serve Cone	145	4	22	31	5	2	15	70
Sundaes								
Strawberry	285	6	48	22	7	3	25	85
Hot Fudge	315	7	50	26	9	5	30	160
Hot Caramel	345	7	58	24	9	4	35	160
McDonaldland Cookies	290	4	47	28	9	2	0	300
Chocolaty-Chip Cookies	325	4	42	44	16	5	5	280
Apple Pie	260	2	30	52	15	5	5	240

SALADS (WITHOUT DRESSING)	CALS.	PRO.	CAR.	%CALS. FAT	FAT	SF	CHOL.	SOD.
Chef Salad	230	21	8	55	14	6	150	490
Shrimp Salad	105	14	6	34	3	1	195	480

McDonalds (cont.)

SALADS (WITHOUT DRESSING)	CALS.	PRO.	CAR.	%CALS. FAT	FAT	SF	CHOL.	SOD.
Garden Salad	110	7	6	57	7	3	105	160
Chicken Salad Oriental	140	23	5	26	3	1	0	230
Side Salad	55	4	3	66	3	1	55	85
Croutons	50	1	7	36	2	0	0	140
Bacon Bits	15	1	0	60	1	0	0	95
Chow Mein Noodles	45	1	5	40	2	0	0	60

DRESSING (1 TBSP.)	CALS.	PRO.	CAR.	%CALS. FAT	FAT	SF	CHOL.	SOD.
Bleu Cheese	70	1	1	40	2	1	5	150
French	60	0	3	75	5	1	0	180
Ranch	85	0	1	95	9	1	5	130
1,000 Island	80	0	2	90	8	1	10	100
Lite Vinaigrette	15	0	2	60	1	0	0	60
Oriental	25	0	6	0	0	0	0	180

DRINKS	CALS.	PRO.	CAR.	%CALS. FAT	FAT	SF	CHOL.	SOD.
Vanilla Milk Shake	355	10	56	25	10	5	40	170
Chocolate Milk Shake	390	11	63	25	11	5	40	240
Strawberry Milk Shake	385	10	63	23	10	5	40	170
2% Milk	120	8	12	38	5	3	20	130
Orange Juice	80	1	19	0	0	0	0	0
Grapefruit Juice	80	1	19	0	0	0	0	0
Coca Cola								
12 oz.	145	0	40	0	0	0	0	15
16 oz.	190	0	50	0	0	0	0	20
22 oz.	265	0	70	0	0	0	0	25
Orange Drink								
12 oz.	135	0	35	0	0	0	0	10
16 oz.	175	0	45	0	0	0	0	15
22 oz.	245	0	60	0	0	0	0	20

INDEX